Sexual Murder

Sexual Flutter

Sexual Murder

Catathymic and Compulsive Homicides

Second Edition

Louis B. Schlesinger

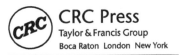

CRC Press
Taylor & Francis Group
Boca Raton London New York

CRC Press is an imprint of the
Taylor & Francis Group, an **informa** business

Second edition published 2021
by CRC Press
6000 Broken Sound Parkway NW, Suite 300, Boca Raton, FL 33487-2742

and by CRC Press
2 Park Square, Milton Park, Abingdon, Oxon, OX14 4RN

© 2021 Taylor & Francis Group, LLC
First edition published by CRC Press 2003

CRC Press is an imprint of Taylor & Francis Group, LLC

Library of Congress Cataloging-in-Publication Data

Names: Schlesinger, Louis B., author.
Title: Sexual murder : catathymic and compulsive homicides / Louis B. Schlesinger.
Description: Second edition. | Boca Raton, FL : CRC Press, 2021. | Includes bibliographical references and index. | Summary: "Sexual Murder: Catathymic and Compulsive Homicides is the culmination of the author's 45 years of experience with, and studying, sexually motivated homicide. Recent advances in empirical research in sexual murder-including findings from the joint research project between John Jay College of Criminal Justice and the FBI Behavioral Analysis Unit in Quantico-has published many important studies. These include such topics as necrophilia, foreign object insertions in sexual homicide, ritual and signature and temporal patterns in serial sexual homicide, mass murder, crime scene staging in homicide, and undoing (symbolic reversal) at homicide scenes. All such research will be included and incorporate into this fully updated Second Edition, including approximately fifty new clinical case studies"-- Provided by publisher.
Identifiers: LCCN 2020042114 (print) | LCCN 2020042115 (ebook) | ISBN 9780367860233 (hardback) | ISBN 9781003143727 (ebook)
Subjects: LCSH: Forensic psychology. | Sex crimes. | Murder. | Homicide. | Women--Crimes against. | Violence. | Sex offenders.
Classification: LCC RA1148 .S48 2021 (print) | LCC RA1148 (ebook) | DDC 614/.15--dc23
LC record available at https://lccn.loc.gov/2020042114
LC ebook record available at https://lccn.loc.gov/2020042115

ISBN: 978-0-367-86023-3 (hbk)
ISBN: 978-1-003-14372-7 (ebk)
ISBN: 978-0-367-71157-3 (pbk)

Typeset in Minion
by Deanta Global Publishing Services, Chennai, India

Contents

Foreword

When I received my doctorate in clinical psychology in 1981, I was already enamored with the world of criminal forensics. The popular television fare of *Investigative Reports*, the *New Detectives*, *Forensic Files*, and *CSI* were still years away, but I picked up a book that profoundly shaped my intellectual journey: *Psychopathology of Homicide* by Eugene Revitch and Louis B. Schlesinger. It was a classic.

Drs. Revitch and Schlesinger had set aside descriptive diagnoses and instead developed a motivational model to help understand why people intentionally kill each other. The reasons for murder are always overdetermined, but here were two gentlemen who proposed an elegant schematic that ranged from purely situational causes for killing to the unconscious psychodynamics of certain murders which appear, at first glance, to be inexplicable. I soon came to learn that Dr. Revitch was a distinguished forensic psychiatrist and had pioneered some of the earliest investigations of the sexual killing of women. One of his first papers, "Sex murder and sex aggression," was printed in 1957 in the *Journal of the Medical Society of New Jersey*.

I was equally impressed with the work of Dr. Schlesinger, a student of Dr. Revitch's, and my propensity to idealize authorities in the field as a young psychologist was bolstered by his subsequent work, particularly in the area of "catathymia," a word quite foreign to me at the time. Dr. Schlesinger does not know this, but I was deeply honored when I finally met him several years ago when he attended a workshop I was giving. We are great sources of intellectual stimulation for each other, and our mutual respect continues.

Sexual Murder: Catathymic and Compulsive Homicides will take its place alongside Cleckley's *Mask of Sanity*, Krafft-Ebing's *Psychopathia Sexualis*, and Ressler et al.'s *Sexual Homicide: Patterns and Motives* as a classic in our specialized field of criminal forensic psychology. This is not marketing hyperbole, and as an expert witness, I hope the foundation for my opinion is persuasive.

Unlike most contemporary forensic psychiatry and psychology research, which is largely descriptive and behavioral, Dr. Schlesinger is interested in the *inner life* of the sexual murderer. Although his internal world may be populated by sexually violent and bizarre fantasies that are anathema to the conscious sensibilities of most individuals—although they are readily sought by many of these same people in their local cinema—an in-depth understanding of the sexual murderer depends on our ability to tolerate and explore his subterranean landscape. If we have no understanding of his drive derivatives, affects, defenses, and compromise formations, how can we fathom his acts?

Our present psychological operations, however, do not function in a vacuum. They are a product of *history and development*, and this is another area in which Dr. Schlesinger finds answers to questions that disturb and frighten most people: Why would anyone be sexually aroused by violence? How could anyone contemplate, let alone commit, such horrendous acts? We live our histories, whether we are the products of healthy parents who do not abuse, neglect, or sexually titillate, or we are the products of the so-called parents who do.

Dr. Schlesinger also emphasizes the importance of *psychological testing and measurement* among those who commit sexual murder. Although sometimes derided, particularly by some forensic psychiatrists who may find test data threatening, standardized measures provide for us an objective reference point with which to compare the results of our individual subject. This is the only truly scientific way in which we can speak to abnormality as deviation rather than a moral failing. One of our Rorschach discoveries, when we studied a large sample of sexual murderers, was the inordinate number of feral movement responses they would give. These responses have been validated as measures of nonvolitional ideation in response to physiological arousal in other populations, but it became for us another way of defining obsessional thought in response to aggressive and sexual feelings among sexual murderers. We thus discovered, quite serendipitously, the first standardized psychological data that supported the clinical finding which had been noted over the past century of obsessional thinking in some sexual murderers.

Data without a theory, however, are just numbers. Dr. Schlesinger's writing in this book also emphasizes the importance of *theory* in understanding sexual murder. Theory shapes the pursuit of data, and data in turn modify theory. This is the scientific dynamic that is kept alive by nurturing a theory of mind, along with the collection of empirical measures. Dr. Schlesinger and I share the same perspective. The most comprehensive theory for understanding sexual murder is psychoanalytic, which, in its many contemporary forms, still acknowledges two fundamental tenets of Freud: human behavior is overdetermined and often motivated by unconscious aspects of the mind. How can we understand sexual murder if we assume all human behavior is rational and cognitive?

Throughout this book, Dr. Schlesinger underscores the importance of *case studies*. The individual case study holds an honored position in psychiatry and psychology, and most of the important discoveries in our field began with the observation of one individual doing something that caught a researcher's eye. Comparative group studies usually follow, but now most of our journals err in relegating the case study to a "letter to the editor." As Hans Eysenck, the great British psychologist, noted half a century ago, idiographic and nomothetic approaches share equal importance in the study of human behavior. Without the case study, we cannot appreciate the uniqueness of each individual. In my forensic evaluations of sexual murderers over the years, I have always been struck by how different each case is, yet how homogenized the public perception of the sexual murderer is. The brilliance of Anthony Hopkins notwithstanding, most sexual murderers would not stand out in a crowd, yet they each bring their own unique and private fantasies and perversions to the crime.

The final aspect of Dr. Schlesinger's work that is most enviable is his development of a *motivational model for understanding sexual murder*, which depends on his earlier work with Dr. Revitch on compulsive and catathymic homicides. This book, *Sexual Murder: Catathymic and Compulsive Homicides*, is a brilliant integration and application of previous theory and research and advances the field of criminal forensic psychology. Amidst the words and images that follow, we move closer to grasping the mystery posed by William Shakespeare over four centuries ago: "One sin, I know, another doth provoke; murder's as near to lust as flame to smoke" (Pericles, I, 1).

J. Reid Meloy, PhD
San Diego, California

Acknowledgments

I would like to express my appreciation to all colleagues, friends, and students who have supported my work, either directly in discussions of the material or indirectly by their encouragement and patience. Special thanks go to Mark Listewnik, Senior Editor at Taylor & Francis Publisher, who was very helpful and encouraging throughout the entire project. I am indebted to Ellen Sexton and Maria Kiriakova, John Jay College's librarians extraordinaire, who—at a moment's notice—are able to obtain any article or book ever published, and even some that were not. Maria was especially helpful in translating Hans Maiers' papers from the original German. I also want to particularly thank Navis Edwards, my longtime friend and assistant, who did her usual excellent job in typing, as well as deciphering my dictation. Also many thanks to my new friend Vivienne (Madge) Lowe, who has excellent computer skills and did all the typing for the final copy. Finally, I want to express my gratitude to my wife Beth, who has always put aside many of her own pursuits to listen to my endless tales of sexual murder cases—even during dinner!

About the Author

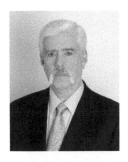 **Louis B. Schlesinger**, PhD, is Professor of Forensic Psychology at John Jay College of Criminal Justice, City University of New York, a Diplomate in Forensic Psychology of the American Board of Professional Psychology, and a Distinguished Practitioner of the National Academies of Practice. He served as president of the New Jersey Psychological Association in 1989 and as a member of the Council of Representatives of the American Psychological Association from 1991 to 1994. Dr. Schlesinger is a Fellow of the American Psychological Association and was the 1990 recipient of the New Jersey Psychological Association's Psychologist of the Year Award, Distinguished Researcher Award in 2014, as well as a recipient of the American Psychological Association's Karl F. Heiser Presidential Award (1993). He was appointed by the Governor of New Jersey and the commissioner of corrections to be a member (and later served as chair) of the Special Classification Review Board at the Adult Diagnostic and Treatment Center (1980–1987), the state's forensic facility; he was also appointed (2001) by the president of the New Jersey State Senate and acting Governor to serve as a member of a Senate task force that rewrote Megan's Law. Dr. Schlesinger is co-principal investigator of a joint research project between John Jay College and the FBI Behavioral Analysis Unit at Quantico, studying various types of violent crime including sexual and serial murder, rape, bias homicide, suicide-by-cop, and other extraordinary criminal behaviors. Dr. Schlesinger has testified in numerous forensic cases and has published many articles, chapters, and eight other books on the topics of homicide, sexual homicide, and criminal psychopathology.

About the Author

Introduction

It has been over 15 years since *Sexual Murder: Catathymic and Compulsive Homicides* was published. A lot has happened in the past decade and a half in the areas of research, theory, and clinical practice, which has made a second edition a necessity. Over the years, I have been encouraged by many colleagues to write a second edition. I resisted, based mainly on time constraints, but there reached a point where I just sat down and did it. The second edition is now up to date with best practices, new clinical case analyses, recent empirical research, and the latest thinking in the field, including my own.

So many people have asked me how I got started in this rather unique sub-specialty. Here's how: during graduate school, I had planned on a career in professional psychology with an emphasis on evaluating and treating children and adolescents. After a 2-year traineeship at a state hospital, I was ready to begin my clinical internship at the New Jersey Neuropsychiatric Institute in Princeton. Due to an administrative snafu, however, I was unable to go there and had to choose another site. The director of training recommended I consider the Menlo Park Diagnostic Center, the state's forensic facility. I was not exactly sure what forensic psychology was since there were hardly any forensic psychologists in 1974. But I had to go somewhere, so I decided to give it a try. I certainly did not realize that the administrative foul-up that resulted in my placement at the Diagnostic Center would so profoundly change my life and professional career.

While at the center I met Eugene Revitch, one of the country's leading forensic psychiatrists, who not only provided exceptional training in assessment but allowed me to participate in sodium amytal interviews, hypnoanalytic sessions, evaluations in state prison, and consultations with law enforcement officers, as well as to observe court testimony. I became so interested in forensic psychology that I signed up for the second half of my internship at Trenton State Prison. My fellow interns all thought I was out of my mind for pursuing forensic psychology as a specialty since the opportunities back then seemed so limited. In the mid-1970s, in order for psychologists to get involved in a forensic case, they had to be invited by a psychiatrist and their role was usually limited to psychological testing. I never dreamed that 20 years later the professional status of psychologists would change so dramatically and that we would have such a major impact on legal decision making.

Dr. Revitch and I became close friends, and over the years, we collaborated on many forensic cases and several books. In 1981, we coauthored *Psychopathology of Homicide*; in 1983, we coedited *Sexual Dynamics of Antisocial Behavior*; and in 1989, we wrote *Sex Murder and Sex Aggression*. Although Dr. Revitch (who died in 1996) had no direct involvement in writing the original volume or this second edition, his influence is present on almost every page.

The second edition of *Sexual Murder: Catathymic and Compulsive Homicides* is the culmination of my 45+ years of experience with, and thinking about, sexually motivated homicide. Sexual murders are generally of two types—catathymic and compulsive.

Catathymic homicides are caused by a breakthrough of underlying sexual conflicts. They can be unplanned, explosive (acute) attacks or planned murders, stemming from a chronic obsession with, or disturbed attachment to, the victim. In compulsive homicides, a fusion of sex and aggression results in a powerful internal drive which pushes the offender to seek out victims to kill—and the killing itself is sexually gratifying. These murders also may be planned or unplanned. In compulsive homicides that are unplanned, the urge breaks through and disrupts the offender's controls when a victim of opportunity crosses his path. The compulsive offender who plans his crimes often eludes law enforcement, and as a result, he can have multiple (serial) victims over extended periods of time. Both forms of sexual murder—the catathymic and the compulsive—are presented in this volume, primarily from a clinical-descriptive perspective, encompassing case studies with analysis.

Sexual murder is a low base rate crime, and, as a result, it has been exceptionally difficult to research empirically. Most of our knowledge about sexual murder, over the past century, has come from the clinical case analysis. There have, however, been recent advances in empirical research, including findings from the joint research project (where I am a co-principal investigator) between John Jay College of Criminal Justice and the FBI Behavioral Analysis Unit in Quantico. Our team has published many important studies on topics such as necrophilia and foreign object insertions in sexual homicide, ritual and signature and temporal patterns in serial sexual homicide, and papers in related areas such as mass murder, crime scene staging in homicide, and undoing (symbolic reversal) at homicide crime scenes. All of this research, as well as research of others, are included in the second edition, along with many new clinical case studies used to illustrate various points.

Chapter 1 covers the many problems encountered in studying sexual murder. Homicide and sexual homicide cannot be understood in isolation. Just as physicians who want to specialize in cancer cannot limit their education to oncology but must first study general medicine, professionals who want to understand sexual murder cannot limit their study to this one criminal behavior. Sexual murder must be understood within the general context of criminal behavior, crime theory, and crime and homicide classification. Accordingly, this chapter, as with other chapters throughout the book, presents sexual murder within the context of nonsexual homicide and crime.

Chapter 2 covers forensic assessment, with a focus on the evaluation of the sexual murderer. Here, distinctions are drawn between the clinical and the forensic approach to the assessment of criminal defendants. Various aspects of the forensic evaluation, including psychological testing, narcoanalysis, hypnosis, and neurodiagnostic assessment, are reviewed, and several complicating factors in the assessment of offenders are discussed, as well as new research on various types of crime scene behaviors that forensic practitioners need to become familiar with. Theories of crime and various systems of classification of homicide are covered in Chapter 3, along with a detailed presentation of Dr. Revitch's and my method of classifying antisocial behavior along a spectrum of motivational dynamics. Throughout this chapter, distinctions are drawn between killings (mostly of women) that are not sexually motivated and killings that are sexually motivated. Finally, the place of sexual murder in the overall classification of crime and homicide is explained.

Chapters 4 through 6 present catathymic homicides. The discussion of catathymia from a historical perspective includes a detailed review of Hans W. Maier's papers, which were published in the early years of the 20th century, and a description of the seminal work of Fredric Wertham. Acute (unplanned) catathymic homicides and the more protracted or chronic catathymic process, which involves a planned murder and an obsession with the future victim, are differentiated and illustrated with many case examples.

The compulsive murderer is the focus of Chapters 7 through 9. Following a presentation of compulsive homicides in historical context, the compulsive murderer who plans his crimes is contrasted with the compulsive murderer whose killings are unplanned. Their different psychological makeups and crime scene patterns are among the topics covered. Finally, Chapter 10 considers prediction, disposition, and possibilities for preventing sexual murder.

The cases reported in this book have been adjudicated and are a matter of public record. Nevertheless, the identifiers—but not the underlying facts—have been altered to add a measure of confidentiality. At times throughout the book, some discussions may seem to stray from the central topic of sexual murder. I hope that the reader will bear with me because I strongly believe that a full understanding of the psychopathology of nonsexual homicide is necessary in order to fully understand sexual homicide. Some details that at first may seem unrelated to the topic (for example, the discussion in Chapter 1 of lunar cycles and homicide) will become clear in later chapters (Chapter 7 in this case) as these various elements are eventually tied together.

My central aim throughout this book is to enlarge the reader's view of sexual murder and to modify some preconceived ideas. If, after finishing this book, readers have broadened and varied their understanding of sexual homicide, my effort will have been successful.

Louis B. Schlesinger, PhD
Maplewood, New Jersey

In the intercourse of the sexes, the active or aggressive role belongs to man. ... This aggressive character, however, under pathological conditions, may likewise be excessively developed, and express itself in an impulse to subdue absolutely the object of desire, even to destroy or kill it.

Krafft-Ebing
Psychopathia Sexualis

The history of human civilization shows beyond any doubt that there is an intimate connection between cruelty and the sexual instinct; but nothing has been done towards explaining the connection, apart from laying emphasis on the aggressive factor in the libido. According to some authorities this aggressive element of the sexual instinct is in reality a relic of cannibalistic desires—that is, it is a contribution derived from the apparatus for obtaining mastery, which is concerned with the satisfaction of the other and, ontogenetically, the older of the great instinctual needs. It has been maintained that every pain contains in itself the possibility of a feeling of pleasure. All that needs to be said is that no satisfactory explanation of this perversion has been put forward and that it seems possible that a number of mental impulses are combined in it to produce a single resultant.

Freud
Three Essays on the Theory of Sexuality

Anyone who has once experienced this power, this unlimited control over the body, blood, and spirit of a man like himself, a fellow creature, his brother in Christ—anyone who has experienced this power to inflict supreme humiliation upon another being, created like himself in the image of God, is bound to be ruled by emotions. Tyranny is a habit; it grows upon us and, in the long run, turns into a disease. I say that the most decent man in the world can, through habit, become as brutish and coarse as a wild beast. Blood and power intoxicate, callousness and vice develop; the most abnormal things become first acceptable, then sweet to the mind and heart. The human being, the member of society, is drowned forever in the tyrant, and it is practically impossible for him to regain human dignity, repentance, and regeneration. One such instance—the realization that such arbitrary power can be exercised—can infect all society; such power is seductive.

Dostoyevsky
The House of the Dead

Understanding Sexual Murder
Problems and Approaches

1

The image of the sexual murderer—especially the murderer with multiple victims—has always aroused concomitant feelings of horror and fascination in the general public. Today, his exploits are graphically reported in the press and on television, in "psycho-thriller" films, and in various "true-crime" books (e.g., Rule, 1983, 1988; Ryzuk, 1994; Schechter, 1989, 1990). As a result of all this attention, some sexual killers, such as Ted Bundy, Jeffrey Dahmer, and the Boston Strangler, have almost become household names. Of course, sexual homicide—homicide motivated primarily by a breakthrough of underlying sexual conflicts or where the killing itself is sexually gratifying—has also been studied by behavioral scientists, sociologists, forensic specialists, and the like. Yet, in contrast to the voluminous research literature on (nonsexual) homicide from psychiatric, psychological, sociological, legal, and investigative perspectives, a solid body of scientific literature on sexual murder is only beginning to be accumulated.

There are a number of problems that make research in the area of sexual murder very difficult: (1) There is no generally agreed-upon definition of sexual homicide; instead, a number of different definitions have been offered, and different terms are used for what seems to be similar criminal behavior. (2) Many murders that might appear to be sexually motivated are actually not sexually motivated. (3) Many murders that are not overtly sexual are sexually motivated. (4) The distinction between a sexual homicide, or a sexually motivated homicide, and a homicide associated with sexual behavior is often blurred. (5) National or state crime statistics on the number of sexual homicides have not been kept. (6) There are a number of practical impediments to carrying out research with these offenders, such as incomplete and inaccurate background histories and the lack of interdisciplinary cooperation. Each of these obstacles, listed in Table 1.1, makes sexual murder a crime that is not only difficult to understand but also very difficult to study.

1.1 The Problem of Definition and Terms

In the FBI's *Uniform Crime Reports* (*UCR*), which provides annual summaries of crime statistics, homicide is defined as the willful (nonnegligent) killing of one human being by another. Deaths caused by negligence, accidents, suicide, or justifiable homicides are not categorized as murder. The level of intent (as in the legal system's classification of homicide into first-degree and second-degree murder, manslaughter, etc.) is also not considered. The *UCR* definition, which is based on findings reported by police investigators, is reasonably clear-cut. It does not take into account an offender's internal state or such issues as blame or moral responsibility. These matters, which are difficult to assess objectively, are left to lawyers, judges, mental health experts, and jurors.

The definition of sexual homicide, on the other hand, is not at all clear-cut. Sexual homicide is not defined by statute as are the illegal paraphilias (such as pedophilia) and

Table 1.1   Problems Encountered in the Study of Sexual Murder

- No generally agreed-upon definition.
- Many seemingly sexual murders are not really sexually motivated.
- Many sexual murders are not overtly sexual.
- Distinction between a sexual homicide, or a sexually motivated homicide, and a homicide associated with sexual behavior is often blurred.
- No national crime statistics exist.
- Practical impediments—such as incomplete and inaccurate background histories and lack of interdisciplinary cooperation—are common.

other sex crimes (such as rape), and the *Diagnostic and Statistical Manual of Mental Disorders* (in any of its editions) has never defined sexual homicide as a specific paraphilia, nor has the *International Classification of Diseases*. Moreover, inherent in the definition of sexual murder is the issue of intent, which adds to the definitional problems. For example, Ressler, Burgess, and Douglas (1988) generally define sexual homicide as "the killing of a person in the context of power, sexuality, and brutality" (p. 1). Almost all killings, however, involve some degree of power and brutality. How do these characteristics distinguish a sexual homicide from a nonsexual homicide? And what is the meaning of "sexuality" in this definition? Does it refer to actual sexual behavior? To render the killing a sexual murder, must there be intercourse, attempted intercourse, a desire for intercourse, or just an internal feeling of arousal? How can an investigator determine whether an offender's arousal was sexual arousal or merely a general arousal (a heightened emotional state) felt by someone who has committed a crime and risks apprehension? In many cases, a clinician will decide that a murder is a sexual murder because it appears to be a sexual murder (Prentky et al., 1989; Swigert, Farrell, and Yoels, 1976). But what appears to be a sexual murder to one practitioner may appear otherwise to someone else.

Along with differences in definitions, many different terms have been used to describe sexual murder, including lust murder (Krafft-Ebing, 1886), sadistic lust murder (De River, 1958), sadistic murder (Brittain, 1970), lust killing (Malmquist, 1996), and even erotophonophilia (Money, 1990), among others (see Table 1.2). Sometimes the same term, such as lust murder, is defined differently by different authors (Hazelwood and Douglas, 1980; Krafft-Ebing, 1886). Reid (2017a) has documented 43 different conceptualizations of sexual and serial murder, some operationalized and some vague descriptions of behavior. Greenall (2012) has described four different scenarios that could define a sexual homicide. Kerr, Beech, and Murphy (2013) listed 13 different definitions of sexual murder. Higgs, Carter, Tully, and Browne (2017) reviewed empirical studies of sexual murder between 1970 and 2016 and reported three types of offenses: "sexualized murder" involving sadism, "grievance murder" involving anger, and "rape murder." While all of these definitions and approaches have merit, the issue of what constitutes a sexual murder remains unsettled.

Many, but not all, researchers agree that serial murders are sexual murders with multiple victims (Schlesinger, 2000a). Some define serial murder as literally the killing of multiple individuals, rather than viewing the crime more narrowly as a subtype of sexual murder (Egger, 1990a). For example, Dietz (1986) distinguishes five separate types of serial murderers: psychopathic sexual sadists, crime spree killers, organized crime multiple murderers, custodial prisoners and serial asphyxiators, and supposed psychotics

Table 1.2 Various Terms, Descriptions, and Definitions of Sexual Murder

Author	Year	Term	Description/Definition
Krafft-Ebing	1886	Lust murder	"The connection between lust and desire to kill" (p. 62); "The sadistic crime alone becomes the equivalent of coitus" (p. 64)
De River	1958	Sadistic lust murder	"After killing the victim, the murderer tortures, cuts, maims, or slashes the victim ... on parts [of the body] that contain strong sexual significance to him and serves as sexual stimulation" (p. 40)
Brittain	1970	Sadistic murder	Offers no specific definition but provides a nine-page description of personality traits and characteristics of sadistic murderers; differentiates from a murderer who kills in a sexual setting (such as one who silences a victim of rape)
Hazelwood and Douglas	1980	Lust murder	"Distinguished from the sadistic homicide by the involvement of a mutilating attack or displacement of the breasts, rectum, or genitals" (p. 1)
MacDonald	1986	Sex murder	"A sexual factor is clearly apparent ... or deeper study will sometimes reveal that sexual conflict underlies the act of aggression" (p. 164)
Ressler, Burgess, and Douglas	1988	Sexual homicide	"Murder with evidence or observations that indicate[s] that the murder was sexual in nature" (p. xiii)
Money	1990	Erotophonophilia	Murder associated with sexual sadism as defined in *DSM* (p. 26)
Douglas et al.	1992	Sexual homicide	"Involves a sexual element (activity) as the basis for the sequence of acts leading to death" (p. 123)
Douglas et al.	1992	Sadistic murder	"The offender derives the greatest satisfaction from the victim's response to torture" (p. 136)
Grubin	1994	Sexual murder	"The killing may also be closely bound to the sexual element of an attack ... the offender's control of his victim, and her pain and humiliation, become linked to his sexual arousal" (p. 624)
Malmquist	1996	Lust killing	"The primary goal is to kill the victim as part of a ritualized attack ... the motivation ... is the enactment of some type of fantasy that has preoccupied him or her for some time" (p. 295)
Beech, Fisher, and Ward	2005	Sexual murder	"[Killing] where there is ... a sexual element ... or sexual component admitted or suspected" (p. 5)

who kill multiple victims. Only the first type is sexually motivated. In an attempt to add definitional precision, Jenkins (1988, 1989) specifically excludes politically motivated and professional contract killers, thereby adhering more to the traditional sexual view of serial murder. The FBI (Morton and Hilts, 2005) recently updated their definition of serial murder to include two or more victims, in separate events at different times. The term "spree murder" (involving a cooling-off period between murders) was essentially eliminated as a separate category.

These differences in terminology and definitions, although they often make communication regarding the meaning of findings difficult, are to be expected in the developing stages of scientific inquiry.

1.2 Many Seemingly Sexual Murders Are
Not Really Sexually Motivated

In cases where there is an overt manifestation of genitality (e.g., a woman's genitals are cut out or mutilated), a determination that the murder is a sexual murder would seem warranted. However, a closer examination reveals that many of these cases are not always that straightforward, and in some instances, the conclusion that the crime is a sexual murder is incorrect. Consider, for example, a person who responds to auditory hallucinations commanding him to kill women and cut out their genitals in order, perhaps, to save the world. Should a murder of this type be considered a sexual murder? There is certainly a sexual element to the offender's delusions, possibly stemming from underlying sexual disturbance, but the primary motivation for the homicide is a response to psychosis.

The notorious and complex case of Richard Trenton Chase, dubbed the "Vampire Killer" (Ressler and Shachtman, 1992), is an example. Chase had a delusion that his blood was evaporating and that he therefore needed to drink the blood of others in order to continue to live. Following his release from a convalescent center (where he was sent after killing small animals and drinking their blood), he began breaking into homes in order to obtain human blood and hence preserve his life. Chase wound up killing ten people in response to this delusional belief, as well as to auditory hallucinations commanding him to kill. His behavior was consistent with, and an outgrowth of, his obvious psychosis. Ressler and Shachtman (1992) considered Chase a serial sexual murderer mainly because some of his female victims had been subjected to genital mutilation. However, Chase also killed without evidence of sexual motivation. For example, he killed a 22-month-old infant by shooting him in the head—behavior atypical of a sexual murder. He also killed men, a child, and animals. There was undoubtedly a sexual element in this complicated case, but the main impetus for the homicides appears to have been a response to a delusional belief. It is likely that multiple motives were operative with Chase: both a psychosis and perhaps a secondary sexual component. But without the psychosis, it is doubtful Chase would have killed.

1.3 Many Sexual Homicides Are Not Overtly Sexual

Many attacks and murders that appear on the surface to be motivated by monetary gain may, in fact, be sexually motivated, although the sexual dynamics are covert (Schlesinger and Revitch, 1997b). Revitch (1957) first reported the case of a man who attacked a woman with a blackjack and was subsequently arrested and charged with assault and attempted robbery. The offender told the police that he needed money and that a woman was an easier victim than a man. When examined carefully, however, he revealed that his long-standing fantasies of tying women's legs had prompted the attack. His initial stated motive of robbery (given to the police) was, then, a rationalization or simply a lie. In accepting his statement at face value, the police had ignored a noose, a rifle, and a copy of Krafft-Ebing's (1886) classic text *Psychopathia Sexualis*—all found in the trunk of the offender's car. Revitch (1965) concluded that, contrary to popular belief, erection, ejaculation, and intercourse do not necessarily accompany a violent (sexually motivated) assault or murder, since the brutal attack may be a substitute for, or take the place of, the sexual act.

Other investigators have reached similar conclusions—namely, that aggressive behaviors with a sexual motive may manifest themselves in symbolic acts of a nonsexual nature

(Davidson, 1952), and that overtly nonsexual crimes (such as burglary, arson, assault, or stealing) may be motivated by hidden sexual forces that are not, at first, obvious even to a trained observer (Banay, 1969). Banay reported several cases of assaults, stabbings, and murders, where significant underlying sexual dynamics were present but had not been initially detected. "Since the individual is seldom completely aware of the motives for his actions, it is natural that a criminal should deny and disbelieve that certain behavior, seemingly nonsexual, could be sexually inspired" (p. 94). He concluded that "crimes are classified more for purposes of orderly enforcement than for a precise identification of their source and essential nature" (p. 91). In fact, Schlesinger and Revitch's (1997a) compendium of various forms of sexually motivated antisocial behavior includes many nonovertly sexual acts such as vampirism, burglary, fire setting, and theft. Many sexual murderers have a history of what would appear to be nonsexually motivated crimes. If the sexual dynamics of these offenses are not recognized, the potential dangerousness of the offender is missed.

Do these conclusions confirm Freud's (1905) hypothesis that "nothing of considerable importance can occur in the organism without contributing some component to the excitation of the sexual instinct" (p. 137)? That is, are we to regard all murders as sexual murders—at least at some level? Such a notion might possibly be correct from a psychoanalytic perspective, but from the perspective of a researcher, an investigator, or a practicing forensic clinician, it is impractical and seems incorrect. There *are* differences between sexual murders and nonsexual murders; it is just hard to specify exactly what the differences are.

1.4 Distinction between a Sexual Murder and Murder Associated with Sexual Behavior Is Often Blurred

Grubin (1994) lists a number of ways in which a homicide and a sexual offense may become linked: a sexual offender may murder his victim in order to silence a potential accuser; he may become angry and kill his victim in response to her resistance; he may panic and accidentally kill his victim; or he may participate in a rape-homicide as a result of group pressure (which sometimes occurs with military troops on a rampage in an occupied territory). Although murder and sex are connected in these instances, the murders were not sexually motivated, and we agree with Grubin who believes that they should not be considered sexual murders. Greenall (2012) describes four different scenarios involving sex and murder: sexual violence then homicide; sexual violence with homicide; homicide then sexual violence; and homicide containing covert sexual dynamics.

The blurred distinction between a sexual murderer and a sex offender who commits a murder is illustrated in a study conducted by Firestone, Bradford, Greenberg, and Larose (1998). In their comprehensive research project involving 48 "homicidal sex offenders," they used various diagnostic tools, including phallometric readings, to help them understand their subjects. However, the circumstances surrounding the homicides are not exactly clear. Many of the offenders seem to have been motivated by one of the scenarios outlined by Grubin (1994). It is not known whether any of the murders were actually sexually motivated and to what group of offenders the results apply.

Meloy (2000) also notes the distinction between sexual murder and murder associated with sexual activity. Nevertheless, he attempted to estimate the incidence of sexual homicides by examining reported homicides that the *UCR* categorize as murders associated with rape, other sex, or prostitution. He points out that these *may* be sexual homicides since sexual murderers often do kill prostitutes or rape and then kill their victims. However, there is an equal probability that many of these crimes were not sexual homicides. All that we can say about these cases is that homicide and sex were related; we cannot say with certainty that the homicide was sexually motivated.

1.5 Absence of National Crime Statistics on Sexual Murder

The actual base rate of sexual homicide is uncertain. The *UCR* do not collect data on the number of sexual murders in the United States, nor does any reliable state database exist. The FBI has never officially estimated the number of sexual (or serial) homicides occurring within the United States, despite hearsay to the contrary (Wilson, 2000). The only country that collected data on sexual murder—and no longer does so—was Canada, under the auspices of the Centre for Justice Statistics, a part of Statistics Canada. However, their definition of sexual murder had been a homicide occurring during the commission of a sexual offense. However, these homicides are not always sexually motivated; rather, they are murders (as Grubin [1994] and Greenall [2012] pointed out) that occur in connection with a sex crime. In fact, the Canadian definition excluded numerous cases of homicide that are sexually motivated—such as those involving strangulation, or multiple stab wounds, without an overt expression of genitality—because of the absence of a sex offense. The prevalence of sexual murder in Canada is estimated to be about 4% of all homicides—which amounts to about 20 cases per year—and has been fairly consistent over time. However, the number of sexually motivated homicides still remains unknown. Given the multiple complex problems with definition, it is easy to understand why accurate statistics on the incidence of sexual murder would be very difficult to calculate. Taking these complexities into account, Beauregard and Martineau (2012) analyzed a database operated by the Canadian Royal Mounted Police and identified 350 cases of sexual homicide that occurred between 1948 and 2010, using Ressler et al.'s (1988) criteria: evidence of the victim's attire or lack of attire, exposure of the victim's sexual parts, sexual positioning of the victim's body, insertion of an object, sexual penetration, or evidence of substitute sexual activity or interest or of sadistic fantasy.

In an attempt to estimate the incidence of sexual homicide in the United States and in other countries, some researchers have made use of indirect data sources—with their inherent problems. For example, Chan and Heide (2009) reported an estimated 4% of incarcerated murderers in the United Kingdom to be sexual murderers. Ressler et al. (1988) took a different approach. They reviewed available U.S. crime statistics and concluded that, although the base rate of serial (sexual) homicide is unknown, there are signs that it is actually increasing. They based their reasoning on two sets of statistics in the *UCR*: (1) the dramatic decrease in the clearance (arrest) rate for homicide over the past 40 years and (2) the concomitant dramatic increase in the number of murders with unknown motives.

Since crime-solving techniques (e.g., DNA, cameras) have become more sophisticated and the number of police officers per capita has increased since the 1960s, we would expect the homicide clearance rates to increase or, at the very least, stay the same. In 1960, for example, 93.1% of homicides were cleared by law enforcement. The clearance rate declined steadily to 63% in 2000 and 63.2% in 2018. It has been argued that sexual murderers, particularly serial sexual murderers, are hard to apprehend because they frequently kill strangers (Godwin, 2000; Langevin, 1991; Meloy, 2000). In addition, some sexual murderers, particularly those with multiple victims, are often geographically mobile (Dietz, Hazelwood, and Warren, 1990; Rossmo, 2000), and that mobility increases the difficulty in apprehension. At first glance, these findings seem to support the conclusion that the decline in homicide clearance rates is attributable to an increase in sexual homicides.

Homicides with unknown motives (i.e., the motivation for the murder is uncertain and does not fit into any of the categories used by the *UCR*) have increased significantly for several decades. In 1976, 8.5% of murders were committed for unknown motives. This figure has risen steadily over the years so that in 1998, the number of murders committed for unknown motives reached 38% and 39% in 2018. Because sexual killings often appear to be motiveless (and, therefore, would be placed in this category), Ressler, Burgess, and Douglas (1988), as well as other researchers, have reasoned that the number of sexual homicides has also increased.

Schlesinger (2001a) has argued that a close examination of the available crime data reveals little scientific support for the view that sexual homicide is increasing. For example, clearance rates have declined not only for homicide but also for rape (72.6% in 1960, 50% in 1998, and 33.4% in 2018) and for (nonsexual) assault (78.7% in 1960, 59% in 1998, and 52.5% in 2018). The increase in murders with unknown motives could be attributable to an increase in other types of homicide such as contract murder, where the motive is not obvious and thus is placed in the unknown motive category.

Most significantly, a close examination of crime-victim data does not support the conclusion of an increase in sexual or serial murder. If sexual homicides were actually increasing, we would expect to see a proportionate increase in the number of female murder victims, since sexual murderers are overwhelmingly men who kill women (Brittain, 1970; Myers, Reccoppa, Burton, and McElroy, 1993; Revitch and Schlesinger, 1989). In fact, the overall percentage of female homicide victims actually dropped by 10% from 1960 (33%) to 2000 (23%) and 22.7% in 2018. In addition, Zahn and Sagi (1987) have demonstrated that victims of stranger homicides are overwhelmingly (85%–92%) males. This finding strongly suggests that the increase in stranger homicides does not signify an increase in sexual homicide, since sexual murderers, who are also often strangers to their victims, mainly target women. Thus, the crime-victim gender data, as well as the declining clearance rates for nonhomicidal violent crime and the increase in murders with unknown motives, does not support the contention that sexual homicide is increasing. In fact, recent research by Myers, Chan, and Mariano (2016) found that for the years 1976–2007, the number of U.S. sexual homicides actually decreased from an estimated prevalence rate of 1.4% of all homicides to 0.4%. However, these researchers used a definition of sexual homicide similar to the former Canadian definition—homicide in conjunction with rape or "other sexual offense." Since the number of rapes has declined dramatically, these results are not surprising. Accordingly, the number of sexual homicides in the United States remains unclear.

1.6 Practical Impediments to Research

Empirical research on sexual murderers (unlike research on sexual offenders, mentally disordered offenders, and other types of criminals) is very difficult to carry out due to several practical impediments. Dietz (1986) has suggested that the dearth of scientific papers on (serial) sexual homicide is largely attributable to its extreme rarity, which does not permit ordinary behavioral science research methods to be easily employed. Comparatively few cases are available to most mental health researchers because the offenders are incarcerated at different institutions, even in any given state. It is not hard to get subjects to study depression, substance abuse, or posttraumatic stress disorder. The researcher can easily go to a psychiatric hospital, rehabilitation program, or veteran's hospital. But it is not easy to get sexual homicide cases since it is a low base rate crime.

Unlike sex offenders, they are not labeled (either legally or institutionally) as sexual murderers, so that their identification for research purposes becomes even more difficult. For example, prison officials can easily identify the numbers and location of incarcerated rapists or child molesters; they can also identify the number of murderers. But they cannot tell a researcher how many sexual murderers are in the institution because they are not labeled as sexual murderers; they are labeled only as murderers. And when a potential offender is identified, perhaps because he expresses a desire to commit a sexual murder (Johnson and Becker, 1997), the homicide itself might not occur for many years—30 years in one case (Revitch, 1957).

When a sexual murderer is evaluated, his background history, vital for a full understanding of his motivation, is often incomplete and inaccurate. Sexual murderers frequently lie and manipulate, not only to escape responsibility for wrongful behavior but also to gain an inner sense of domination, mastery, and control over others (Douglas and Olshaker, 1995), including researchers and clinicians. Such offenders frequently lie and manipulate when they do not have to, and even when it is to their ultimate disadvantage to do so. They use their tactics in order to abduct a victim and, after they are apprehended, often continue to use them on their attorneys, experts, prison officials, media, family members, and others. As one offender stated, "I feel I have to lie. Why tell you the truth and let you know what's happening and where I'm at? I'll lie and hold it over you without you ever knowing" (Schlesinger, 2001b, p. 54).

In carrying out research with sexual murderers, therefore, investigators must always be aware that these offenders' self-reported histories are frequently inaccurate. They probably will deny, minimize, or rationalize their antisocial behavior, even when that behavior has been well documented and corroborated by multiple sources. When confronted, they might say that the sources are inaccurate or only partially true. Moreover, some important background information, such as instances of sexual abuse, may not have been documented and must be elicited from the offender's self-report. The investigator cannot assume that the offender's account is completely or even partially accurate. An offender might lie about abuse to help him in mitigating a sentence; he might lie about abuse because he does not want to be seen in a weak or victim position. In short, a complete understanding of the sexual murderer—especially his motivation and psychodynamics—is dependent on an accurate background history, which is very difficult to obtain.

In some instances, the offender may be willing to cooperate in all aspects of the evaluation but is advised by his attorney not to do so. The attorney may demand to be present during the examination and may limit inquiries to the specific legal issues being raised. In one recent case, a sexual murderer who killed at least four women in a repetitive, ritualistic manner was being evaluated for competency to waive his *Miranda* rights. The attorney would not let her client speak about the homicides or offer any relevant background information that did not relate directly to the *Miranda* issue. Although that attorney was doing her job, rich information that might greatly enhance our understanding of sexual murder became lost. When such offenders go to prison, they also may be advised by counsel not to discuss anything in their background that is not already known. Any new revelation, in an attorney's view, might jeopardize a client: additional charges might be brought, or the parole board might use such information to keep the offender incarcerated longer.

The lack of interdisciplinary cooperation is yet another practical impediment to the full understanding of the sexual murderer. Until very recently, professionals in various disciplines of clinical and forensic psychiatry and psychology, criminal justice, criminology, and criminal investigation worked independently of one another. As noted by Hazelwood (1989)

> for too many years, the various disciplines concerned with homicide refused to acknowledge that significant expertise existed outside of their own communities. The prevalent attitude has been "what can I possibly learn from them?" Fortunately, over the past ten years, a greater willingness to share, accept and jointly develop information of multi-disciplinary interest has been observed. (p. vii)

Only rarely did mental health professionals collaborate with members of law enforcement, even though criminal investigators sometimes have more experience in cases of sexual murder—at least from their investigative perspective. Information still remains scattered in different professional periodicals sponsored by the host profession.

Without professional collaboration, different perspectives remain unintegrated and complete understanding elusive. Criminologists and sociologists often study criminal behavior from a statistical-epidemiological perspective. Criminal investigators study criminal behavior from the perspective of crime scene analysis. Psychiatrists and psychologists are concerned mainly with the offender's mental state at the time of the crime, as well as underlying psychopathology, usually related to a traditional *DSM* diagnostic category, or sometimes risk assessment or potential for rehabilitation. Since the determinants of sexual homicide are multidimensional, lack of interdisciplinary cooperation significantly reduces complete understanding.

1.7 Phenomenological-Descriptive vs. Statistical Approaches

Empirical phenomenology is a type of qualitative analysis that has had a long and distinguished history in psychological research (most notably used by Freud) and is particularly well suited for new areas of study or areas such as sexual murder that are difficult to research. This approach enables psychologists to categorize and classify their observations in order to study certain conditions that cannot otherwise easily be quantitatively assessed. Skrapec (2001), for example, has used the phenomenological approach from an existential perspective in her study of the personal meanings of the experiences of sexual murderers. Milsom, Beech, and Webster (2003) have used qualitative analysis in a study of sexual murderers, and others have recognized the value of this approach (Safarik and Jarvis, 2005) with certain areas of crime research. Hein and Austin (2001) note that

> there is no single so-called correct way to conduct phenomenological research. Rather, the specific method used depends, to a large extent, on the purposes of the researcher, his or her specific skills and talents, the nature of the research question, and data collected. (p. 3)

Hein and Austin also note that the specific phenomenological method chosen may need to be modified and adapted to meet the needs and characteristics of the particular investigation.

Phenomenological-psychological research has also been called "descriptive" research (Giorgi, 1977; Valle, King, and Halling, 1989) or "qualitative" methodology (Camie, Rhodes, and Yardley, 2003; Silverman, 2011) which includes the case study approach. Morgan and Morgan (2001) have reported the history and advantages of the "single-participant research design," a type of phenomenological research for use in clinical settings. They argue that such an approach is flexible enough to satisfy the requirements of basic science and also enables investigators to study events in a nonlaboratory difficult-to-control environment.

Some psychologists (e.g., Pallone and Hennessey, 1994) advocate a more traditional statistical approach as a means of securing empirical validation. However, that type of analysis, with which most behavioral scientists are familiar, has been questioned in the contemporary methodological literature. Those who have questioned it (e.g., Abelson, 1997; Chow, 1998; Cohen, 1994; Estes, 1997; Loftus, 1996) argue that traditional statistical methodological types of analysis using traditional statistical inference may not be appropriate in many areas of study. The traditional statistical study still, nevertheless, seems to be favored among behavioral scientists. However, the American Psychological Association's new journal *Qualitative Psychology* indicates an increasing appreciation for this approach. We agree with Litwack's (2002, p. 175, 176) observation:

> If descriptive studies ... were done, even with some reasonable assurance of the veridicality of the descriptions involved, would our [leading journals] publish them? Or is our field still somewhat trapped in what I believe to be the erroneous and harmful illusion that, in social science, only what can be quantified is worth studying—or publishing?

In the study of sexual murder, we are not yet at the point where highly quantified validation studies are always appropriate. Since researchers can hardly agree on what constitutes a sexual murder, it seems preposterous to only accept as credible a detailed empirical analysis of its nature. Moreover, highly quantified results tend to lend an aura of scientific respectability, which, in some instances, may be actually pseudo-science (Rozeboom, 1970). Empirical statistical validation is certainly a goal, but we first need to agree on the behavior we are attempting to validate.

There is also the risk that premature quantification could actually impede rather than enhance understanding. For example, reliance on a strict definition could potentially limit one's ability to see new relationships, especially at an early stage in the development or understanding of a disorder. The phenomenological-descriptive approach, although it lacks quantitative precision, does allow a certain degree of freedom to reframe and reorganize observations and rethink the meaning of unique cases, whereas a strict definition might exclude such possibilities.

Accordingly, the approach of this book is largely phenomenological-descriptive; it is an attempt to take a fresh look at sexual homicide by categorization and classification of observations. Thus, we will rely heavily on case studies with analysis, but not to the exclusion of empirical studies where appropriate.

1.8 The First Case of Murder: Forensic vs. Clinical Psychological Approaches

At an early stage in the development of the science of homicide, the study of cases is a necessary first step. But if the study of murder is the study of cases, what case is best to begin with? Should we first attempt to analyze a complex case of sexual homicide with multiple victims or would a more appropriate starting point be a "typical" case of murder? In fact, the first reported murder—the biblical Cain–Abel murder—is instructive in this regard, since it contains most of the elements of the typical contemporary homicide. Since sexual murder is a subtype of homicide, it is impossible to fully understand the former without an understanding of the latter. In addition, the Cain–Abel murder illustrates the significant distinctions between the forensic and clinical psychological approaches used by present-day practitioners when they are asked to evaluate a homicide, a distinction that will be covered more thoroughly in Chapter 2.

> And the Lord had respect unto Abel and to his offering.
> But unto Cain and to his offering he had not respect. And Cain was very wroth, and his countenance fell.
> And the Lord said unto Cain, Why art thou wroth? and why is thy countenance fallen?
> . . .
> And Cain talked with Abel his brother: and it came to pass, when they were in the field, that Cain rose up against Abel his brother, and slew him.
> And the Lord said unto Cain, Where is Abel thy brother? And he said, I know not: am I my brother's keeper?

> *Genesis* **4: 4–9**

Let us assume that the body of Abel is discovered by a passerby who then calls the local police. At this point, the offender is unknown, and an investigation begins. Since this is his first homicide, and the detective has no experience in such matters, he contacts two professionals—a clinical and a forensic psychologist—who deal with human behavior. Even though they also have no experience with homicide, the detective hopes that they can provide some direction to the investigation.

At a meeting, the detective explains the facts of the case to both psychologists. He reports that the deceased has a brother named Cain, but the detective quickly dismisses Cain as a possible suspect because "brothers love one another; it could never be a family member." Both psychologists, however, remark that in their experience, contrary to popular belief and to the impression that most people would like to project, family members often do not love one another. In fact, both psychologists explain, it is quite common for a family member to feel deep jealousy, resentment, anger, and hatred toward another family member. The detective then decides to call in Cain for questioning, and Cain quickly confesses. At this point, the approaches taken by the forensic and the clinical psychologist diverge.

The clinical psychologist meets with Cain in order to learn as much as he can about him. He approaches the task from the traditional perspective of clinical psychology (not different from the approach used in general psychiatry). In the clinical psychological (or psychiatric) approach, the mental health professional conducts an evaluation of the patient, arrives at a diagnosis, and develops a treatment plan based on the diagnosis. Thus, the clinical psychologist interviews Cain, takes his (background) history, asks him to explain the homicide, administers a battery of psychological tests, and arrives at a diagnosis.

The clinical psychologist concludes that Cain—primarily since he seemed to have acted impulsively—must have an impulse control disorder. As a result of his testing and observations, he also determines that Cain has a borderline personality disorder, along with low self-esteem. The clinical psychologist entertains the possibility that Cain may also have a bipolar disorder (somewhat of a diagnostic fad that leads to overdiagnosis) but reserves judgment on this diagnosis for now. Thus, the clinical psychological (or psychiatric) approach to evaluating a homicidal defendant is basically the practice of clinical psychology (or general psychiatry) in a legal context. The case is approached in the same manner as the mental health professional would approach a patient in a hospital, a mental health center, or a private office setting. There is a search for a diagnosis to explain behavior.

The forensic psychologist approaches the Cain–Abel murder case from a distinctly different perspective. He does not want to interview Cain immediately as the clinical psychologist did; instead, he asks for a detailed description of the criminal act itself, as found in the police reports, autopsy report, witness statements, and crime scene findings. What the offender actually did—not just what he said he did—is of primary concern to the forensic psychologist; it is of much more concern, at this point, than his diagnosis. The forensic psychologist believes that if one wants to understand the mind of the criminal, one must first study his crimes. After carefully studying the Cain–Abel homicide, he arrives at a number of findings:

- Cain was angry and jealous just prior to the murder; apparently God favored Abel's offering more than his.
- The killer was the victim's brother and, therefore, had a close relationship with him.
- There was an apparent swiftness to the act. The Bible does not say exactly what transpired, except that "Cain rose up," implying that it was an explosive attack.
- The method of killing was direct violence. The Bible indicates that Cain "rose up and slew him," suggesting that the violent act was not only sudden but also direct and effective.
- The location of the homicide was close to home base. In the biblical premodern society, people spent time in open spaces, or "in the field," as opposed to contemporary places of congregation, such as homes or taverns.
- There was a conversation prior to the murder, perhaps an argument. The Bible reports that "Cain talked with Abel," but it does not say exactly what they spoke about. An angry dispute, however, seems likely, given Cain's apparent jealousy and discontent.
- The offender lied when confronted with the offense. The Lord asked Cain where Abel was, and he responded, "I know not."
- The question of the victim's possible role in the homicide is raised (Wolfgang, 1969). Did Abel play any part in bringing about his death, or was he just a totally passive victim of circumstances?

Each professional submits a report. The clinical psychologist begins with a self-report description of the homicide as recounted by Cain. It seems that Cain was unable to recall a lot of details. He did, however, manage to give several versions of what occurred, all at variance from a statement he gave to the police when arrested—a statement which he now claims was forced. Cain first told the clinical psychologist that he was provoked; next, that Abel's death was an accident; and finally that he was protecting himself from Abel, who actually threatened him. The forensic psychologist has not yet interviewed Cain, so he writes an initial report detailing the eight points he learned from the study of the homicide itself.

The following month, another person is found dead, a victim of an apparent murder. The same detective calls on the clinical and forensic psychologists for assistance in solving the crime. All three professionals now have had some experience in homicide. The clinical psychologist, relying on his evaluation of Cain, says to the detective, "Look for an individual with a borderline personality, low self-esteem, and an impulse control disorder." The forensic psychologist, relying on what he learned from his study of the homicide itself, tells the detective that he should look for a family member or someone who had a close relationship with the victim. He predicts that the murder was probably sudden, perhaps triggered by jealousy or anger; the offender and the victim may have had an argument just before the murder. It is likely that the killing was the result of a direct assault and took place close to where victim and offender typically congregate. He continues that the offender may not be truthful once he realizes he is a suspect. The forensic psychologist is not yet certain what role, if any, the victim may have played.

The clinical psychological approach to the homicide was of little help to law enforcement in this case. The suggestion that the murderer is someone with a borderline personality, low self-esteem, and has an impulse control disorder does not enable the detective to narrow the field of possible suspects, nor does it explain what occurred. On the other hand, the suggestion that he should look for a family member or close associate who was jealous of, or arguing with, the deceased is of practical help to the detective. And examining exactly what transpired, utilizing information from multiple credible sources provides a more solid foundation for drawing conclusions about the offender's state of mind than simply relying on the accused person's version(s) of what occurred.

1.9 Epidemiological Aspects of Homicide: Sexual Murder Must Be Understood in Context

Before we can study sexual murder further, an understanding of the epidemiology of homicide is necessary since sexual homicide cannot be studied or understood in isolation. To study only sexual murder is comparable to a physician who only studies one disease. Many of the characteristics of the nonsexual murderer are the same as the sexual murderer, but some traits and behaviors do differ. Thus, sexual homicide is a subtype of homicide, and in order to fully understand sexual murder, it must be viewed in context.

1.9.1 Incidence of Crime and Homicide

A review of the *UCR* reveals that the majority of all present-day murders are basically of the Cain–Abel type. The patterns of homicide have also been fairly consistent over extended periods of time. For example, from 1837 to 1901, most murders were domestic, followed in frequency by murders committed during the course of another felony (Attick, 1970), a pattern that holds up to the present. However, in order to estimate and understand the prevalence of sexual murder, we first need to place it in proper context—not only its incidence in relation to nonsexual homicide but its incidence in relation to all crime.

Approximately 85% of all reported crime is property crime which includes offenses such as larceny, motor vehicle theft, and burglary. About 12% of all crime is a violent crime such as aggravated assault, robbery, forcible rape, and murder. Among violent crimes, murder is the least frequent offense, accounting for only 1.3% of violent crime.

In 2018, assault accounted for 66.9% of all violent crime, followed by robbery (23.4%) and rape (8.4%). There were 7.2 million property crimes (17.6% clearance rate) and 1.2 million violent crimes (45.5% clearance rate). And while the statistics for crimes such as motor vehicle theft, burglary, and larceny may be inaccurate (due to a variety of reporting problems), the statistics regarding homicide may also be somewhat misleading, even given the unambiguous nature of the act. For example, because of recent advances in emergency medicine, or due to particular circumstances or interventions, some intended murders wind up as assaults, whereas some intended assaults may end up as murder (Doerner and Speir, 1986).

Although murder occurs least frequently in comparison to other offenses, the clearance (arrest) rate for murder is higher than the rates for all other crimes. Murder is generally not a difficult crime to solve (Geberth, 1996), since most homicides involve family members, friends, and acquaintances, similar to Cain and Abel. However, sexual homicide may be an exception, since many sexual murders are not of the Cain–Abel variety; sexual murderers sometimes kill strangers, making apprehension much more difficult. Even with the absence of hard data, most experts (Meloy, 2000; Swigert, Farrell, and Yoels, 1976) believe that sexual homicide is extremely rare. Of those who murder once, only a small fraction murder again—for example, in the form of serial sexual homicide (Busch and Cavanaugh, 1986). Thus, when one examines the crime statistics as a whole, it is clear that sexual murder is an extremely rare occurrence.

1.9.2 Historical Patterns

Over the years, the incidence of homicide has fluctuated. At the beginning of the 1900s, the homicide rate was rather low, with the first peak reached in the Depression years of the 1930s (Holinger, 1987). The homicide rate dropped during World War II, probably because most men (the most frequent perpetrators of homicide) were overseas. There was a slight increase in homicide in the late 1940s and early 1950s. By the end of the 1950s, the homicide rate had dropped somewhat, but it increased again in the 1960s and climbed steadily since then so that by the 1980s, the murder rate in the United States was the highest of the 20th century. Most U.S. citizens by the late 1980s were convinced that the crime and homicide rates in America were on a steady increase, with little hope that the trend would alter. Nevertheless, consistent with fluctuating historical trends, throughout the entire decade of the 1990s, crime, as well as murder, decreased continuously, and then began to increase again in the 2000s.

1.9.3 Age Patterns

The age patterns for homicide in America have been fairly steady over the years. Very few children commit homicide but, contrary to popular belief, homicide committed by children has always occurred. For example, in 2018, there were ten homicides committed by children of ages 9 to 12. As adolescence begins, the homicide rate picks up considerably. Most homicides are committed by young adults (20–24 years old). After age 35, homicide rates decline, but there were still 92 murders committed by offenders over age 75. Murder victims are also about the same age as the offenders. The vast majority of victims are 20–40 years old and then decline proportionately.

1.9.4 Additional Findings

A review of the *UCR*'s supplemental homicide data confirms some generally suspected findings. Firearms, especially handguns, were the weapon of choice in 72% of murders in 2018. Knives and personal weapons (such as hands, fists, or feet), blunt objects (clubs, hammers), and other dangerous weapons (poisons, explosives) in the remainder. Since most homicides occur when people are close to each other and likely to get into arguments, most murders occur during the summer and the (holiday) month of December (Chertwood, 1988). Additionally, the homicide rate is highest on Saturday evenings or early Sunday mornings (Hagan, 1994), possibly reflecting not only interpersonal contact but the use of alcohol as well. In fact, Wolfgang (1958) first established that about half of all offenders, as well as victims, were under the influence of alcohol at the time of the homicide, a finding that holds up today.

It has long been suspected, even since premodern times, that there is a relationship between lunar cycles and homicide. Police officers and hospital emergency room personnel have consistently reported an increase in interpersonal violence during a full moon. One study (Lieber, 1978) did, in fact, seem to show a correlation between the moon and homicide rates, although Schafer, Varano, Jarvis, and Cancino (2010) dispute this finding. It has been theorized that since the human body is about 80% water, the moon's influence is similar to the impact it has on tides.

Among industrialized nations, the United States seems to have one of the highest homicide rates; Japan and Austria seem to have the lowest rates (Fingerhut and Kleinman, 1990), but comparisons between countries are very difficult to make given the vast differences in so many factors. Explanations for the comparative frequency of homicide in the United States include American tolerance of aggression, access to firearms, and the impact of the media (social media) and television (Malmquist, 1996). Some researchers have even speculated that the United States leads the world in the number of sexual murders (Hickey, 1997; Newton, 1992; Norris, 1998), but there is really no scientific support for this assertion (Schlesinger, 2001a). In fact, sexual murder has been documented since premodern times in every country and every culture, and its occurrence has always been very rare, with no signs it is increasing (Schlesinger, 2000a).

1.10 Victimology: Dynamics of Victim and Offender

What role, if any, did Abel play in the Cain–Abel homicide? Was he, as Wolfgang (1969) asks, an "unsuspecting, helpless, passive victim stalked by a cold, calculating killer," or does the victim play "an active part in a surprisingly large number of cases, so active that he seems deliberately to have brought about his own death" (p. 55)? This question must be asked, no matter how difficult and unsettling the answer may be. Unfortunately, some (partially informed) individuals regard victimology as an attempt to blame victims or to encourage people to see themselves as victims. In fact, the study of victims is undertaken not to assign blame or to provide rationalizations but to help investigators understand the interpersonal dynamics involved in certain types of crimes (Karmen, 2001).

Some research findings strongly suggest a close connection between victim and offender. In Wolfgang's (1958) classic sociological study of 588 murders that occurred in Philadelphia between 1948 and 1952, 25% of victims and offenders were relatives, 28%

close friends, 14% acquaintances, and about 20% husbands and wives. Forty-one percent of all women killed were killed by their husbands, but only 11% of husbands were killed by their wives. Wolfgang concluded that a woman who commits a homicide is more likely than a man to kill her mate; when a man is killed by a woman, he is most likely to have been killed by his wife.

A review of the *UCR* over the past 40 years shows relative stability in these findings. Most contemporary murders are committed by men (87%), and most victims are also men. Almost half of all murder victims knew their assailants with less than 10% killed by strangers. Husbands or boyfriends were identified as the murderer in about a third of the time when the victim was a woman, but less than 5% of male victims were slain by wives or girlfriends.

Since the majority of murderers and victims know each other well and associate with each other frequently, it is not surprising that most homicides are intraracial. Since victims and offenders are closely connected, it is logical that arguments would trigger about one-third of the murders, since familiarity often results in animosity. Other close victim–offender connections have been documented by the *UCR* over the years, including homicides as a result of romantic triangles, parents killing children, children killed by babysitters, and arguments between victims and offenders over money or property.

The same statistics that show a close connection between victim and offender in the United States have also been duplicated in research conducted in different countries, in different cultures, and at different time periods. For example, Svalastoga (1956) studied 172 murders that occurred in Denmark. In this study 90% of the victims were relatives, friends, or acquaintances. The 52 female murderers in his sample rarely went outside the family to commit a homicide, and none had killed a stranger. Similarly, East (1950) found that only 6% of 300 murderers who were judged to be insane, and only 16% of 200 murderers found sane, killed strangers. The vast majority killed family, friends, and acquaintances. Bohannan (1960) found the same offender–victim relationship pattern in homicides among various African tribes.

On the basis of his findings, Wolfgang (1958) ultimately concluded that about 26% of the victims appeared to precipitate their own death and did so not by subtle or covert signs but by some overt physical (usually aggressive and provocative) behavior. He cited many examples to demonstrate his contention. A man who repeatedly beat and threatened his wife finally invited her to stab him with a knife, and she did so. In another case, a man who repetitively beat his wife handed her a knife and dared her to use it. She said she would if he hit her again. He slapped her in the face, and she stabbed him to death. In still another case, an intoxicated man got into an argument with another man and brandished a knife. The other man displayed a gun, the victim dared him to shoot, and he did. Wolfgang (1969) concluded that, in these and many similar cases, the victims were (unconsciously) attempting to commit suicide—a view also held by others (Ellenberger, 1955; MacDonald, 1986). More recently, the phenomenon of suicide-by-cop (wherein a person seriously threatens a police officer, who then shoots him) is receiving a great deal of attention and is thought to involve similar (but perhaps not unconscious) suicidal dynamics (Dewey, Allwood, Fava, Arias, Pinizzotto, and Schlesinger, 2013; Pinizzotto and Davis, 1999).

Even before Wolfgang's study, Von Hentig (1941) had published an article focusing on the interaction (sometimes symbiosis) between victims and offenders. He concluded that the victim is one of the causes of a crime: "In a sense the victim shapes and molds the criminal … to know one, we must be acquainted with the complementary partner" (p. 12).

Several years later, Mendelsohn (1956, 1963) coined the term "victimology." He illustrated his concept (Mendelsohn, 1963) by discussing the case of a man who killed his wife and her paramour after he found them together in bed. Mendelsohn concluded that the wife's "perverse" and provocative conduct had prompted the homicide. The history of victimology, which is now a well-recognized interdisciplinary specialty, has been reviewed recently by Karmen (2012) and Doerner and Lab (2012).

In addition to the sociological studies of von Hentig and Mendelsohn, the contributory role of the victim in criminal acts has been recognized in poetry and literature. For example, poet and philosopher Kahlil Gibran (1923) wrote in *The Prophet*, "The murdered is not unaccountable for his own murder, and the robbed is not blameless in being robbed" (p. 41). In Franz Werfel's (1920) novel *Not the Assassin but the Victim Is Guilty* (discussed by Ellenberger, 1955), a young boy kills his cold and tyrannical father after years of coping with the father's obnoxious behavior which left the son hating him bitterly. Following the murder, the young man stated, "I, the assassin, and he, the victim, are both guilty! But he is a little more guilty than I." The contributory role of the victim is more subtly explored in Shiga Naoya's (1993) short story *Han's Crime*. In this story, the protagonist's wife becomes pregnant by her cousin, a close friend of the husband, and then kills the baby in order to hurt her husband even more. Despite the deterioration of their marriage and "amazingly cruel" relations between the two, she continues to serve as her husband's assistant in his circus knife-throwing act. Ultimately, he severs her carotid artery with the knife during a performance.

Victims also have been studied from a psychodynamic point of view. MacDonald (1986) argues that some people become victims as a result of various unconscious needs and conflicts: "Just as there are accident prone persons, so also there are persons who are prone to become victims. Thus, there may be a symbiotic relationship between the criminal and his victim" (p. 59). According to MacDonald, the types of individuals especially susceptible to becoming victims are depressives, masochists, and tormentors. Depressed individuals often seek punishment and frequently get killed in the process—behavior that can be viewed as fundamentally suicidal. Neustatter (1957) cites the strange case of a depressed psychiatric patient who repeatedly asked other patients to kill him; eventually one did. Masochists derive pleasure from being abused and thus constantly place themselves in dangerous situations. MacDonald cites the case of a young woman who consistently returned to her abusive boyfriend and eventually was killed by him. This author describes the tormentor as a person who usually dies at the hand of a family member whom he has persistently badgered. As an example, he reports the case of a woman who suffered for years from the behavior of her alcoholic husband. Provoked beyond all measure, she impulsively killed him during an argument.

Perhaps the most practical approach to victimology—an approach that has the most relevance to understanding sexual murder—comes from law enforcement. Mental health professionals seek to explain the personality and behavior of a murderer through psychological concepts, whereas law enforcement officers seek to apprehend unidentified offenders through investigative concepts (Douglas, Ressler, Burgess, and Hartman, 1986; Geberth, 1981; Jackson and Bekerian, 1997; Rossi, 1982). Since it has long been recognized that there is usually a close relationship between offender and victim, a study of the victim may unearth clues to the identity of the offender. Even in cases where a murderer does not know his victim, his selection of that victim rarely is random (Lunde, 1976). Thus, from an investigative perspective, information about the victim is as essential as any other type of information obtained from a crime scene.

Table 1.3   Background Information Needed to Assess Level of Victim Risk

- Lifestyle
- Employment
- Personality
- Friends (type, number)
- Income (amount, source)
- Family
- Alcohol/drug use or abuse
- Normal dress
- Handicaps
- Transportation used
- Reputation, habits, and fears
- Marital status
- Dating habits
- Leisure activities
- Criminal history
- Assertiveness
- Likes and dislikes
- Significant events prior to the crime
- Activities prior to the crime

Source: Adapted from Douglas, J.E., Burgess, A.W., Burgess, A.G., and Ressler, R.K., *Crime Classification Manual*, Jossey Bass, San Francisco, 2013, pp. 17–18.

Investigative profilers and behavioral analysts therefore attempt to gather a complete history of the victim (see Table 1.3), including background, habits, and resistance ability, in an attempt to answer a central question: Why did this person become the victim of a sexual murderer? Key to the answer is an assessment of victim risk: the level of risk (high, moderate, and low) in which the victim placed herself (either intentionally or unintentionally) prior to becoming a victim (Douglas, Burgess, Burgess, and Ressler, 1992). For example, some sexual murderers seek high-risk victims (such as hitchhikers or prostitutes), whereas others seek out low-risk victims (e.g., people whose habitual lifestyles, such as a preference for staying at home, make them relatively inaccessible as targets). Thus, information on victim risk, as well as on the level of risk the offender takes to commit the crime, helps investigators generate a profile of the unidentified offender being sought.

1.11 Comment

Despite the many problems involved in the study of sexual murders and despite their relative rarity, the tragedy they cause and the potential for repetition make them too important to ignore. Although we might not be at a level of understanding where advanced statistical analysis can be employed, case studies, as well as descriptive statistics and qualitative research designs, are credible and heuristic (Camie, Rhodes, and Yardley, 2003). Gradually, by comparing and grouping cases, identifying commonalities, and discovering unique qualities, we are increasing our understanding of this form of criminal behavior.

Not only can our findings help us further understand sexual homicide (as well as various forms of sexually motivated antisocial behavior), but there is a practical application for this knowledge base. Psychologists and psychiatrists have customarily been used as forensic specialists in matters such as criminal responsibility, competency, sentencing, risk assessment, and parole. In addition to these traditional areas, new areas of forensic practice are emerging that require extensive knowledge of criminal psychopathology such as consultation to nonforensic mental health professionals and law enforcement, government, and industry. Although, admittedly, we often lack statistical validation studies, it is simply incorrect to conclude that we know too little about sexual murder, for example, to be of help to other professionals and the criminal justice system.

In the past 30 years, the explosion of knowledge in the mental health field has been phenomenal. No longer can one be in general practice; instead, specialization in one or several areas is required if one is to practice ethically at an acceptable level of competence. Forensic psychologists and psychiatrists with knowledge of criminal psychopathology may be a great resource to nonforensic mental health professionals seeking consultation on a treatment case. For example, a nonforensic general psychiatrist or clinical psychologist may encounter a patient whose behavior (e.g., hatred for cats or obsessive interest in detective magazines) raises issues of (forensic) concern (Schlesinger, 2001b). Forensic professionals (with expertise not only in law and legal standards but also in the psychopathology and psychodynamics of crime) can be of great practical help, providing information on a patient population that is often foreign to the general clinical practitioner.

The practice of psychological (criminal or investigative) analysis, used mostly by law enforcement officers today (but also by industry in terms of threat assessment of troubled employees), actually had its beginnings with mental health professionals. By the late 1950s, most states had initiated specialized programs to evaluate and treat repetitive sex offenders or sexual psychopaths (Friedmann, 1948; Vuocolo, 1969). When law enforcement officers became stymied in an investigation—as it often occurs with sexual crimes, including sexual murder—they would typically call staffers at their local sex offender program for assistance. Primarily, they would request a "profile" of the unidentified offender, based on the staff member's experience with such cases. The profile was frequently very general, filled with psychological jargon, and usually unhelpful.

In 1957, psychiatrist James Brussell consulted with New York law enforcement on the notorious "Mad Bomber" case. Here, an individual planted bombs throughout New York City, remaining undetected for over 16 years. With Brussell's uncannily accurate profile—including the offender's style of dress, religion, and living arrangements—the range of suspects the police were considering narrowed, and an arrest was made. Brussel (1968), in explaining his profiling technique, said that he had simply reversed the process routinely used by mental health professionals. The psychiatrist, for example, evaluates a person and then makes predictions about how this individual might behave. The psychiatrist might predict, for instance, that the person would get depressed, make suicide attempts, or have problems with authority. In drawing a profile of an unidentified offender, Brussell explained, he already knows what the offender did as he can examine crime scene information; then he attempts to deduce what type of person would have committed the crime in this particular manner.

In the 1970s and 1980s, members of the FBI Behavioral Science Unit developed and refined the technique of criminal profiling (Pinizzotto, 1984; Pinizzotto and Finkel, 1990), discussed further in Chapter 7. They attempted to describe unidentified offenders by analyzing the behavioral significance of these offenders' conduct at the crime scene. Psychiatrists and psychologists who have extensive backgrounds in behavioral science and criminal psychopathology should surely be able to make a contribution to law enforcement in this regard (McGrath, 2000). Psychological profiling (or behavioral analysis) has been used in cases of sexual murder, other types of sexual offenses, hostage taking, arson, and anonymous letter writing (Douglas et al., 1986). Although profiling techniques have not, for the most part, been statistically validated (Pallone and Hennessey, 1994), recent research has come a long way in demonstrating moderate to strong accuracy rates with the method (Fox and Farrington, 2018). Behavioral analysis has also been considered helpful not only as an investigative tool (Ressler, Burgess, Douglas, and Depue, 1991) but as an aid in threat assessment for patients and disturbed employees (Davis, 2001), as well.

Forensic Assessment
Evaluation of the Sexual Murder

2

2.1 Background

The method of evaluating criminal defendants in order to determine their state of mind, dangerousness, competency, or—in the case of a sexual murderer—to simply understand the criminal act is fundamental in forensic practice. In Chapter 1, the Cain–Abel murder case was used to illustrate the distinctions between a clinical assessment (as routinely performed in hospitals, mental health centers, and private offices) and a forensic evaluation. In this chapter, a more detailed comparison of the two types of evaluations will be presented as this is critical in understanding the criminal offender, in general, and the sexual murderer, in particular.

Mental health practitioners such as psychiatrists and psychologists are generally taught to evaluate their patients by first interviewing them, perhaps utilizing additional psychological or neurodiagnostic testing, and sometimes requesting supplementary interviews with family members. Hospital, school, and medical records or perhaps reports from prior therapists are also frequently reviewed. Following the evaluation, a diagnosis is made and a treatment plan developed. Clinicians are taught to listen to their patients. If a patient says that he feels depressed, anxious, or agitated, or that he has suicidal thoughts, the mental health professional usually accepts the patient's symptom description as valid unless there is a good reason not to believe him. Lying, deceit, exaggeration, and malingering do occur and may be explored in clinical practice, but generally the main emphasis is on diagnosis and treatment.

Melton, Petrila, Poythress, Slobogin, Otto, Mossman, and Condie (2018) describe various differences between a forensic and a clinical (or what they refer to as a therapeutic) assessment (see Table 2.1). They note differences in the scope of the evaluation, the client's perspective, voluntariness, autonomy, threats to validity, relationship and dynamics, and pace and setting. The fundamental distinction, however, is that, in forensic assessments, there is a high likelihood that the defendant will not always be truthful as he has an obvious motive to lie, exaggerate, or distort symptoms and events. Thus, the traditional clinical approach (in which mental health professionals have been trained) cannot be used for forensic assessments. Forensic psychology (or psychiatry) is not simply the practice of clinical psychology (or general psychiatry) in a forensic setting (Schlesinger, 2003, 2005). Forensic psychology is a separate specialty that requires a modification of the traditional clinical approach. Unfortunately, this distinction is not stressed enough in books on forensic psychology/psychiatry. In fact, several well-known texts do not even mention the basics of a forensic examination (Blau, 1998; Bluglass and Bowden, 1990; Cook, 1980; Gunn and Taylor, 1993; Guttmacher and Weihoffer, 1952; Hess and Weiner, 1999; Irvine and Brelje,

Table 2.1 Dimensions Distinguishing a Therapeutic from a Forensic Assessment

Assessments	Results
Scope	Clinical assessments stress diagnosis or treatment needs; forensic evaluations more commonly address narrowly defined events or interactions (such as criminal acts) of a nonclinical nature. In forensic assessments, diagnosis and treatment needs are in the background.
Importance of the client's perspective	In a clinical setting, the focus is on understanding the client's unique view of the situation or problem. In a forensic setting, a more "objective" appraisal is necessary because the forensic examiner is concerned primarily with accuracy; in a forensic evaluation, the client's view, although important, is secondary.
Voluntariness	Persons seeking mental health therapy commonly do so voluntarily. Persons undergoing forensic assessments commonly do so at the behest of a judge or an attorney.
Autonomy	In the clinical setting, patients have greater autonomy and input regarding objectives and procedures. The objectives in a forensic evaluation are determined by the relevant statutes or legal "tests" that define the legal dispute.
Threats to validity	Although unconscious distortion of information is a threat to validity in both clinical and forensic contexts, the threat of conscious and intentional distortion is substantially greater in the forensic setting.
Relationship and dynamics	Treatment-oriented interactions emphasize caring, trust, and empathic understanding as building blocks for developing a therapeutic alliance. Forensic examiners may not ethically nurture the client's perception that they are there in a "helping" role. In forensic settings, there are divided loyalties and limits on confidentiality. Concerns about possible manipulation of defendants in the legal context dictate more emotional distance between forensic examiner and subject.
Pace and setting	In a clinical-therapeutic setting, evaluations may proceed at a more leisurely pace. Diagnoses may be reconsidered over the course of treatment and revised well beyond the initial interviews. In a forensic setting, a variety of factors, including court schedules and limited resources, may limit the opportunities for contact with the client and place time constraints on completing the evaluation or reconsidering opinions.

Source: Adapted from Melton, G.B. et al., *Psychological Evaluations for the Courts*, 4th ed. Guilford Press, New York, 2018, pp. 43–46.

1972; Power and Selwood, 1987). Instead, these volumes focus on various laws, legal tests, and legal standards that forensic practitioners need to know.

As the criminal defendant's version of events (as well as background information and symptom description) has to be corroborated, a review of the facts of the case is fundamental to a forensic assessment. This is very important with all criminal defendants and sexual murderers in particular because they are notorious for being untruthful (Schlesinger, 2001b). Earlier books on forensic psychiatry do recommend the use of corroborative information in conducting assessments. For example, Davidson (1965) cautions that one should not attempt to evaluate a criminal defendant before reading witness statements and investigative reports. Otherwise, the examiner

> will certainly be embarrassed if he examines a defendant in the absence of the whole story. He then has to rely on the patient's own explanation of events, and, as often as not, this explanation is factually incorrect. Many defendants are psychopaths, and many psychopaths tell untruths with glibness and assurance, so that only a naive examiner accepts as fact the information furnished by the patient. (p. 38)

MacDonald (1969) urges examiners to obtain information from outside sources such as family, employers, military personnel, police, probation officers, and hospitals. Sadoff

(1975) advises a first interview without review of corroborating information, followed by a second interview after the review of such material:

> By obtaining statements of confessions read to the police, by examining others who may have seen the defendant at the time of the alleged offense, or near that time, by discussing the problem with mother, spouse, or other close family members, the psychiatrist will have the ability to corroborate certain information received from the patient or to negate it by inconsistent material from others. Certainly, inconsistencies in what was obtained in the clinical interview, and what [the defendant] allegedly told the police or authorities, should be checked into in close detail during the second interview. Methods by which the patient handles this direct assault on his credibility should be noted and forms a part of the examination. (pp. 27–28)

Many mental health professionals who practice in a forensic setting do not follow these recommended procedures or may not even be fully aware of the distinctions between a clinical and forensic assessment. They conduct a forensic evaluation in the same way as they would evaluate a patient in a hospital, mental health center, or private office. They rely on what the criminal defendant tells them about the offense as well as their symptoms. In their study of forensic assessments, for instance, Heilbrun, Rosenfeld, Warren, and Collins (1994) found that most of the evaluators they questioned said that they did "incorporate" third-party information, but they did not explain how or whether they made use of this information in the process of arriving at conclusions and opinions. To the extent that they relied largely on the defendant's own reports, the validity of their conclusions must be called into question; moreover, such an approach does not contribute to our understanding of rare crimes such as sexual murder in which every case needs to be thoroughly and competently examined.

The following case exemplifies the improper way to conduct an evaluation of a man charged with murder.

Case 2.1: Expert Relied Solely on Defendant's Statements

While fishing after school, two adolescent boys detected several partially wrapped packages which had washed ashore. With a stick they rolled one package a short distance from the river, opened it, and found two plastic bags that appeared to contain the torso of a human. The boys immediately went home and notified their parents, who called the police. A search of the area turned up additional bags containing an arm, legs, and a human head.

The medical examiner determined that the deceased was a woman in her 50s with a deformed left hand, the result of a birth defect. The authorities released this information to the media, hoping that the deformity could serve to identify the victim. After hearing the story on the evening news, a friend of the deceased (B) called the authorities. The victim's 66-year-old common-law husband (AA) was arrested after he gave the following statement to the police:

> I was living with her. I couldn't take her anymore. She was senile and I cracked up. We had a fight. I stabbed her two or three times. I don't remember where. It was a kitchen knife that I used to stab her with. I chopped her up. I used an axe. I put the pieces in plastic bags and then put portions of the body into the refrigerator. I left them there a couple of days. Then I threw them off the Smith Street Bridge. I took the pieces there in a shopping cart. I then moved out of the apartment and got a new apartment in the next town. I changed my name. I threw all

her clothes out in the garbage. I wiped up the blood with a rag. I don't remember if I painted the apartment or not, but I think I did. She was always screaming at me. I just couldn't take it anymore. It shouldn't have happened, but I just couldn't take her anymore. She was falling down all the time. If anyone asked, I just told them B went to a nursing home.

To evaluate his client, the defense attorney retained a hospital-based general psychiatrist who had substantial experience in conducting forensic assessments. The psychiatrist first took the offender's history and then conducted "a psychiatric examination and a mental status examination." He reported the following findings:

> The defendant attributed a considerable amount of his difficulties to a mugging which occurred some years ago and he pointed to a scar on his scalp, on the back of his head. Actually, AA did not know whether or not he killed B, but he ultimately was arrested and incarcerated. Here is a man who is thoroughly confused and is suffering from obvious organic brain disease (brain tissue injury) which has produced memory loss, both for recent and remote events. He has little recall of any events, no less the ones that caused him to be incarcerated. He has a long history of alcoholism and was institutionalized at a rehabilitation program on at least one occasion. He is poorly oriented as to time. He does not know the exact hour of the day or the date. However, he did know the year and month. Associative thought processes are in question. He did not answer questions without prodding, nor did he answer them directly and relevantly. Affective behavior was also unusual. Insight as to how he affects others is impaired. Reality-testing functions, however, appeared to be intact, in that he is not overtly hallucinating or delusional.

The psychiatrist offered a diagnosis of "organic brain syndrome due to alcohol (toxic)" and gave the following final opinions and recommendations:

> Here is a man who has actual physical brain impairment and it is extensive. Moreover, AA is very credible in his replies (whatever they may be), inasmuch as he frankly stated that he did not know whether he killed B or not. He has no recollection of it. This examiner is of the opinion that he certainly falls within the purview of the M'Naughten Rule and that he did not know the nature and quality of his acts by reason of his brain disease.

Here, the psychiatrist disregarded the facts of this case (although his report indicated that he had read all the police and witness reports) and relied totally on what the defendant told him. He evidently ignored AA's statements to the police that he had killed B following an argument, dismembered her, packed the body parts in a methodical fashion, placed them in his refrigerator, and then, over the course of a week or so, dropped the various body parts off a bridge, hoping that they would drift out to sea. AA then cleaned the apartment, painted part of it, changed his name, and moved. When examined, the defendant told the psychiatrist that he had no idea what had happened, and the psychiatrist evidently believed him.

When the prosecution expert evaluated AA, he was uncooperative and unpleasant, with anger right at the surface. He reported that he never had arguments with anyone and that he had never previously been in trouble with the police. When it was pointed out to him that he had been arrested several years earlier for armed robbery, he denied any knowledge of such an incident. He said that he did not remember murdering anybody and that he had never heard of B, even though he had lived with her for 8 to 10 years. He also insisted that he did not remember disposing of the evidence, moving to a new location several miles away, changing his name, and telling those who inquired about the victim that she had gone to a nursing home.

The defendant was also uncooperative with psychological testing and refused to do many of the tasks. When asked to name the three colors of the American flag, he said, "Red, white, that's all I know." He also stated that the shape of a ball is "square." When asked to name four recent U.S. presidents, he said, "The hell with the presidents, they never gave me nothing." He did, however, provide an interesting response to Thematic Apperception Test (TAT) card 13MF, which gives some inkling of the possible motivation for the homicide:

> He is standing there, or maybe he killed her. Maybe they were fighting or something. Maybe he just hit her or stepped on her. He killed her, that's all I know. Maybe she kicked him or something like that. They had a fight, she kicked him, and then he killed her, I guess.

The psychiatrist retained by the defense attorney approached this case as if the defendant were a newly admitted patient in the hospital, in which case the psychiatrist would seek to describe the presenting problem. Although the psychiatrist indicated in his report that he had reviewed the various police reports, he did not explain why the defendant gave a detailed statement to the police but told him that he had no memory of the events. The psychiatrist concluded, as a result of the defendant's reported lack of memory, that the offender had an organic brain syndrome caused by alcoholism. Evidently, this psychiatrist believed that anyone who would have killed his lady friend in such a manner must have been insane; he thereby demonstrated his lack of understanding of the legal standard, as well as his general uninformed approach to the evaluation. The prosecution expert, by contrast, relied on the facts of the case and integrated these facts with the offender's responses. The defendant eventually pleaded guilty, and in a statement to the court, gave a detailed account of the murder and surrounding events. Complete neurological evaluation was negative.

Case 2.2: Multiple Experts Relied Solely on Defendant's Statements

A 55-year-old male became involved in a long-term tumultuous relationship with a woman a few years younger. He was jealous, argued, and fought with her, had two arrests for domestic violence, and stalked her.

The defendant described the homicide as follows:

> Wednesday morning, that evil day. A. was lying in bed. I leave, gone for a good four to five hours. I came home through the door. I heard A. in the kitchen, beer on the table. I got angry at that: "Why are you drinking?" A. snapped, "You lying bastard." She grabbed the big knife in the kitchen. We spinned, and whatever happened, happened. It was nothing but the devil. … I caught her arm, we spun around, and wound up in the bathtub.

At this point in describing what happened, the defendant became agitated and angry. He yelled, ranted, screamed, and carried on in an animated way. He would not answer or discuss anything about the homicide itself. He just yelled, "Whatever happened, happened." He screamed so loudly that he actually broke one of the speakers in the room where the evaluation was being monitored for security purposes. His yelling and screaming went on for about 45 minutes; he then calmed down and participated in all other parts of the evaluation. J.A. was evaluated multiple times by at least six different mental health experts. In fact, the defendant testified in a pretrial court hearing and provided the same account of what happened. "She grabbed the big knife in the kitchen. We spinned, and whatever happened, happened."

The problem with this case is that the six experts relied solely on what the defendant told them. However, what the defendant told them did not at all accord with the behavioral evidence. For example, there were multiple knives used, not just one: three bloody, broken knives were found in the kitchen sink. When the prosecution expert asked about the three knives, the defendant did not answer but just began to yell and scream, "Whatever happened, happened." In addition, the defendant said multiple times that A. came at him with the knife, he caught her arm, they spun around and wound up in the bathtub. However, this description also did not agree entirely with the crime scene evidence. Specifically, there was extensive blood throughout the kitchen—on the table, chair, floor, cabinets, countertop, and walls. Accordingly, it would seem that the victim was stabbed for the most part in the kitchen because that was where all the blood was (as well as in the bathroom) with her body finally winding up in the bathtub.

Text messages sent by A. to a friend just weeks before the homicide were illuminating. A. wanted to call a victim hotline. She said the defendant stole money from her. She wanted a police escort because J.A. was following, stalking, and harassing her (when she left their apartment) with accusations about infidelity. She wanted to move out. On one occasion, J.A. went to the laundromat and brought A.'s clothes back to his apartment. When asked whether he, in fact, stalked or followed A., the defendant responded, "No, no, I wouldn't stalk her. For what? How come she didn't call the police and put a restraining order on me?" When asked about text messages indicating that she wanted to move out, the defendant said, "Why didn't she go then?" And he essentially did not respond to other assertions in A.'s text messages.

The defendant was also probed regarding his desire to marry the victim. "I fell in love with A. I was trying to prove my faithfulness and friendship." When asked why he wanted to marry someone he previously had called a Jezebel, the devil, and evil, J.A. offered no response other than to get angry and start yelling. And when asked about other aspects of the homicide such as the cuts on his hands and why he did not leave the apartment once he gained control of the knife (as he claimed), he just kept yelling and screaming.

Reasonable mental health professionals can disagree—and very often do—about diagnoses. The problem, in this case, was that the six defense experts relied solely on what the defendant told them. The offender was a religious individual and a deacon in his church. He had a strong religious background and referred to hearing God's voice, Satan, the Holy Spirit, and the like. Forensic examiners must be culturally competent in taking factors such as this into account in arriving at an accurate diagnosis. The six experts, including the judge, incorrectly believed that the subject's reference to hearing God's voice was evidence of a psychosis, rather than being part of a religious experience. The defendant never experienced auditory hallucinations or any other symptoms of psychosis.

The primary defense psychiatrist who testified at the trial concluded that the defendant was psychotic and found "his mental distress contributed to an inability to form a requisite knowing and purposeful state of mind. Taken in conjunction with each other, the burden of incapacitation appears readily reached" (a phrase that he used in almost all his reports, notwithstanding the facts of the case). In fact, there was no evidence of any psychotic-level disorder, but there was evidence of depression caused by J.A.'s circumstances and of a personality disorder with antisocial and borderline traits (following *DSM-5* criteria).

Many forensic experts believe that if they diagnose a psychotic-level condition such as schizophrenia or any form of psychosis, the defendant is incompetent in all areas and meets the standard for either diminished capacity or insanity. Nothing could be further from the truth. An incorrect diagnosis is not the only issue. The *DSM-5* (2013) makes it clear that "the clinical diagnosis … of a mental disorder … does not imply that an individual with such a condition meets legal criteria for the presence of a mental disorder, or a specified legal standard" (p. 25). Yelling, screaming, calling A. the devil, and referencing the Bible are not, in themselves, evidence of psychosis, most notably when it occurs in selective circumstances.

J.A. testified at his trial, along with the primary defense expert; it did not go well for either individuals. The jury convicted the defendant in a record 44 minutes. There had been a 7-year delay since the time of the homicide as they found J.A. incompetent, a result of (a) various examiners' incorrect belief that if you say you hear God's voice—no matter what the circumstances or your cultural background—it is a psychotic symptom, and (b) the examiners' reliance solely on what the defendant told them, not on a careful examination of the behavioral evidence.

The next case raises another important issue frequently encountered in forensic work. A defense attorney, for example, will retain an expert who has extensive knowledge and experience with a particular condition such as substance abuse, sex offenses, eating disorders, juvenile delinquency, or posttraumatic stress disorder. But this expert may not understand the basics of conducting a forensic examination and, therefore, as in the preceding examples, approached the case as if the defendant were a patient being evaluated in an office setting or a hospital.

In Case 2.3, the defense-retained psychologist had extensive expertise (obtained through the treatment of patients in her private practice) in battered woman syndrome. She also had served as a consultant in numerous court cases addressing the issue of battered woman syndrome, but unfortunately she approached all her assessments from a traditional clinical, as opposed to a forensic, perspective.

Case 2.3: Expert Practiced Clinical Psychology in a Forensic Setting

A 38-year-old female (B), with a 20-year history of drug abuse and drug-related offenses (including drug selling and prostitution), rented a room in a boarding house occupied mainly by other drug addicts. There she met a 42-year-old drug dealer (A) and began a 5-month intimate relationship with him. A continued to sell drugs, and B became known as his "enforcer." She carried a gun and was frequently observed intimidating other drug buyers. On several occasions, she hit buyers over the head with a pipe for not paying A on time. She pistol-whipped at least one drug user in front of others and routinely threatened almost everyone who frequented the boarding house, a known location for buying and using drugs.

Two drug users (C and D), who frequented the house regularly, owed A $600. B decided to look for the couple in order to get the money. She asked several drug addicts if they had seen C and D in the local area. One addict said she has seen them and B convinced A, after some arguing, that they should follow this individual who would take them to C and D. According to one witness, A was not greatly concerned about the money owed him and did not really want to look for the couple, but B convinced him to do so. When A and B located C and D, B forced both into their car at gunpoint, according to another witness.

Once back at the boarding house, A and B took C and D into a room. There, according to several individuals who were in the hallway at the time, B slapped D. One witness heard D "beg, for her life. D said she had a 13-year-old daughter to live for, and she also said, 'Please don't kill me.'" A held his gun on C while B shoved newspapers down his throat, which eventually caused his death. B then slowly strangled D with a stocking, causing her death; she also stabbed C multiple times with her knife. A and B then took both bodies to the basement. The next morning, they moved the bodies to a field several miles away and set them on fire.

Several days later, A and B were arrested. A refused to provide a statement, but B gave the police four different statements. First, she denied any knowledge of the murders. Then she implicated someone else who lived in the boarding house. Then she accused A. Finally, she admitted that both she and A were involved but said that A had killed the victims and that she had merely acted as his assistant. She did not say that she was afraid of A but explained that she had assisted him out of loyalty.

The defense attorney retained a psychologist with expertise in the treatment of battered women. Due to lengthy legal maneuvers, the psychologist first interviewed B in jail 3 years after the murders. Her conclusions were based solely on what the defendant told her. She did not rely on any of the relevant police reports, witness statements, or autopsy findings.

The psychologist began her interview by asking B to describe her relationships with prior boyfriends, including her relationship with A. B told her of numerous relationships, all of which she claimed involved abuse. She went into great detail explaining the abusive relationship she had with A. She said that A hit her when he was angry, knocked her down, slapped her, and struck her in the face with his fist. She described the violence as frequent and occurring in "cycles"; following the violence, A would make up to B by buying her flowers and expensive gifts. Upon questioning, B also reported being psychologically abused by A and said that he had even raped her on several occasions. She explained to the psychologist that she was "terrified" of A and believed that if she did not participate in the murders, A would have killed her as well: "I was petrified; I was scared I'd be next." B then, upon questioning, "described becoming isolated in the relationship, which reinforced her sense of helplessness and A's power and control over her. According to B, A would not allow her to see her friends or family members." B's account of events to the defense expert was at variance with witness statements, as well as her own statements given to the police.

The defense psychologist administered the TAT, wherein B gave repetitive stories of "women being beaten by the men, or even killed, and the women taking the men back with a promise that it will not happen again." According to the psychologist,

> B does not report the traditional signs of trauma associated with battered woman syndrome, although, based on B's history, one would not expect to see signs of psychological trauma. In persons who have a history of abusing substances, the trauma is obscured by the drug use. In fact, it is likely that the alcohol and drug use were B's way of coping with the psychological pain and trauma of her abuse.

The report continued:

> The relationship B described with A is consistent with what occurs in battered woman syndrome. B was dependent on A both psychologically and economically. A had been

violent with her and had manipulated her into compliance and submission. B was passive and compliant in interpersonal relationships, and she had no self-worth. Coupled with both her personality makeup and the abuse she suffered, plus B's history of drug abuse, she had no options other than to remain passive and compliant and to continue to cope with whatever troubled her by using drugs and numbing the pain. She didn't consider disobeying A. Further, in her mind she knew A was upset with both C and D, but she had no idea he would murder them. B has now learned by her attendance at a jail-sponsored domestic violence support group that hitting is always wrong and that she is beginning to understand what happened to her and the mistakes she made. When she stabbed C, she was following A's orders. She was terrified. She heard C and D plead for their lives, and she was also afraid for her life at that time.

Her report concluded:

> B was intimidated at the time of the murders into helping A, and this fear would be considered reasonable for any person in that situation, even more so for someone who was battered and who was passive and compliant. In a sense one can accrue to her the status of being a kidnapping victim, or the victim of a terrorist. She was his victim and had to comply in order to save her own life. What was apparent to this examiner, over the 7-month period in which B was evaluated, was that she is benefiting from the services in the jail and is moving herself to a psychologically new place. Over the past 7 months, she has changed considerably.

Unfortunately, this psychologist, who had considerable experience in treating patients with battered woman syndrome, relied only on what the defendant told her. She did not question the defendant about contradictory witness statements which indicated that B took the leading role in the murders. Apparently, she also did not question B closely about specific symptoms of battered woman syndrome (or posttraumatic stress disorder). She simply assumed that the symptoms would be "obscured" by B's substance abuse. Therefore, she diagnosed the disorder as battered women syndrome, even though B did not display the characteristic symptoms and had not used substances in 3 years.

When B was evaluated by the prosecution expert, she was uncooperative and hostile, especially when she was asked about the facts of the case or about prior statements that were inconsistent with what she had told the defense psychologist. B explained her relationship with A, stating,

> He was good to me. He showed me nice things. I felt that he loved me. Now that I am clean and sober today, I realize he used me to make money. Standing at that door selling his drugs all day, all night, non-stop. I realize A used me. I realize now if someone loves you, they don't beat you up, knock your teeth out, blacken your eyes. When he got angry he'd tear me up. When he got angry, at least once or twice a week, this happened.

When asked why she did not leave him, B responded, "I don't know. I was caught up into the drugs and him. After he'd hit me or twist my arm, he'd always buy me something real nice." However, she could not explain why, over a 5-month period, nobody saw or heard any of this alleged violence, even though the rooms in the boarding house were described as "paper thin." The person who roomed next to A and B said, "I could hear everything. I heard them argue and I heard them have sex, but I never heard any violence between them at all. If anything, B was the violent one toward everyone else. A was real laid back."

B's arrest record showed that she had a long history of violence, but when asked about these incidents, she "could not remember." When asked why she did not leave the abusive relationship, she stated, "I never thought about leaving, because he'd buy me flowers. I liked the relationship. A took me from the streets. I really ran the drug business. I was in charge and liked it." She stated that she did not feel "psychologically trapped" and had no flashbacks, numbing of emotions, or other symptoms typical of battered women or of those who have experienced a trauma. B claimed that the people who gave statements indicating that she was the one who was violent, "the enforcer," and the instigator of the murders were simply being untruthful.

When asked why she did not mention being frightened of A when she was initially arrested, B responded, "I don't know why I didn't mention it. Everyone knows I was scared. People knew A was in control." Even after A was arrested and was unable to hurt her, B was still unable to explain why she expressed no fear of him; the reported fear of A supposedly experienced by B only emerged 3 years after their arrest during the defense expert's evaluation.

Psychological test findings were helpful in understanding some of the dynamics of the case. For example, the Rorschach showed mild anxiety and depression, inner conflict, and a very severe personality disturbance, characterized by weak controls and lack of solid integration and cohesiveness. There were a number of aggressive, as well as regressive, perceptions, such as the following: "Looks like two people pulling the person in the middle apart. The person is holding someone's hands up and pulling them. Separating him. It looks like blood 'cause it's red. Maybe their legs are bleeding." "Looks like a sword separating something, splitting something in half. Splashed or splotched paint on the wall." Her most primitive Rorschach response suggested that her functioning could become very regressive: "A monster. A big ugly monster. Claws and big feet; he is dropping something out of him. Maybe he is shitting, I don't know what all that is, coming out of him." The Minnesota Multiphastic Personality Inventory (MMPI) profile reflected a broodingly resentful person, who is angry and ruminates about real or imagined injustices done to her.

The jury found B responsible for both murders. They found no evidence of battered woman syndrome or anything even closely connected to it. The defense psychologist was not incompetent or untruthful; she simply did not know how to conduct a forensic evaluation. She was basically practicing clinical psychology in a forensic setting by interviewing the defendant in the same way she would interview a patient who came to her for treatment. Although this psychologist, like the defense experts in Cases 2.1 and 2.2, said that she had read the legal discovery, her final conclusions demonstrate that she ignored these findings or, at the very least, believed that her own interview with the defendant was more valid. Neither of these experts helped the defendant or provided much understanding of the offenders or their crimes.

2.2 Psychological Testing

Psychological testing is a quantitative or quasi-quantitative method of evaluating personality, psychopathology, and mental functioning. It has been used for many years to supplement information obtained through the clinical interview and review of various background records. Testing has always had general appeal because its purpose, in part, is to reduce much of the subjectivity of the clinical evaluation, as well as to assess the

Table 2.2   Sampling of Conventional Psychological Assessment Tools

Structured diagnostic interviews:
- Mini-International Psychiatric Interview for Children and Adolescents (MINI-KID)
- Structured Clinical Interview for DMS-5 (SCID-5)

Checklists and rating scales:
- Behavior Assessment System for Children, Third Edition
- Brief Psychiatric Rating Scale—Anchored (BPRS-A)
- Child Behavior Checklist (CBCL)
- Hamilton Depression Rating Scale (HAM-D)
- Psychopathy Checklist—Revised (PCL-R)

Personality inventories:
- Beck Depression Inventory-II
- Miller-Forensic Assessment of Symptoms Test (M-FAST)
- Millon Clinical Multiaxial Inventory-IV (MCMI-IV)
- Minnesota Multiphasic Personality Inventory-2—Restructured Form MMPI-2-RF)
- Personality Assessment Inventory (PAI)
- Personality Assessment Inventory—Adolescent (PAI-A)
- California Psychological Inventory (CPI)
- NEO Personality Inventory—Revised (NEO PI-R)
- 16PF Questionnaire

Projective personality tests:
- Rorschach Inkblot Technique
- Thematic Apperception Test (TAT)

Tests of intellectual functioning:
- Reynolds Intellectual Assessment Scales Second Edition (RIAS-2)
- Stanford–Binet Intelligence Scales, Fifth Edition (SB5)
- Wechsler Adult Intelligence Scale—Fourth Edition (WAIS-IV)
- Weschler Intelligence Scale for Children—Fifth Edition (WISC-V)

Tests of memory functioning:
- Test of Memory and Learning Second Edition (TOMAL-2)
- Wechsler Memory Scale—Fourth Edition (WMS-IV)

Source: Adapted from Melton, et al. *Psychological Evaluations for the Courts* (4th ed.) Guilford Press, New York, 2018 p. 48.

individual from a different perspective. Since psychological testing is an aid in the process of diagnostic (and psychodynamic) formulation, it has been widely used in forensic assessments, where the need for objectivity and accuracy is paramount (Heilbrun, 1992). Table 2.2 lists a number of traditionally used psychological tests.

Melton et al. (2018), in criticizing the use of psychological testing in a forensic context, point out that "most [traditional] tests have neither been developed nor validated specifically to inform judgments about legally relevant behavior" (p. 49). Thus, they argue, such tests are largely unnecessary because (1) they do not directly address the specific legal question that the evaluation is to supposed to answer; (2) they represent compilations of characteristics found in groups of individuals and therefore may not apply to a particular offender being evaluated; and (3) they measure current psychological functioning, whereas legal questions often relate to the defendant's psychological functioning at a prior time.

We believe that these views are too narrow and somewhat off the mark. As a practical matter, testing has never been designed, nor should it be used, to address a specific legal standard per se. However, an accurate psycholegal assessment almost always requires a complete understanding of the individual being assessed. As Heilbrun (1992) points out, psychological testing often can reveal and clarify an underlying psychological problem that was not initially recognized (such as organicity, sexual preoccupation, or subtle thought disorder). (Such problems often are detected only after a complete assessment, which includes testing, has been performed.) The argument that testing has no value because it is normed by aggregate data makes little sense; that is the point of psychometric testing. If norms were not used, it could be said that the assessment is too idiographic. Lastly, although some testing measures current functioning, some tests also assess more stable traits and characteristics. If a thought disorder or, for that matter, antisocial personality, is present at the time of testing, it probably was present at the time of the offense. The value of testing and its use in the legal arena depends largely on the psychologist's skill in making test findings understandable and relevant to those with no background in behavioral science such as the attorneys, judge, and jury (Schlesinger, 2003).

2.2.1 Rorschach Test

The various methods of personality assessment that have become known as projective tests developed slowly over an extended period of time (Rabin, 1968). A projective technique "evokes from the subject what is in various ways expressive of his private world and personality process" (Frank, 1948, p. 47). Perhaps the most widely used projective test is the Rorschach, developed by Swiss psychiatrist Hermann Rorschach in 1921 and brought to the United States by David Levy around 1924 (Klopfer and Kelly, 1942). Although the efficacy of the test has been questioned mostly by nonclinical researchers, its sustained popularity for over 80 years has been well documented (Bornstein, 2001; Piotrowski and Keller, 1992). The Rorschach is regularly utilized in both clinical and forensic settings. And contrary to the popular myth, the Rorschach is welcomed in the courtroom and its scientific validity has only been attacked very infrequently (Meloy, Hansen, and Weiner, 1997; Weiner, Exner, and Sciara, 1996). In fact, the Society for Personality Assessment (2005) published a statement on the status of the Rorschach in clinical and forensic practice. Having reviewed the scientific evidence, they concluded: "the Rorschach possesses reliability and validity similar to that of other generally accepted personality assessment instruments" (p.219).

The Rorschach is invaluable in understanding the psychopathology of criminal offenders, in general, and sexual murderers, in particular (Revitch and Schlesinger, 1981 Gacono and Meloy, 2013; Gacono, Evans, and Viglione, 2002). In a series of empirically based studies (Gacono, 1992a,b; Gacono Meloy, and Bridges, 2000; Meloy Gacono, and Kenney, 1994), researchers compared the Rorschachs of sexual murderers to those of nonsexually offending (but violent) male psychopaths and (nonviolent) pedophiles. They found a number of personality characteristics that shed light on the psychological makeup of the sexual murderer. For example, traits such as attachment abnormality, characterological anger, pathological narcissism, formal thought disorder, borderline reality testing, and obsessional thoughts differentiated the sexual murderers from the two control groups. On the basis of these findings, Gacono, Meloy, and Bridges (2000) developed a model of sexual homicide.

In attempting to gain a full understanding of the psychological makeup of an offender, one must look beneath overt traits and behaviors to the basic personality structure or framework on which these traits are fixed. The psychologist must ascertain how strong or weak the framework is and where the vulnerable areas are. Just as a structural engineer inspects a building by examining the strength and composition of the beams and underpinnings (rather than the color or type of siding), the psychologist must accurately and inclusively describe the structure of the subject's personality.

By focusing simply on overt traits and behaviors, we overlook an important aspect of the assessment. Understanding what is beneath traits and behavior leads to a much different understanding of the offender. For example, two individuals may present with impulsivity as a problem, but one of these individuals may have a weakened borderline-like structure, whereas the other may be structurally more intact. The extent of structural weakness has major implications for treatment as well as prognosis, particularly in differentiating individuals who may act out from those who do not. That is, an individual who harbors disturbed, sexually aggressive fantasies but does not act on them may have more structural integrity than someone who has similar fantasies but cannot control the urge to act.

An individual's level of structural integration, as well as his level of inner cohesiveness, is assessed by an analysis of the formal characteristics of the subject's Rorschach responses, and also by a practical commonsense view of the content of what is perceived. For example, one (serial) sexual murderer gave many primitive Rorschach perceptions suggesting severe inner disorganization and structural weakness which might account, in part, for some of his behavior: "A bug somebody stepped on, squashed, blood, it's blood." "An explosion like a war movie." "A slide under a microscope smeared under glass, all spread out, trapped under glass." "An X-ray of twins being born. Pink little babies crapped up." "Someone could have hemorrhoids and this is a piece of toilet paper. It's what the person was eating to make him shit like that. I don't know what he ate. The green is spinach, the yellow is corn not digested." "Somebody vomited. The colors. The way it's all splattered out." In contrast, another individual, who had elaborate fantasies of keeping women captive and torturing them but was able to control any inner urge to act, gave relatively clear responses, the most disturbing being "the stump of a tree gnawed off" (given to card IV). Certainly, the mere presence of bizarre, aggressive, and primitive content does not—by itself—suggest the potential for violence (or sexual homicide) if an individual is not otherwise predisposed to commit such acts.

Revitch and Schlesinger (1981) reported the case of a 19-year-old boy who murdered his mother by stabbing her repeatedly while she slept. This boy, who had a history of sadistic acts toward animals, gave the following extremely aggressive and primitive Rorschach content: "A cockroach crushed. The guts are pouring out. The stomach, the blood, the insides, it was killed violently and smeared around." "This is a lady with her head chopped off. The blood is flying all over the place." "A butterfly with his head bashed in and his feet are bleeding." "Two rabbits bleeding. They were shot in the body and out the mouth." "Two native ladies fighting over something. The loser is gonna die and bash her head against this." "A gigantic cockroach shot in the back. Here is all the blood." "A deformed bug with his guts on the side." "A dead horse drowning in its own blood." "Insects fighting over the blood of losers." This young man was not overtly psychotic but, instead, appeared withdrawn; he was diagnosed as schizoid and evidenced paranoid ideation periodically. He had fantasized for years about committing a sexual homicide but finally committed a matricide. His Rorschach illustrates the enormous amount of anger, primitive aggression, and inner disorganization that contributed to his loss of control.

Psychodynamic inferences come from an analysis of Rorschach content, with special attention given to the specific stimulus pull of the various inkblots. Although content analysis has always occupied an important place in Rorschach interpretation (Aronow, 1994; Lane, 1984; Lindner, 1946, 1950), it has fallen out of favor in recent years in preference to structural analysis that is more empirically based (using the

Exner [1974] system). Nevertheless, we have found dynamic interpretation, although perhaps not empirically anchored, to be very useful. For example, the dynamic significance of the following Rorschach responses of several sexual murderers is too important to ignore: Card IV (male card): "Ovaries of a woman." "A monster, he looks like he is defecating. It's diarrhea coming out of him." Card VI (sexual card): "It looks like a gun. Here's the barrel, here's the trigger. It's a gun with a bullet coming out." "Vagina exploding, all in pieces." Card VII (female card): "Scum from a pond, spread out." "A woman with her legs spread open. Her legs are all mutilated. Something up her vagina and it's broken off, a piece right here."

An individual's ability to empathize, which is fundamental in a psychological evaluation, is illuminated by the Rorschach. Schaefer (1959) defines empathy as "the inner experience of sharing in and comprehending the momentary, psychological state of another person" (p. 345). In other words, empathy is the ability to put oneself in the position of another, so that he can experience how the other person feels. Empathic capacity is obviously important in understanding sexual murderers (many of whom torture their victims); moreover, the ability to empathize may also help to distinguish those who act out their fantasies from those who do not. Gacono, Meloy, and Bridges (2000) refer to entitlement and grandiosity, as well as abnormal bonding, as characteristics important in the psychodynamic understanding of sexual homicide; these traits are clearly related to empathy. A careful assessment of Rorschach human movement perceptions is enormously helpful in assessing the level of empathic capacity. Miller and Looney (1974) studied Rorschachs of murderers who dehumanized their victims and found that such offenders did not regard these victims as people: "There is a paucity of images that would suggest a stance that other people are full, warm, and alive" (p. 191). Lack of empathy, revealed by an absence of human perceptions on the Rorschach, was also noted by De Bousingin (1971) in a study of six cases of murder. Thus, empathic capacity assessed clinically and bolstered by Rorschach findings is an important aspect to be considered in any assessment of the sexual murderer's personality.

2.2.2 Thematic Apperception Test (TAT)

The TAT has had a long and distinguished history, beginning with the seminal work of Murray (1938, 1943, 1951), and continues to be a widely used and widely respected projective technique (Alvarado, 1994; Geiser and Stein, 1999; Jenkins, 2014; Jenkins, 2017; Lundy, 1988). Perhaps the main appeal of the TAT is its simplicity:

> The manifest material yielded by the TAT is not mysterious in appearance. The comparatively untrained person can appreciate fabricated stories … he needs no acquaintance with technical symbols and test scores to obtain at least a superficial feeling for the moods and perspective of the subject who produced the stories, and even the experienced tester profits from this property, which differentiates the TAT from other tests. (Rosenwald, 1968, p. 172)

We have found that the TAT (which involves the creation of fantasy stories) is critical in helping to understand the sexual murderer, as his acts are a direct outgrowth of fantasy (Ressler, Burgess, and Douglas, 1988; Schlesinger, 2000a). Through the TAT the offender may reveal levels of motivation that he might deny when questioned directly (Porcerelli, Abramsky, Hibbard, and Kamoo, 2001). Satten, Menninger, and Mayman (1960) found that the murderers in their study almost always denied conscious ideas of killing, but their TAT stories revealed preconscious homicidal fantasy or ideation.

The following are examples of the value of the TAT in illuminating the dynamics of the homicide:

Example 1

A 16-year-old boy who committed several sexual murders, preceded by voyeuristic burglaries, was unable (or unwilling) to reveal the motivation for his acts when interviewed directly or even when questioned under the influence of sodium amytal. Some of the dynamics of his crimes, however, emerged through the TAT, specifically card 13MF:

> The lady is dying in bed. She is dead. He just killed her. He is crying and saying he is sorry, but it is too late. He calls the cops to turn himself in, he knows he's done wrong. If he lets it go, he might do more. He wanted to go to bed with her; she didn't want to, so he killed her. He'd hope she'd come over and help him with his homework. He'd hope she'd like him a lot enough to go to bed with him. He couldn't have her; he was real hurt, so he took it out on her. He strangled her and then he felt sorry. He might see another girl he liked and she might say no, and he'd end up killing her or somebody else. There is too much anger after the person says no. He just can't stop himself.

Example 2

A 23-year-old sexual murderer gave the following story in response to TAT card 13MF:

> He just killed that girl. He didn't mean to, but he lost control. She is naked. He attacked her. It puts him in control. When he attacked her, she was scared. He raped her. Maybe he had a crush on her. He felt rejected and turned down. He is ashamed of what he did. He wanted her all to himself, so he killed her to possess her completely.

Example 3

A 32-year-old man (Case 9.9), who committed a planned and brutal sexual murder, first denied guilt, but several of his TAT stories revealed his fixation on violence and his resentment of women. On card 3BM, the offender stated,

> Her husband beat her up. She verbally talked back. He assaulted her. He assaulted her because she protested and spoke out against him. He doesn't feel. He has no feelings at all. He liquidated the situation. He resolved it the way he saw fit. He beat her up. He was hurting inside. He disregards everybody else but himself. He doesn't really care about anyone.
>
> He sees things the way he sees it. The situation goes on and on and on. No ending. She is battered until he makes her lose her will. He just doesn't care. He is a very cruel person. He doesn't know why he is like that. He's been asking himself that for a long time.

To card 4 he responded, "Things are going to get hectic. She is trying to corner him and he is going to come out fighting against her because she is the predator at that point. He comes out fighting."

To card 14GF, he created the following story:

> It looks like a mother abusing her child. The mother is trying to kill him. She is going to extremes with the child. The child hates his mother. He just hates her. He has bitter feelings when he thinks of her. As far as he is concerned, she doesn't exist. He finds it hard to understand women. He is suspicious of women because of his mother. He is aware that women can act like his mother. They can become real confused. They can get kind of evil.

Interestingly, on card 13MF, he created a nondescript story of an individual "who is married and feels bad because he was with another woman." This type of response is not uncommon in individuals who sometimes detect the purpose of the test and resist giving a story that might in some way directly implicate them or reveal their motivations.

Example 4

A 15-year-old boy, who committed a murder following a sexual assault, revealed some important dynamics through TAT card 13MF:

> This is a sex crime. A rape crime. He feels sorry. He forced her. She didn't want to do it and he did.
> He liked the woman. He then kills the woman so she doesn't go and talk to the police. He chokes
> her. He didn't have a weapon. He thought he'd be in jail for rape, so he decided to choke her. He
> thinks nothing will happen to him. He already killed her and nobody knows he was with her.
> He thinks she'll tell the cops he raped her. So he killed her because he didn't want his wife and
> children to know he raped a woman. He feels sad all his life. He'll remember that. He doesn't get
> caught because the police don't have any proof who killed her. He wanted her. He liked that girl.
> He liked killing her too.

A subject may sometimes not reveal much about the dynamics of his crime through the
TAT, since he makes a conscious attempt not to implicate himself (as noted in Example 3).
In addition, McKie (1974) found that some murderers "block out" unpleasant emotions
and create bland, nondescript stories because they "fear that their feelings or impulses will
overwhelm them" (p. 29). But even in these cases, the subject usually cannot help revealing
something about himself which may be of great significance in understanding the case. For
example, the 16-year-old cited in Example 1 (who committed sexual murders) revealed his
inner thoughts and feelings through his story given to TAT card 14:

> It's a man and in a dark room looking out and he feels all alone. Nobody to love him. Since
> he was a child he was abandoned. He grew up in an orphanage with no education. He figures
> he can't make it in the world because no one will give him a chance. He stays in his room by
> himself. He doesn't eat or drink much. He just thinks nobody will help him.

It must be emphasized that the mere production of a violent or sexually aggressive TAT
story does not mean that the individual has acted out in this way or, in fact, will act out
in this manner. The relationship between fantasy and violence is not always direct and
obvious (Jensen, 1957). Clearly, the number of people with disturbed fantasies is much
greater than the number who actually act out. However, in a population of offenders
who committed a sex murder, the examiner's main purpose is not to speculate on the
meaning of the fantasy production in order to make a prediction; instead, the examiner
seeks to understand the motivation of an individual who has already acted out his fantasy. Some studies have shown that TAT stories of murderers as a group tend to be more
disturbed, with more themes of gratuitous violence, than the stories of nonmurderers
(Fujita, 1996; Saito, 1995).

Thus, any method of eliciting an offender's fantasy life is of great help in understanding his crime. One such method—a test similar to the TAT—is the Criminal Fantasy
Technique (CFT) (Schlesinger and Kutash, 1981). This test is comprised of 12 cards, each
of which depicts a crime that is about to occur, is now occurring, or has just occurred. The
subject's task is to create a story based on the crime depicted. The CFT has proved to be
quite useful with various types of offenders, especially sex offenders and sexual murderers
whose crimes are direct outgrowths of pathological fantasy (Deu, 1998). For example, one
such offender who killed six women created a fantasy of a man

> who must be in control. Power and control is everything. There's lots of ways to feel in con-
> trol, but killing is the most control. Slow deliberate killing is what makes him feel great. He
> thinks about it and he does it. He doesn't mean to hurt anyone, but he doesn't care.

A 24-year-old serial rapist provided insight into his sexual burglaries by the following CFT fantasy production:

> He takes women's clothes … he likes feeling and smelling them. Can't feel a woman, so he feels her clothes … the woman who lived there wouldn't go out with him, so he broke in to take her clothes … he had intentions of killing the girl with a crowbar and raping her.

2.2.3 Projective Drawings

Projective drawings have long been utilized as a supplement to other projective techniques in the traditional psychological assessment battery (Handler and Thomas, 2013; Kaufman and Wohl, 1992; Leibowitz, 1999). The test can be administered in a variety of ways: the subject is asked to draw a person; a house, a tree, and a person; a family; an animal; the worst thing imaginable; or other topics, such as a person in the rain. Projective drawings are perhaps the least sophisticated of the various projective tests, since there is no established standardization for them, and interpretation is often highly subjective. In fact, Uhlin (1978) has noted that "in order for projective drawings to function alone in criminal proceedings, they must be powerful and descriptive [enough] to … touch the sensitivity of the untrained layman and overcome what may be strong personal subjectivity" (p. 63). We therefore eschew "wild" methods of interpretation based on clinical lore (e.g., interpreting a hole in the trunk of a tree as representing the developmental stage of childhood trauma). Hammer (1997a,b) advises taking due caution in interpreting drawings, but he firmly believes that violent acts including murder, rape, and exhibitionism can be greatly understood by a subject's illustrations. Meloy (2000) notes the usefulness of figure drawings and reproduced an interesting drawing by an offender who committed a sexual murder as an example.

Often, however, an offender's drawings reveal very little that enhances our understanding of the case because the offender may be resistant and exert little effort. For example, a sexual murderer who bit his victims on the chin while strangling them was guarded throughout the entire evaluation, and his drawings were almost completely noncommittal (see Figure 2.1). The same level of resistance was found in a 23-year-old who abducted females at amusement parks and killed them by ligature strangulation. His nondescript drawings are displayed in Figure 2.2. In other cases, the subject's conflicts are simply not revealed on this test. For example, Figure 2.3 displays the drawings of a 19-year-old who killed his mother by strangulation, followed by necrophilia. The offender whose drawings are printed in Figure 2.4 had as his life's goal "to rape and kill a woman." This Ivy League college student did so after first killing his parents. The drawings in Figures 2.3 and 2.4, however, are not overtly disturbed and do not demonstrate sexual disturbance at a level of face validity, although they are rather strange and seem to reflect the general interpersonal conflict.

In other cases, more revealing material is depicted by offenders' drawings. Drawings in Figure 2.5 were done by a 26-year-old who killed prostitutes by strangulation. Compare his drawing of a female to the other sketches. The drawings in Figure 2.6 were rendered by a 24-year-old who killed a 16-year-old female acquaintance by smashing her head with a pipe. His superior intellect is suggested by the careful details of his house and tree; his conflicts with people are indicated by the relatively poorly done human figures.

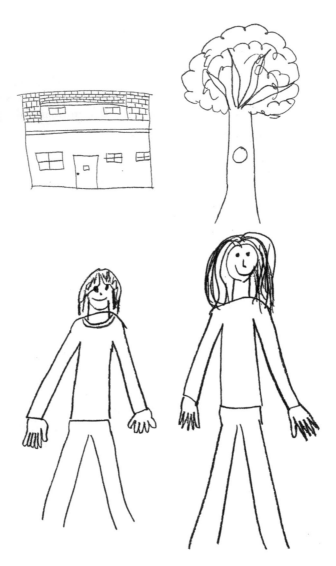

Figure 2.1 Drawings by a sexual murderer who was guarded throughout the examination.

Figure 2.7 denotes drawings produced by an adolescent who attacked a pregnant woman without provocation. Notice the line quality of the stick in comparison with the rest of the drawing. Figure 2.8 shows drawings by a 16-year-old who committed sexual burglaries, once defecating on the bed of a 15-year-old girl, whom he eventually assaulted while she was asleep in her bed. His feelings of inadequacy are obvious in his sketches.

Projective drawings are especially useful with children and adolescents, who may be less inclined to cover up their underlying motivations. The drawings in Figure 2.9 were made by a 13-year-old who was preoccupied with his undescended testicle. He sexually assaulted several female classmates. A 9-year-old who killed several cats, dressed in girls' clothes, set fires, and sexually assaulted a 7-year-old female neighbor produced the drawings in Figure 2.10. An 8-year-old who "loves violence" and expressed a desire to kill girls created the drawings in Figure 2.11. The drawings in Figure 2.12 were produced by a 9-year-old who was preoccupied with fire and obsessed with "knives and sex." This youngster

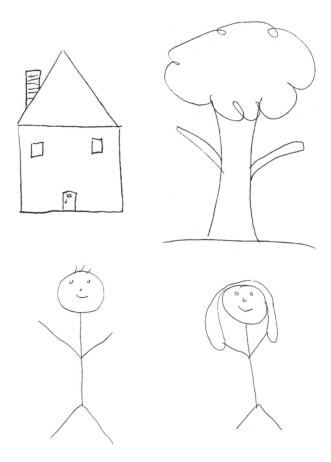

Figure 2.2 Drawings by a sexual murderer who was resistant during assessment.

labeled the last drawing shown as "someone tied to a stake burning alive." The drawings in Figure 2.13 were made by a 13-year-old of borderline intelligence who had a fetish for female underwear, killed cats, and stuck girls with a pencil.

In many cases, random drawings by offenders (not done in the context of formal testing) can also be revealing. Figure 2.14 was made by an individual who had sadistic fantasies but denied engaging in such activity. He considered his drawings a pastime. Figure 2.15 depicts the sketches of a 20-year-old who developed suicidal thoughts following the commission of a brutal sex murder.

2.2.4 Bender–Gestalt

The Bender–Gestalt was first developed as a screening test for organicity (Bender, 1938) and later came to be utilized as a projective technique (Hutt, 1968a,b). For many years this test was widely used, but its popularity has decreased somewhat over the past several decades, but still used and found helpful by many psychologists (Borum and Grisso, 1995; Oas, 1984; Raphael, Golden and Cassidy, 2002). As a test for organicity, the Bender–Gestalt provides objective means of detecting perceptual-motor incoordination and brain damage (Hain, 1964; Hutt, 1968a, 1968b; Koppitz, 1964). Over the past 20 years, however, sophisticated neuropsychological testing has largely replaced the Bender–Gestalt as a screening device.

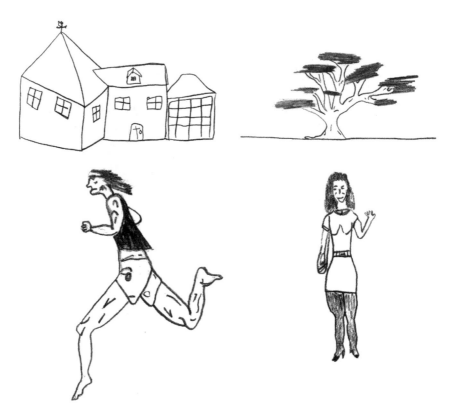

Figure 2.3 Drawings by a young man who killed his mother by strangulation, followed by necrophilia.

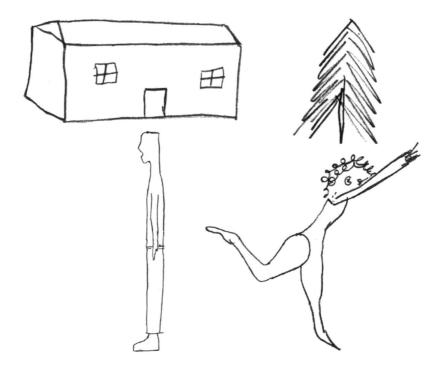

Figure 2.4 Sketches by a man whose life-goal was to "rape and kill a woman."

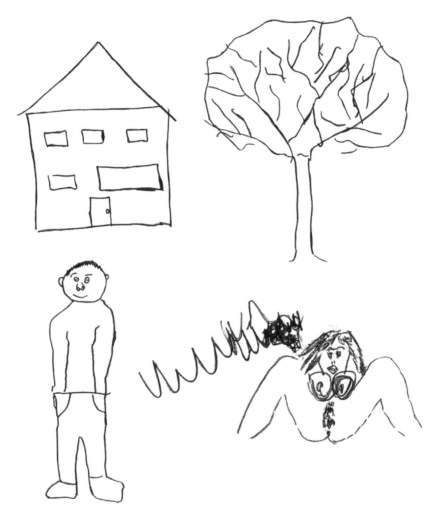

Figure 2.5 Drawings by an offender who killed prostitutes by strangulation.

As a projective technique, the Bender–Gestalt (like the projective drawings test) calls for an interpretation of various drawings by a subject. With this test, also, examiners must use caution and common sense and must avoid speculative determinations (such as interpreting figures that slope down as reflective of depression, or figures sloping upward as reflective of euphoric trends). The Bender–Gestalt has no special value in the examination of sexual murderers and should be used only supplementally. A few findings, however, are worth noting. For example, heavy line pressure and excessive angulation are frequently found in the records of hostile and aggressive individuals (see Figure 2.16) and may have some relevance to homicidal offenders. In addition, examiners have frequently observed that many individuals who act in extremely violent ways (including those who have committed homicide) often draw figures colliding with one another, disregarding obvious boundaries (see Figures 2.17 and 2.18); this observation, however, has not been empirically validated.

2.2.5 Personality Inventories

As part of their test battery, psychologists, particularly forensic psychologists, also use various personality inventories, including the Minnesota Multiphasic Personality Inventory

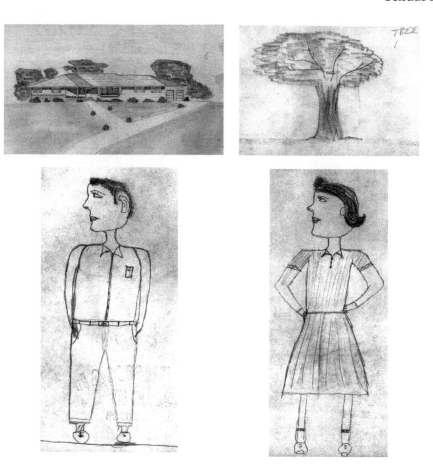

Figure 2.6 Offender's spontaneous drawings while he was serving time for the sexual murder of a 16-year-old girl.

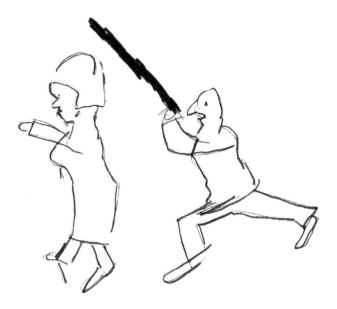

Figure 2.7 Sketch by an adolescent who attacked a pregnant woman without provocation.

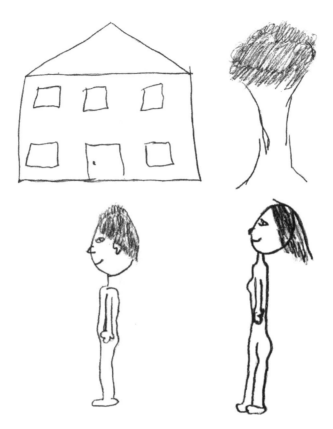

Figure 2.8 Drawings by a 16-year-old who committed sexual burglaries and sexual assaults.

(MMPI/MMPI-2), the California Psychological Inventory (CPI), and the Millon Clinical Multiaxial Inventory (MCMI/MCMI-2-4). These inventories, unlike the projective techniques, are highly standardized and have been empirically validated as instruments for assessing personality traits and characteristics and for providing a general personality profile of the subject. In addition, psychologists sometimes use more specialized instruments such as the Psychopathy Checklist and the Structured Clinical Interview from *DSM-5*. Although these instruments lack the clinical richness of the projectives, they have proved useful in studies of various types of criminal behavior, including homicide (e.g., Fraboni, Cooper, Reed, and Saltstone, 1990; Hare et al., 1990; Holcomb, Adams, and Ponder, 1985; Kalichman, 1988); but few such studies have involved sexual murderers.

Figure 2.18 displays a Bender–Gestalt drawing by a 30-year-old who killed his wife.

Personality inventories, however, can be especially helpful when they are used in conjunction with clinical findings and other projective tests (Ganellen, 1996). Perhaps their greatest value is their capacity to corroborate clinical findings or to detect, by objective means, characteristics that would otherwise not be clearly delineated.

2.2.6 Intellectual, Cognitive, and Neuropsychological Assessment

Intellectual/cognitive assessment is essential in any thorough psychological evaluation, and particularly so in forensic assessments, where such matters as criminal responsibility or competency must be determined. An instrument commonly used for intellectual and

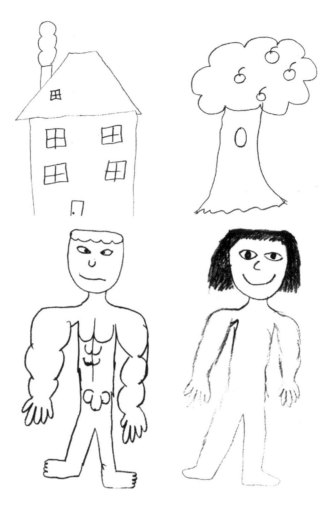

Figure 2.9 Drawings by a 13-year-old who assaulted several female classmates. He was preoccupied with an undescended testicle.

cognitive assessments is the Wechsler Adult Intelligence Scale (WAIS), which emphasizes performance and verbal skills and gives separate scores for vocabulary, arithmetic, memory span, assembly of objects, and other abilities. Some researchers have found differences in overall IQ and in subtest patterning (Dieker, 1973; Panton, 1960; Wagner and Klein, 1977; Weins, Matarazzo, and Gavor, 1959) between controls and various types of offenders. Kahn (1968) has argued that impulsive/violent/antisocial individuals routinely have higher performance than verbal IQ scores because

> verbal functioning requires delay of impulse expression ... performance functioning, on the other hand, is closer to direct impulse expression. Consequently, individuals such as sociopaths ... would have little capacity to delay impulse, and hence, function better on performance than verbal tasks. (p. 113)

This finding, however, has not been corroborated by others (Panton, 1960).

Analysis of an offender's intellectual functioning is particularly important in cases of sexual murder, especially those that have gone undetected for many years. Relevant information sometimes will emerge from an offender's response to a test item or group of items.

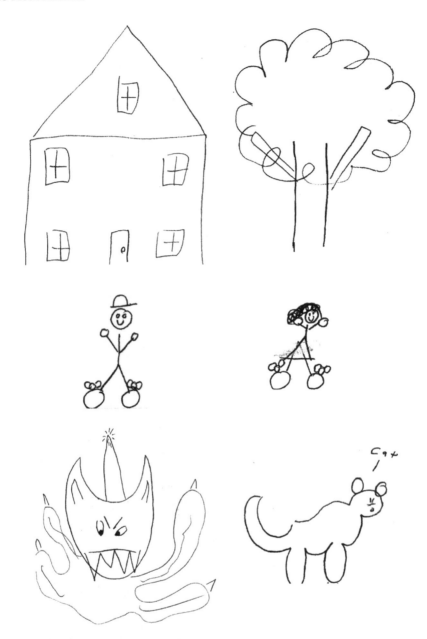

Figure 2.10 Drawings by a 9-year-old who sexually assaulted a 7-year-old female neighbor. He killed cats, set fires, and dressed in female clothes. When asked to draw the worst thing he could think of, he drew a picture of the devil and a cat.

For example, an individual who murdered over 100 victims and remained undetected for 30 years scored a low average in overall intelligence but very high in social comprehension. Clearly, his practical intelligence had helped him elude the police for a long period of time (Schlesinger, 2001c). Brittain (1970) believes that an above-average IQ is related to, and may partly explain, some of the elaborate fantasies found in compulsive repetitive sexual murderers. Other investigators also have concluded that serial murderers as a group have superior intellect (Hickey, 1997); however, this finding has never been substantiated clinically or empirically, and it is contrary to our experience as well. Just as in personality

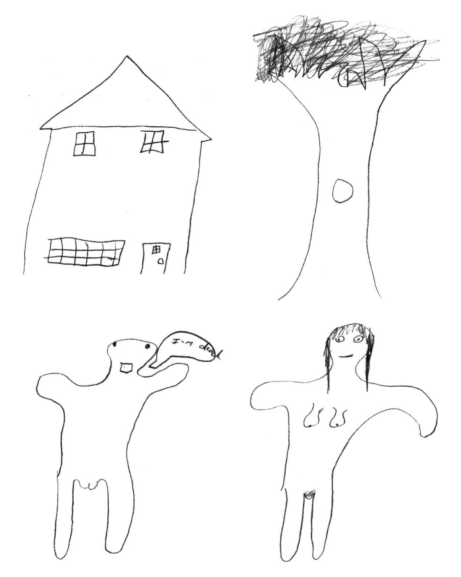

Figure 2.11 Sketches by an 8-year-old who expressed a strong desire to kill girls.

tests and inventories, it is important to understand the applicability of intelligence testing in a forensic assessment. For example, there are some abbreviated tests (e.g., Wechsler Abbreviated Scale of Intelligence-II) which can be used in forensic assessments, but not if the issue before the court is the defendant's intelligence.

As noted in the WASI-II manual (2013), "the WASI-II FSIQ should not be used for legal, judicial, or quasi-legal purposes" (p. 10).

Neuropsychological assessment has been used extensively in forensic assessments where neurological injury is a suspected causal factor in the individual's behavior, particularly if some type of sudden violence has occurred. In fact, many studies have attempted to show that neuropsychological differences exist between normals and criminals. Pontius and Yudowitz (1980), for example, believe that individuals with frontal lobe dysfunction may engage in antisocial acts because they cannot stop their behavior once an action pattern begins. They find support for their theory in neuropsychological test findings which

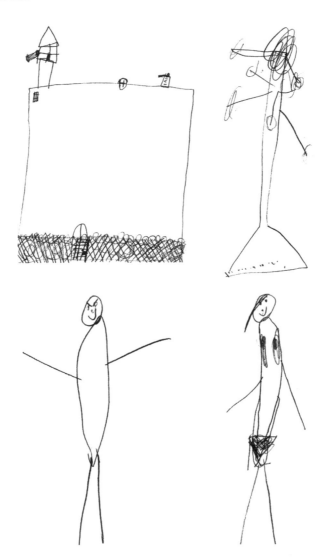

Figure 2.12 Drawings by a 9-year-old preoccupied with knives, sex, and fire. When asked to draw a house, he drew a prison.

show that offenders did poorly compared to controls in their ability to switch cognitive sets. Lewis, Pincus, Feldman, Jackson, and Bard (1986) and Lewis, Shanok, and Pincus (1979) found neuropsychological and neurological deficits in the violent offenders whom they studied; however, other researchers (Nestor, 1992; Nestor and Haycock, 1997) found less clear-cut results. There has yet to be any study of neuropsychological functioning among sexual murderers.

2.2.7 Specialized Forensic Tests

Since traditional psychological tests were not developed to address specific forensic/legal issues, a number of researchers have developed what are sometimes called specialized forensic tests or forensic-assessment instruments. The purpose of these tests is to directly address and elucidate specific legal questions. There are a number of different specialized

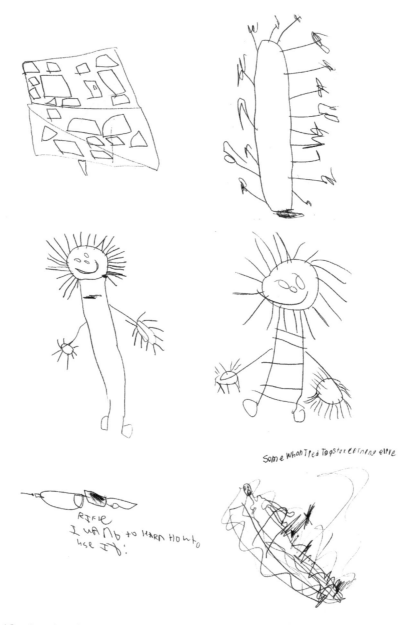

Figure 2.13 Sketches by a 13-year-old (with borderline intelligence) who stuck several girls with a pencil. He killed cats and had a fetish for female underwear.

forensic tests, including those to assess competency to waive *Miranda* rights, competency to stand trial, insanity, etc. (e.g., Goldstein, Romaine, Zelle, Mesiarik, and Wolbransky, 2011; Rogers and Johansson-Love, 2009). Although these specialized tests do have some merit, they often do not add a great deal beyond what can be obtained in a clinical interview that focuses on specific issues. Each case has a unique set of facts and circumstances that cannot always be captured by a particular test. Moreover, and most important, many of the specialized tests do not address the legal standard specific to the jurisdiction, which can vary widely. The court, however, is going to be guided by the criteria used in the legal standard, not the results of a test.

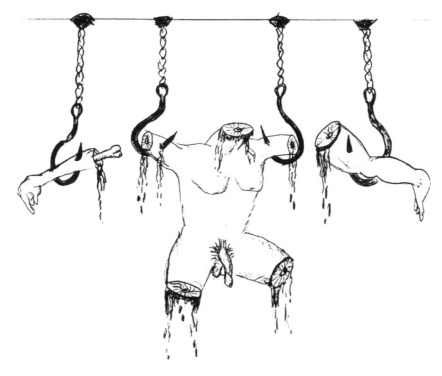

Figure 2.14 Drawings by an inmate who had sexually aggressive fantasies but denied engaging in such activity.

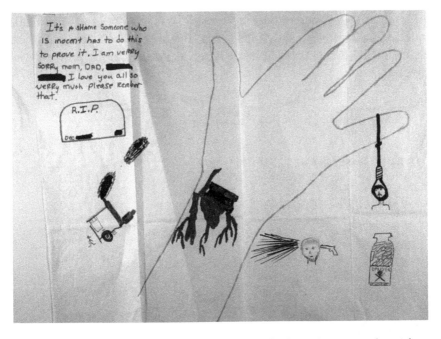

Figure 2.15 Sketches by a 20-year-old who committed a brutal sex murder. After making a confession, he expressed suicidal ideas and later claimed his statement was false.

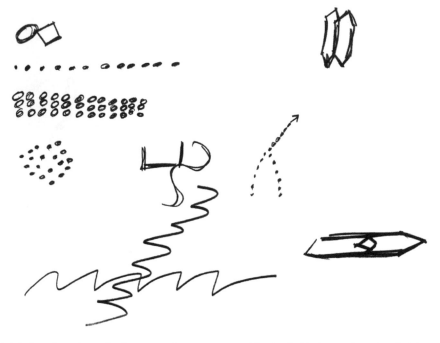

Figure 2.16 Bender–Gestalt drawings by a 28-year-old who killed two female children by beating them with a pipe.

It is usually not difficult to evaluate an offender and address the specific elements of *Miranda*, competency to stand trial, and other legal standards. Psychologists who rely solely on test results are going to miss, or not even address, a lot of the elements specified in the legal standard. Reliance only on test results—specialized or traditional—is never recommended and can prove to be self-defeating. The use of specialized forensic tests without addressing all the elements listed in a particular statute can be problematic when the case goes to court.

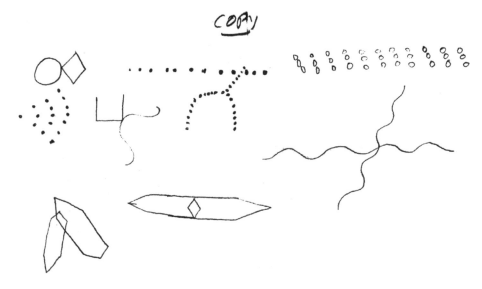

Figure 2.17 Bender–Gestalt drawings by a 16-year-old who killed his mother.

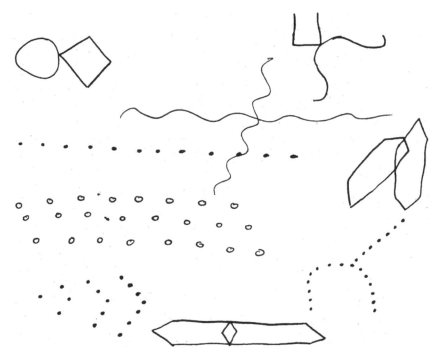

Figure 2.18 Bender–Gestalt drawing by a 30-year-old who killed his wife.

> Although most specialized forensic assessment instruments appear to have face validity, they should be used with caution, in a supplemental way, and never in place of an evaluation of the specific legal standard as outlined in the statute of a particular jurisdiction. (Schlesinger, 2003, p. 502)

In fact, Melton et al. (2018) state that some forensic-assessment tests

> provide some of the trappings of sophisticated normed instruments (i.e., multiple scales and apparently quantified measures) but are conceptually flawed or have little empirical research to validate the author's claims about the instruments' capabilities … An interesting number [of such tests] … are marketed without adequate research and development. (p. 52)

2.2.8 Revised and Updated Tests

Who could argue with the usefulness of revising various tests and inventories so that they are updated and align with current norms, demographics, and the like? This procedure has certainly been followed in the many revisions of the *Wechsler Intelligence Scales* and has proved useful. However, when using a personality test or inventory in a forensic matter—with the stakes being extremely high—one must make sure that the revision is appropriate. For example, a revision of the MMPI—referred to as the Restructured Clinical Scales (RC)—has come under a great deal of scrutiny. In fact, a special issue of the *Journal of Personality Assessment* (October 2006) was devoted to the many problems with these scales. As noted by Nichols (2006),

> as a result of these various problems, the RC scales should be used with caution. The application in medical, chronic pain, personnel, and forensic evaluations may be of particular

concern because of their increased likelihood of forensic challenge. Even within outpatient and inpatient settings, the interpretation of the RC scales may mislead clinical inferences because of their defects in design and composition. (p. 137)

Rogers, Sewell, Harrison, and Jordan (2006) also state, "We caution against the use of the MMPI-2-RC scales in professional settings until these and other issues of test validation are satisfactorily addressed" (p. 146).

These same arguments with respect to test validation and revision have also been advanced for the revisions of the *Millon Clinical Multiaxial Inventory* (Retzlaff, 2010). Some have even suggested that many updates or revisions have been undertaken for nonscientific (e.g., marketing) purposes (Butcher, 2000; Friedman, Bolinskey, Nichols and Levak, 2014; Silverstein and Nelson, 2000). Reliance on quantification at the expense of common sense is becoming more common. Accordingly, caution is advised; new is not always better.

2.2.9 Neurodiagnostic and Biological Testing

The search for biological and neurological causes of crime, violence, and murder has been ongoing for over a century (Koch, 1889). Among the medical measures used for this purpose are the electroencephalogram (EEG), commonly requested in sudden and unprovoked murders; neuroimaging studies (CT scan, PET, and MRI); neuroendocrinological investigations; and assessments of chromosomal abnormalities.

The relationship between abnormal EEG findings and violent behavior has long been noted (Pillman, Rohde, Ullrich, Draba, and Sannemueller, 1999; Silverman, 1943). Researchers (Raine et al., 1998a,b) also have found differences in PET scans between individuals who commit impulsive acts of violence and those who commit premeditated acts. Hormonal differences between offenders and controls have also been found (Horney, 1978). There has even been speculation that chromosomal abnormalities such as an extra male chromosome (XYY) may have some relationship to violent crime (Brown, 1962; Jacobs, Brunton, and Melville, 1965). One investigator (Davidson, 1994) has suggested that an extra female chromosome (XXY, Klinefelter's syndrome) may have been responsible for an 18-year-old man's unprovoked sexual attack on a young woman. The research regarding abnormal medical correlates of crime, taken as a whole, remains unclear, although positive statistical correlations have been reported by many authors.

Researchers to date seem to have found more abnormalities in impulsive/explosive offenders than in individuals whose crimes (including murders) have been planned in advance (Blake, Pincus, and Buckner, 1995; Bricken, Haberman, Berner, and Hill, 2005.) The presence of organic abnormalities suggests that a weakening of inhibitory controls renders the offender unable to resist psychogenically induced impulses to act. In cases where organicity is present or suspected, the forensic psychologist or psychiatrist should discuss findings with a neurologist or a neuroendocrinologist who has experience and expertise in forensic matters, in order to interpret medical findings properly.

2.2.10 Narcoanalysis

Narcoanalysis (interviewing a subject who has been intravenously injected with a substance such as sodium amytal, chloroform, scopolamine, or pentothal) has been used since the early 1930s (Naples and Hackett, 1978). It continues to be used for therapeutic purposes—for instance, in the treatment of conversion disorder (Fackler, Anfinson, and Rand, 1997) or mutism (McCall, Vaughn, Shelp, and McDonald, 1992) or in an attempt to uncover repressed memories of abuse (Piper, 1993). The general theory is that the injected drug will reduce inhibitions and defenses so that a mute patient will talk, a hysterically paralyzed patient will move limbs, and a patient who is amnesic for events will verbalize what had happened (Kavirajan, 1999). The usefulness of narcoanalysis depends on many factors, including the experience of the examiner and goals that are attempted to be achieved. Parwatikar, Holcomb, and Menninger (1985) found amytal to be useful in detecting malingered amnesia, but "not uniformly successful in bringing to recall stressful events preceding alleged crimes" (p.98).

Sodium amytal is not really a "truth serum," as it is sometimes called. Redlich, Ravitz, and Dession (1951) found in some of their cases that fantasies produced under the influence of sodium amytal had the character of a confession. However, these authors, as well as MacDonald (1954), concluded that individuals who were determined to deceive and give false information prior to the narcoanalytic interview also deceived when under the influence of the drug. Melton et al. (1997) offer guidelines in conducting a narcoanalytic (or hypnotic) interview in order to reduce deception. Clinicians should (1) determine whether the amnesia is legitimate and, if so, whether it is potentially recoverable; (2) advise the attorney, prior to conducting the interview, that the subject's report is not necessarily true; (3) avoid asking the subject leading questions during the interview.

A face-to-face interview with the offender prior to narcoanalysis is absolutely necessary. Rapport must also be established, just as in any interview, or very little verbalization will take place. In some cases, offenders under indictment or attempting to prove their innocence demand to be examined under the influence of the drugs in order to "prove" their innocence or to provide a confession where they do not feel able to do so in a direct fashion. Revitch and Schlesinger (1981) cite the case of a serial murderer who confessed to his crimes in considerable detail following a sodium amytal interview. Like any procedure, its value and usefulness depend largely on the skill and experience of the practitioner.

2.2.11 Hypnosis

Hypnosis has been used in criminal investigations and in psychological therapy for many years. Its purpose has been to help a witness recall details of an event. Not everyone, however, is hypnotizable or can be hypnotized to a sufficient depth. A great deal of experience with hypnosis and hypnotic techniques is necessary for a successful result in forensic cases. Zonana (1979) was unable to get a confession or to retrieve the memory of an event with narcoanalysis, but he succeeded with hypnosis. Using hypnosis, Meyerson (1966) was able to recover the memory of two mothers who had killed their children and claimed amnesia for the crimes. Earlier, Izner, Goldman, and Leiser (1953) successfully restored the memory of a person with amnesia who was responsible for an accidental fire setting without any criminal intent.

In other instances, however, hypnosis has been unsuccessful. A professional hypnotist with considerable forensic experience was unable to gain a confession from a serial murderer; in fact, the hypnotist was even misled by this offender and incorrectly concluded that he was not guilty. Relinger and Stern (1983) developed guidelines that were designed to standardize forensic hypnotic procedures and to minimize the possibility of producing inaccurate memories during hypnotic interrogation. But despite the use of guidelines even by well-credentialed and experienced practitioners, many problems occur (McConkey and Sheehan, 1992). In one case, for example, a man accused of sexually abusing his daughters got convinced of his guilt after he recovered what turned out to be pseudo-memories during hypnosis. In a case replete with errors of fact and methodological difficulties, he ultimately—and probably erroneously—pleaded guilty (see Olio and Cornell, 1998). We therefore believe that hypnotic techniques are applicable only in isolated cases for detection. Hypnosis is far more useful for therapeutic purposes or for understanding the complex psychodynamics of offenders, such as in cases of sexual homicide.

2.3 Deception Syndromes

Patients seen in a clinical-therapeutic setting sometimes (consciously or unconsciously) distort information or exaggerate or minimize symptoms. However, most patients who apply for treatment give fairly accurate descriptions of their problems, and most clinical practitioners (unless there is reason to suspect otherwise) accept their patients' presentations as valid. In forensic settings, however, subjects may distort and exaggerate symptoms in the hope that their "aberrant mental condition" will provide an excuse for unacceptable behavior (for instance, in insanity cases), or help them avoid sanctions (in the sentencing phase), or will enable them to obtain entitlements (such as compensation for disabilities or personal injuries) (Melton et al., 1997, p. 54). Malingering, however, is not a black-and-white occurrence. In fact, it can consist of a complex set of behaviors, which may include traditional malingering, pseudomalingering, Ganser's syndrome, rationalization and justification, or just direct lying (see Table 2.3).

2.3.1 Malingering

Malingering (also referred to as simulation) is the conscious attempt to feign an (mental) illness. It should be distinguished from dissimulation or what Rogers (1988) refers to as defensiveness: the conscious and deliberate attempt to minimize or deny symptoms of an

Table 2.3 **Various Types of Deception Syndromes**

Terms	Definitions
Malingering (simulation)	A conscious attempt to feign (mental) illness.
Dissimulation (defensiveness)	A conscious attempt to minimize or deny symptoms of mental illness.
Pseudomalingering	A conscious attempt to feign the illness that the individual actually has.
Ganser's syndrome	A tendency (most often observed in prisoners) to respond to questions with approximate answers, such as $2 + 2 = 5$. Subjects may also manifest a dazed sensorium, hallucinations, and bizarre behavior.
Rationalization and justification	A conscious attempt to make behavior appear reasonable when otherwise its irrationality would be evident; an attempt to give a plausible explanation for what would otherwise seem irrational or inappropriate conduct.
Direct lying	A conscious attempt to falsify, prevaricate, or misrepresent information, usually to avoid punishment for wrongdoing.
Pathological lying	Lying as a result of underlying psychopathology—for instance, lying to enhance one's sense of self (*pseudologia fantastica*) or to gain a sense of domination or control over others.

(mental) illness. There are a number of ways to detect malingering (Drob, Meehan, and Waxmqan, 2009), including structured clinical interviews (Rogers, 1984), psychological testing (Schretlen, 1988), and the use of independent third-party information. In some cases, it is easy to detect malingering on clinical grounds and by listening with the "third ear." For example, offenders who malinger commonly develop symptoms following an arrest but seldom prior to the commission of the crime. The malingerer overreacts and often "sees less than the blind and hears less than the deaf." The simulator believes that the more strangely he behaves, the more psychotic he will look; however, it is very difficult to maintain malingered psychotic symptoms for an extended period of time (Enoch, Trethowan, and Bracher, 1967). Moreover, there are frequent variations in the malingerer's clinical presentation and the actual illness that he is attempting to feign, since he is portraying a layman's concept of how a psychotic individual would act.

The following case is illustrative of a woman who attempted to feign multiple personality disorder in order to avoid criminal responsibility for the murder of a 12-year-old girl.

Case 2.4: Feigning Multiple Personality Disorder

CC, a 38-year-old unemployed woman, lived with her 16-year-old-daughter. The daughter regularly brought a number of her high school friends to CC's apartment where the adolescents listened to music, smoked pot, and engaged in sexual relations. CC began to associate with the teenagers and developed a romantic relationship with an aggressive and sadistic 16-year-old who became her "boyfriend." The boyfriend enjoyed intimidating other adolescents, especially an emotionally weak 12-year-old girl who lived several blocks away. CC and her boyfriend held this child (who was assumed to be a runaway) captive for 2 weeks. During this time period, the boyfriend, along with CC, tortured her. They tied her to the radiator, kept her undressed, forced her to eat feces, hog-tied her, made her kneel on rice, and beat her in front of some of the other adolescents. CC and her boyfriend warned the other teens that if they told anyone about these acts they, too, would become victims of similar cruelty.

One evening, the boyfriend held the 12-year-old by her legs and threw her back and forth, hitting her head and causing her death. Afterward, CC and her boyfriend wrapped the child up with duct tape and nailed her body onto the ceiling rafters in the attic. CC and her daughter then moved out of their apartment, and the group disbanded. A short time later, CC heard (through her daughter) that word of the homicide had spread. She immediately called the police and blamed the killing on her young boyfriend. Nevertheless, she was arrested and charged with murder, kidnapping, terroristic threats, aggravated sexual assault, and a number of other related offenses surrounding not only the 12-year-old's death but also the torture and abuse of a number of other adolescents.

CC was evaluated by two renowned psychiatrists and a clinical psychologist who were on the faculty of a leading medical school. All three experts were well known in their field and periodically took on forensic cases. They evaluated CC in the same way they would evaluate any patient whom they saw in the hospital or in their private offices; that is, they relied solely on what CC told them. During the questioning, CC revealed a dual personality; she claimed that the other personality had participated in the torture and death of the child, although she denied any memory of these events. In addition to multiple personality (a defense that was popular at the time), these experts concluded that CC suffered from a neurological disorder, had been subjected to childhood sexual abuse, and was psychotic.

The prosecution expert found none of these conditions. Although psychological testing revealed some mild organicity, nothing of significance was detected. This expert concluded that CC had a severe personality disorder with inadequate, dependent, and mild borderline traits; but there were no signs, either clinically or on testing, of a psychosis, a thought disorder, or a breakdown in reality testing. There was, however, clear evidence of malingering. CC gave many different versions of the various crimes and was untruthful throughout the interview. She also gave many suspicious test responses that suggested deception. For example, the MMPI showed a very clear attempt to feign and exaggerate psychopathology.

All the defense experts observed displays of alleged multiple personality when they evaluated CC. In fact, one defense expert's description of CC's behavior (contained in the psychologist's report) is typical not of multiple personality but of malingering:

> During the session D [CC's name for her alter ego] commented frequently on the possibility that we are being observed, monitored, or taped. He [the alter ego was a male] mentioned that our examining room was the only room without a camera, and he physically inspected a loudspeaker on the wall. He picked up the telephone on one occasion and listened to the dial tone. He alluded to noises outside the window and several times closed the door to the room, commenting that people may be listening. This hypervigilance led him to inspect the pictures on the wall. During the testing he frequently paced around the room or tapped his fingers on the table.

The prosecution experts did not observe any of this conduct. They also found no signs of true auditory hallucinations. For example, when asked what she meant by "hearing voices," CC explained, "Before you came, a voice told me, 'Don't trust him; he is for them.'" That is not an auditory hallucination. CC also indicated that she was "in touch with reality at all times," but she then recanted and said that during the time when the offenses occurred, "I was not in touch with reality at any period." She also stated upon questioning, "I kept saying to my boyfriend, 'We'll get in trouble and it will most likely be me, because I am the adult.'"

The defense experts all agreed that CC suffered from multiple personality disorder; however, after listening to all the evidence, the jury disagreed, finding her guilty of all charges. This case is an excellent example of three highly respected and competent practitioners who conducted a clinical evaluation but not a forensic evaluation. They relied solely on what the defendant told them. Moreover, they had very little understanding of malingering or deception, as in general clinical practice it does not typically occur. CC displayed the characteristic signs, symptoms, and conduct of a person simulating mental illness; the deception was easily detectable when the examination was approached from a forensic, rather than a clinical, perspective. A 10-year follow-up at prison found CC adjusting relatively well with no signs of multiple personality, psychosis, or brain damage.

2.3.2 Psychometric Assessment of Malingering

A number of useful tests help in the assessment of malingering. Because of the frequency of malingering in criminal defendants, forensic practitioners are admonished to develop a low threshold for suspecting deception in this population. Unlike as in clinical practice, the examiner cannot automatically accept the defendant's description of symptoms or explanation of events because the litigant has an obvious motive to lie and distort. Accordingly, malingering, deception, and direct lying must always be considered—not assumed but assessed.

The *DSM-5* (2013) is clear to point out that "the essential feature of malingering is the intentional production of false or grossly exaggerated ... symptoms, ... motivated by external incentives such as ... evading criminal prosecution" (p. 726). The *DSM-5* also notes that malingering should be strongly suspected if

> (1) the individual is referred by an attorney ... or criminal charges are pending ... (2) [there is] a marked discrepancy between the individual's claimed ... disability and the objective findings and observations ... (3) lack of cooperation during the diagnostic evaluation ... and (4) [there is evidence of] antisocial personality disorder. (p. 727)

Mental health professionals often have difficulty recognizing malingering when they rely solely on clinical judgment. Accordingly, a number of tests specifically designed to assess malingering have been developed. The *Miller-Forensic Assessment of Symptoms Test (M-FAST)* (Miller, 2001) is a well-validated scale designed to provide information regarding the probability that an individual is feigning mental illness. A cutoff score is used to maximize the probability that an individual is correctly classified as a malingerer. Another test commonly used, the *Structured Interview of Reported Symptoms* (Rogers, Bagby, and Dickens, 1992) is more extensive and is designed to detect malingering, deception, and symptom fabrication in a forensic population. This test covers a vast array of symptoms, including very rare symptoms, symptom combinations, improbable or absurd symptoms, blatant symptoms, subtle symptoms, severity of symptoms, selectivity of symptoms, and reported versus observed symptoms. Consistency of the subject's responses is also assessed as malingerers often cannot recall descriptions of feigned symptoms.

It is also not uncommon for a criminal defendant to feign cognitive loss, intellectual disability, and, most commonly, amnesia. The *Test of Memory Malingering* (Tombaugh, 1996) is a well-designed and useful test to assess malingered memory loss. The test initially appears very difficult but is extremely easy; there are cutoff scores to determine whether the subject's memory or cognitive loss is real. In many forensic assessments, the issue of amnesia emerges. The defendant might remember everything with respect to his activities before and following the homicide, but for the brief period where the victim was killed there is a claim of loss of memory. Malingered amnesia is not at all uncommon in criminal cases; it occurs basically for two reasons: (1) many defendants believe that it is to their legal advantage to say they do not remember the offense, and (2) many defendants do not want to remember and discuss what they have done.

Just as it is important to carefully evaluate revised and updated psychological tests, as previously noted, it is equally important to evaluate revised and updated tests for assessing malingering. For example, Rogers, Sewell, and Gillard (2010) updated the *Structured Interview of Reported Symptoms (SIRS)* which would seem to be beneficial. However, the revised *SIRS-2* has come under some criticism, and some researchers have concluded that the original *SIRS* (1992) is more useful than the revised edition (Green, Rosenfeld, and Belfi, 2013; Tarescavage and Glassmire, 2016). As previously noted, test revisions are generally desirable, but to revise tests for marketing purposes or for what some have suggested is an attempt to get practitioners to purchase new tests, or just to revise for the sake of revising, is not appropriate and is often self-defeating.

Case 2.5: Feigning Intellectual Disability

A 31-year-old male was married for about 10 years; he and his wife had two young daughters. The marriage was fairly unstable, with conflict stemming from affairs that both individuals had several years earlier. The defendant was employed as a cook at a well-known restaurant and also worked part-time at another restaurant. His wife was employed as a supervisor for a local business. She met a man at work, had an affair with him, and the husband found out.

After a week or so of arguing, she told her husband she was going to leave him for the other man. They got into a heated confrontation about his wife's desire to leave him, and the husband ended up strangling her to death. He took off her clothes, placed the dead body in the bathtub, turned the water on, and put his wife's clothes in plastic bags in the trunk of his car. He then called 911.

When the police arrived, they found the victim nude, lying on her back, and submerged under water in the bathtub. The defendant told the authorities that his wife accidently drowned, as she liked to take a bath lying on her back with the water running into her mouth. He provided many inconsistent versions of events when interviewed by the police.

The defendant did not have a great deal of formal education, but he always worked, was a well-respected employee, raised two children, and frequently traveled abroad. The defense expert evaluated the defendant and found he had an IQ of 56; he concluded that the defendant was mentally retarded (intellectually disabled) and, as a result, was unable to waive his *Miranda* rights. The psychologist based the diagnosis of mental retardation solely on an IQ score. However, an IQ score is not a diagnosis and is never sufficient for a diagnosis of intellectual disability. An IQ score alone—which represents an averaging of skills—can be easily affected by many factors such as attention, concentration, culture, psychopathological disorders, physical handicaps, and the subject's motivation. As a result, an IQ score can be quite misleading. According to criteria established by the *American Association on Intellectual and Developmental Disabilities*, the *Diagnostic and Statistical Manual of Mental Disorders*, and the *Wechsler Intelligence Scales*, an individual's ability to adapt to the demands of daily life is considered to be a more reliable diagnostic guideline than IQ scores alone. Therefore, a diagnosis of intellectual disability can be properly made if an IQ is below 70 (in the intellectually disabled range), or even above 70, as long as there is an impairment in two areas of adaptive functioning. But if an IQ score is below 70, and there is no impairment in adaptive functioning, there is no basis for a diagnosis of intellectual disability.

In this case, it proved helpful to administer the *Test of Memory Malingering (TOMM)*. Malingerers believe that the test is very difficult for people with genuine memory impairments, and they intentionally perform poorly, while nonmalingering individuals, even those with substantial cognitive impairment (such as dementia and traumatic brain injury), exert their full effort and easily do well. They have high scores on the *TOMM*. Malingerers, however, score very low on the *TOMM*. Any score lower than 45 on the three trials of the test should raise concerns that the individual is malingering. In this case, the defendant scored 8, 10, and 6 on the three *TOMM* trials, a result that suggested he was making an intentional and concerted effort to do poorly for obvious reasons, just as he had done on the IQ test. The documentation of malingering on the *TOMM*—as well as his having intact adaptive functioning—suggested that the defendant was clearly attempting to feign intellectual deficiency for obvious reasons.

2.3.3 Pseudomalingering

Malingering is not limited to the normal; a mentally ill person can also feign mental illness for many of the same reasons a nonmentally ill individual chooses to simulate. For instance, Schneck (1962) describes pseudomalingering as a condition in which a mentally ill individual feigns the mental illness that he or she actually has. One of his patients, for instance, explained his behavior by stating,

> I claim falsely that I am depressed because I do not want to admit to myself that I really am. By deceiving others, I am even more certain of deceiving myself, and I can effectively assure myself that I am well if I can mislead others into believing that I am ill.

Schneck believes that deception through pseudomalingering (a denial of illness through claims of illness) is a temporary ego-supportive device. This condition was graphically portrayed in Leonid Andreyev's short novel *The Dilemma*, published in 1902. The novel deals with a physician who murdered his wife. He was truly psychotic but also feigned psychosis in an attempt to absolve himself of criminal responsibility.

Arieti and Schreiber (1981) and Schreiber (1984) report the case of a schizophrenic who went on a killing spree, accompanied by his young son. Under the delusion that God had ordered him to exterminate the human species, he killed one of his own sons, in addition to killing two other boys and several women. In court, this offender attempted to act in the way he believed a schizophrenic behaves. Thus, he jumped on the floor, barked like a dog, rolled around, etc. He was, in essence, attempting to simulate an illness that he actually suffered from, but he did a poor job at it since he portrayed the layman's concept of schizophrenia.

2.3.4 Malingering-by-Proxy

Various forms of bias and deception can be problematic in clinical as well as forensic assessments. Several forms of bias (and deception) can originate not in the defendant but in the forensic examiner, as examiners can be influenced by various demographics of the subject such as race, gender, age, social class, and prior diagnoses. Gaarb (1998) notes that evaluators often gain a diagnostic impression based on one or more demographic variables and "then ask questions that support the hypothesis rather than questions that would disconfirm the hypothesis or support an alternative diagnosis" (p. 59). MacLean, Neal, Morgan, and Murrie (2019) found that many forensic clinicians are not familiar with various forms of bias and also rely on ineffective bias-mitigation strategies.

In another form of bias, it is not the litigant who fabricates, exaggerates, or distorts symptoms; here, the malingering stems from the examiner. In describing such cases, Schlesinger (2003) notes, "Here, the forensic psychologist finds in the defendant signs, symptoms, or disorders that were initially suggested by the referring attorney." Dr. X. asked the defendant to "take off your jacket." He stated in the report, "I left the room briefly. When I returned, he had taken all of his clothes off, from the waist up, illustrating Mr. A.'s impaired auditory comprehension." The defendant also said throughout the evaluation that he was innocent of the charges. The psychologist interpreted the defendant's protestations as a strong tendency to perseverate mentally, which he considered further support for his diagnosis of mental retardation. When evaluated by another expert, the defendant explained that he took off his shirt because the psychologist introduced himself as Dr. X.

The defendant was ill and had asked the county jail staff to see a doctor, and he thought that the psychologist was, in fact, the doctor who wanted to evaluate him medically.

These types of cases of malingering-by-proxy are not uncommon. For example, a 35-year-old male charged with the murder of a 12-year-old boy was evaluated by a psychiatrist. The defendant explained to the psychiatrist that when he met the boy in a wooded area, he felt that "the devil was with me," implying that his thought to kill and sexually assault the child was the work of the devil. The psychiatrist incorrectly, and deceptively, put in his report and testified that the defendant thought that the little boy was the devil himself. When the defendant was evaluated by another expert, the defendant adamantly refuted the psychiatrist's interpretation of what he had said. Following his conviction, several of the jurors explained that they believed the psychiatrist "twisted" what the defendant said for the psychiatrist's own purposes, which the jurors believed was to help the defense.

It is certainly possible that evaluators who engage in this type of conduct can be incompetent or simply unethical. But it is also possible that they are not fully aware of how vulnerable forensic practitioners can be to various forms of bias, which can result in distortions in a number of different ways. Accordingly, the defendant is not always the malingerer—there are several ways an examiner can malinger (by proxy) for the defendant.

2.3.5 Ganser's Syndrome

Ganser (1898) described a cluster of symptoms that he observed in prisoners. In addition to clouding of consciousness, some somatic conversion, and hallucinations, these prisoners would habitually give approximate answers to simple questions. Examples of questions and approximate answers include:

Question: 2 plus 2 = ? *Answer*: 5
Question: The watch shows 10:15; what time is it? *Answer*: 11:15.
Question: How many legs does an elephant have? *Answer*: 5.
Question: What season is this [actual season is fall]? *Answer*: winter.

Are individuals who respond in this fashion deliberately malingering, or do they have a bona fide disorder? Ganser did not believe that his patients were simulating; however, this conclusion remains controversial (Cocores and Cohen, 1996; Cocores, Schlesinger, and Mesa, 2007). Arguments against malingering are that (1) all patients are in a dissociative state and do not remember giving approximate answers; (2) if they were malingering, they did a terrible job; and (3) Ganser's syndrome has been reported for hundreds of years in different cultures and different continents, all with the same symptom picture. On the other hand, some have argued that approximate answers may have been considered a symptom of mental illness in the late 1800s so that prisoners gave these answers in the hope of being diagnosed as mentally incompetent. But some prisoners still produce approximate answers, and it is unclear why they would consciously choose such a rare symptom pattern if they even heard of it. Although cases of Ganser's syndrome are still found (Sigal, Altmark, Alfici, and Gelkopf, 1992), they are not prevalent, even though the prison population has increased. Cocores and Cohen suggest that approximate answers, a common symptom years ago, have been replaced by more commonly occurring symptoms (e.g., hearing voices) in prisoners who are malingering.

Case 2.6: Ganser's Syndrome

A 68-year-old male was evaluated in the county jail for competency to proceed; he was accused of killing his employer following an argument. The defendant presented himself as frail and disabled, and he walked with two crutches. This was the first time he had ever been incarcerated, and he was totally unprepared for the experience of being in a county jail. The defendant was difficult to evaluate; it took a great time to get a simple answer from him, and the evaluation was held in a room with much surrounding noise and disruption.

The defendant gave a number of answers on an intelligence test that were approximations (i.e., his responses were a little off), such as the date, the time, and the month. When discussing the role of the judge, he appeared confused. When asked the color of the judge's robe, he said, "green." At this point, the evaluation was terminated; the man appeared to be uncooperative, the conditions for an evaluation were poor, and he was obviously not feeling well.

It seemed that the symptoms he displayed did not fit a typical syndromal pattern. Ganser's syndrome did not immediately come to mind because it is not common and is poorly understood. But after going over what he had said, the defendant was seen a second time and asked more specific Ganser-evaluation questions. It became clear that the approximate answers he gave, as well as his dazed sensorium, were not malingering but rather Ganser's syndrome.

The defendant was transferred to a hospital where he spent several months, and his symptoms cleared up. A dazed sensorium is common particularly in elderly inmates, but approximate answers are not and should be an immediate red flag for the possible presence of Ganser's syndrome.

2.3.6 Rationalization, Justification, and Direct Lying

Some offenders who commit pathological acts may claim and actually believe at some level, that they had a rational motive. For example, some sexual predators who break into a home may steal an insignificant object to convince themselves that they are there not for pathological reasons (which they do not fully understand), but actually to commit burglary (Schlesinger and Revitch, 1999) for gain. Offenders who commit homicide may try to justify their behavior by insisting—and sometimes even believing at some level—that the murder was not planned and directed but was an accident, or that it was provoked by the victim. An example of rationalization is provided in Dostoyevsky's classic *Crime and Punishment*. The main character, Raskolnikov, rationalized that by killing the pawnbroker, he could free society of a useless and harmful being and, in addition, his money would be a contribution to the general welfare. Often prosecutors will present what seem to be "common sense" explanations for the most bizarre crimes and murders, or they may accept an offender's logical and "common sense" confession of his alleged motive at face value. In one case, for example, the prosecution claimed that a defendant who admittedly stabbed his victim 150 times had done so to prevent her from identifying him after he stole a small amount of money.

Finally, some offenders will resort to direct lying. Lying is very common among the general population who seek to enhance their self-image, avoid hurting others' feelings, and similar other motives (Lewis and Saarni, 1993; Ford, 1996). Many criminals will lie to avoid responsibility for wrongdoing; they may be pathological liars who seek to enhance themselves (Weston, 1996), or (as sexual murderers often do) they might lie to gain a feeling of power, domination, and control over others (Schlesinger, 2001b). These offenders will lie not only to experts but to their attorneys, police, their families, and everyone else. One serial sexual murder said, "why should I tell you the truth? I'll lie and hold it over you." This individual's father said his son lies about absolutely everything, even when he does not have to lie.

Thus, the evaluation of offenders is a complex, multileveled task that requires a high level of sophistication, understanding, and experience with all the different methods and motives that underlie an individual's explanation for alleged criminal behavior.

2.4 Issues in the Determination of Guilt

Criminal defendants, especially sexual murderers, will frequently deny that they committed the crime for which they are accused. If such an offender actually did commit the crime, an examiner will find it difficult to understand all levels of the criminal psychodynamics as the offender will not discuss the event. In other instances, a criminal defendant who denies guilt may really not have committed the crime, despite eyewitness accounts, a failed polygraph, and even a prior confession. The forensic practitioner, therefore, needs to be familiar with the research in these areas, since the determination of guilt affects the overall forensic evaluation.

2.4.1 Eyewitness (and Earwitness) Identification

Since the early 1900s, psychologists have recognized that the human information-processing system is by no means perfect, and hence significant errors in memory and perception often will be made. Münsterberg (1908) in his classic text *On the Witness Stand* noted that research findings in human perception could be used to inform the criminal justice system about frequent errors in eyewitness identification. About 70 years later, Buckhout (1974) devised a number of compelling studies indicating that eyewitness testimony is highly unreliable. Additional eyewitness identification research (e.g., Loftus and Doyle, 1976; Loftus and Ketchman, 1991; Loftus, 2019; Skeem, Douglas, and Lilienfeld, 2009) repeatedly demonstrated the unreliability of eyewitness testimony—testimony that is heavily relied on by the court.

Besides the inherent unreliability of eyewitness accounts of crimes, some of the procedures used by police to obtain these accounts also create problems. Kassin, Tubb, Hosch, and Memon (2001) point out that many "criminal justice procedures" such as the following can seriously affect an eyewitness' accuracy: wording of questions, line-up instructions, child witness suggestibility, attitudes and expectations, hypnotic suggestibility, alcohol intoxication, cross-race bias, and the forgetting curve.

Despite such confounding factors, the courts have been reluctant to accept the research evidence that eyewitness identification is unreliable. Recently, however, they have been confronted with numerous cases where individuals who had been convicted as a result of eyewitness testimony—particularly uncorroborated eyewitness identification—were exonerated through DNA evidence. As a result of such cases, the U.S. attorney general, after examining the relevant literature, ordered the National Institute of Justice to come up with national guidelines for the interrogation of eyewitnesses (Wells et al., 2000).

The same type of research is beginning to be collected with earwitness testimony (Wilding, Cook, and Davis, 2000; Yarmey, 1995; Bull and Clifford, 1999). Some investigators (Olsson, Juslin, and Winman, 1998) have found that earwitness accuracy is even poorer than eyewitness accuracy, possibly because earwitnesses have more confidence than the eyewitness in their inaccurate identifications.

2.4.2 Polygraph Findings

Cesare Lombroso's (1876/1911) observation of a correlation between deception and changes in pulse and blood pressure laid the basis for the development of the lie detector test. The polygraph is based on the assumption that if a person lies in response to critical questions, an identifiable pattern of changes in respiration, heart rate, blood pressure, and skin resistance can be elicited. Lee (1953) considers the polygraph a useful shortcut that saves time and effort in obtaining a confession from guilty offenders. He cites a number of instances where an offender denied guilt but then confessed after being shown results of a failed polygraph test. According to Lee, "the mere threat of a test accomplished in ten minutes what the sheriff and his deputies were unable to accomplish in 12 days of grilling" (p. 163).

However, Smith (1967) is skeptical of the accuracy of polygraphs, citing many cases of false confessions elicited after positive polygraph findings. He believes that the physiological changes reported are caused by stress rather than deception and that variables such as the examiner's experience, self-confidence, and attitude play an essential role in the results. Perhaps the most ardent critic of the polygraph is Lykken (1998), who believes that far too many people have been fooled into accepting polygraph findings blindly. Lykken considers the polygraph to be nothing more than pseudoscience, with accuracy no greater than that achieved by the tossing of coins. There is a little dispute that the polygraph measures something; the controversy is whether it detects lying. The consensus in the scientific community is that it is not a reliable and valid measure of lie detection, but it is certainly used frequently to assist in hiring decisions and other types of evaluations where the credibility of a person is in question.

Despite false positive and false negative test results caused by personality and procedural factors, many believe the polygraph can be a useful adjunct in the work of detection when used properly by highly skilled examiners (Yankee, 1995). Infact, Grubin (2010) concludes that "given what we know about the efficacy of polygraph testing with sex offenders, one might argue that it is no longer a question of why we should use it in forensic psychiatry, but why we don't" (p. 450). The polygraph is not very different from medical instrumentation used in clinical diagnosis; no instrument is perfect, and all laboratory findings must be interpreted and incorporated into the total picture. When medical instrumentation was becoming popular 85 years ago, Cushing (1933) expressed an opinion that is still relevant today and can be applied to the polygraph, namely, that medical findings from instrumentation should be "supplementary [and subordinate] to … the careful study of the patient by a keen observer" (p. 1571).

2.4.3 False Confessions

Not all confessions can be taken at face value. False confessions—in which individuals admit to having committed crimes that they did not commit—have been recognized for many years. False confessions can be classified in several ways, but the most generally accepted and most useful system was delineated by Kassin and Wrightsman (1985). They group false confessions into three general categories: (a) spontaneous-voluntary false confessions, in which individuals—on their own accord—come to authorities and admit to having committed crimes that they did not commit; (b) coerced-compliant false confessions, in which suspects confess to crimes in order to achieve a specific goal, such as bringing a lengthy and stressful police interrogation to an end; and (c) coerced-internalized false confessions, in which suspects come to believe—during the interrogation—that they are guilty of a crime that they did not commit and did not initially remember committing (a phenomenon similar to false-memory syndrome, see Pope, 1996).

Freud (1916) discussed false confessions and believed that unconscious guilt feelings might induce certain individuals to commit crimes in order to be punished, and some false confessions may be connected to similar psychodynamics. Some believe that false confessions, which were rampant during the 16th and the 17th-century witch hunts, can be explained by fear or the effect of torture, mass hysteria, delusions, and implanted beliefs. But even without cruelty and torture, false confessions that are later recanted—or denial of guilt with a later confession—seem to be more common than was previously thought.

Because a confession may have more impact on a jury verdict than any other type of evidence (Driver, 1968), correctly identifying a false confession is important. In fact, it has been known for years that the likelihood of gaining a conviction in a case in which the defendant has confessed is extremely high (Sutherland, 1965) since it is hard for a jury to understand, as a matter of common sense and human nature, why people would admit to committing crimes unless they were guilty.

For the past 25 years, there has been an explosion of research on false confessions (e.g., Gudjonsson, 2018; Kassin, 1997, 2008; Lassiter and Meissner, 2010). The findings have shown that there are internal and external factors that can contribute to a false confession. Internal factors involve psychological vulnerabilities of the suspect such as juvenile status, presence of mental illness, or borderline or lower intelligence. The common denominator among the internal psychological factors is that such vulnerable individuals may be susceptible to becoming confused, as well as to being easily manipulated, especially by authority figures such as the police. And because of their vulnerability, they cannot stand up for themselves and may yield to police pressure or may shift their answers during an interrogation. External factors involve the process of the interrogation itself (e.g., length, trickery, deception, threats, and coercion) and other tactics that might be used to get the subject to confess.

One of the most controversial methods of eliciting a confession is the well-known Reid Technique (Inbau, Reid, Buckley, and Jayne, 2004) which involves a nine-step method of interrogation. Given the controversy surrounding the Reid Technique—specifically the possibility of inducing false confessions—it has been prohibited in several countries but is still allowed in the United States. This technique, as well as other methods of interrogation, are sometimes based on police officers believing that they know the truth of what happened, and they increase pressure on the defendant to confess to what the authorities believe actually occurred. Many police officers believe that they can detect lying in a suspect by such behaviors as eye blinks and turning one's head right and left, although these methods of detection are not generally taught today.

False confessions, in general, are complicated because the suspect can have all the above-noted vulnerabilities—and might even be an intellectually disabled (mentally retarded) psychotic adolescent—and still give a true confession; an individual without any such vulnerabilities can give a false confession, and even a known and proven false confessor can give a true confession. False confessions are only beginning to be understood. The research on false confession is relatively recent (since the 1990s) compared with the research on other psycholegal processes such as the reliability of eyewitnesses (which began around the early 1900s). And the various research studies of false confession are complex, nuanced, and involve issues of methodology, sampling, inferential statistics, and varying interpretations and generalizability of the findings.

There is no generally accepted estimate of the prevalence of false confessions; its prevalence, in some respects, may even be unknowable. Those individuals critical of police interrogations believe false confessions are common, while others have a much different point of view. It is not known exactly how many documented false confessions there have been in homicide cases (well over several hundred), but there are approximately 25,000 homicides a year in the United States, and many of the documented cases of false confession extend back to the 1970s.

What exactly constitutes internal psychological vulnerability also lacks consensus and clarity. For example, an individual who is overtly psychotic and becomes confused during an interrogation is different from an individual who is depressed and makes a spontaneous-voluntary false confession possibly to relieve guilt feelings. Ongoing research in this area has studied the relationship of false confessions to various internal psychological factors such as anxiety, impulsivity, social desirability, assertiveness, and self-esteem, but none of these findings and conclusions are settled or generally accepted. And a close scrutiny of much of this research—such as the relationship of false confession to a personality disorder or depression—reveals that it is unknown and has never been determined (by the researchers themselves) whether their subjects' reported false confessions were really false or just a claim of false confession (and the subject actually committed the crime).

Given the amount of research on false confessions, it is surprising that there is relatively little research on the confession process itself. Deslauriers-Varin, Lussier, and St. Yves (2011) are an exception. These researchers studied how individuals decide to confess, and they found that those who had no prior experience in the criminal justice system, lacked social support, and believed that evidence against them was strong were most likely to confess to the authorities. Wetmore, Neuschatz, and Gronlund (2014) found that secondary confessions—an admission of guilt by the subject to a third party such as a jailhouse informant—often had as much weight with juries as primary confessions, notwithstanding their frequent unreliability. Other studies have researched confessions; however, most of these studies are in some way related to false confessions (e.g., DeClue, 2005), the effect of confessions on judgments of guilt, and the like.

A recent study (Feliciano, Robins, Fletouris, Felps, Schlesinger, and Craun, in press) examined confessions in intimate partner homicide. The purpose was to study the confession process itself; specifically, the different ways individuals admit their guilt because a confession is not always made to the police. In their nonrandom national sample of 70 intimate partner homicides, the most common method of confession was to a non-law-enforcement individual (e.g., a family member or an emergency medical technician); the second most common method was a voluntary-spontaneous confession to a member of law enforcement without being challenged; the third most common was an evidence-based confession during an interrogation. Seven of the intimate partner homicide offenders confessed in a suicide note. Some offenders confessed but, at the same time, provided a defense, such as acting in self-defense or in response to psychotic delusions. The researchers are currently studying confessions in sexual murders and in other types of homicides because it seems clear that the way individuals confess depends on the type of offense they committed. Preliminary findings indicate that over one-third of sexual murderers do not confess at all. It is hoped that these findings will help us to gain a better understanding of the way people confess in general, in order to place false confession in context.

Many researchers have reported interesting and illuminating cases of false confessions. For instance, Kennedy (1961) reported the case of a false confession, which was later retracted but that nevertheless resulted in the execution of an innocent man. The man was convicted of murdering his wife and daughter, who had actually been killed by a sexual murderer. The accused—illiterate and confused—explained that he had confessed because he was upset and fearful of the interrogation process. This case illustrates how, during an interrogation, perhaps because of fatigue or anxiety, a suspect may suddenly blurt out a confession, and investigators (also fatigued) may convince themselves that the confession is genuine. In another case, reported by MacDonald (1961), 30 men spontaneously falsely confessed to the murder of a young woman, whose nude body had been cut in half at the waist and mutilated with multiple stab wounds. Revitch and Schlesinger (1981) reported three cases of false confession; one was described as coerced, one as internalized, and one as spontaneous—descriptions that coincided with the Kassin and Wrightsman (1985) classification system published several years later.

Just as subjects may temporarily delude themselves into believing they are guilty when they are not, they may also delude themselves into believing they are not guilty when they actually are, particularly if the homicide was ego dystonic and explosive. It is, therefore, critical that the forensic examiner be aware of the various forces, both within the person and in the interrogation process itself, that can lead to false confessions.

Case 2.7: Coerced-Compliant and Internalized False Confession

B.H., 24 years old, had been living for about a year with a young woman and her two children (a boy and girl) aged 7 and 8. It was a tumultuous relationship: B.H. was described as having a violent temper directed toward the woman and sometimes toward the children. The defendant was known to the police for fighting and other types of disorderly conduct, and he also had served a prison sentence for burglary.

The bodies of both children were found in the basement of their apartment building by a tenant. The 8-year-old girl was found bound, naked, with her underwear shoved in her mouth. The little boy was killed by the offender banging five long nails into his head. The children's mother told the authorities that she thought B.H. was capable of carrying out the homicides. During the course of the investigation, B.H. gave three statements to the police. The first statement was a detailed denial of guilt. The next day, he gave a second statement and changed some of what he had previously told the police but continued to deny involvement in the murders. Later that same day, B.H. gave a third statement implicating himself in the two murders and the sexual assault on the female child. B.H. then denied guilt when he was brought to the county jail within hours after he implicated himself.

The defendant was found guilty by a jury of aggravated manslaughter although the trial began as a capital murder case. It became clear that members of the jury found problems in the defendant's statements and the investigation itself, but they nevertheless convicted him of the lesser charge of aggravated manslaughter.

B.H. underwent extended periods of interrogation. He was interrogated on the first day for about 14 hours after not having slept the prior night. On the second day of questioning,

B.H. was with the police for about 16 hours and was interrogated for about 12 hours. His five-page typed statement, in which he implicated himself, took 5 1/2 hours for the officers to complete. The specific questions B.H. was asked are not known, and neither are the answers he gave over the lengthy period of interrogation, as his statement and the police reports are not a verbatim question-and-answer account of what was said.

It seems that the detectives believed that the defendant was guilty because of what they considered to be signs of deception including eye blinks, grinning, and "lack of appropriate emotional response." Although B.H. did not know certain facts about the crime, the interviewers concluded that the suspect was being "deceptive" and not forthcoming. Rather than concluding that B.H. may not have known the facts because he was not involved in the murders, the interviewers incorrectly concluded that the suspect was simply lying or "playing games."

The police were certain they knew exactly what happened. For example, when asked how the nails were driven into the child's head, the suspect first said, "Crowbar?", "Hammer?" and then said "chair." When the police pointed to a rock they had placed on a table, B.H. said a rock was used to bang in the nails. The detectives assumed that B.H. knew the correct answers because he committed the crime. When B.H. asked the officers what would happen if their investigation determined that someone else committed the crime, the police told him no one else was involved. Many individuals, while giving a statement that turns out to be a false confession, often try to elicit the "correct" answers from the police; in retrospect, B.H. seems to have been attempting to elicit answers. But the detectives thought "he was testing our knowledge of the crime."

In many false confession cases, detectives believe that the suspect is guilty, and findings that point toward innocence (or absence of guilt) are often minimized or rationalized. This minimization occurred on a number of occasions with B.H. For example, B.H. gave two different versions of how the children were killed. This discrepancy was not considered a red flag to be further investigated. Only the "facts" linking him to the murders were the focus of the questions. In addition, the suspect said he did not use any electrical wire, while the autopsy showed electrical wire was used. B.H. also said that he vomited and left a Canadian Club bottle close to the crime scene, but neither was ever found.

And when B.H. asked the detectives what would happen if the FBI analysis of forensic evidence showed that he did not commit the crime, he was told that the analysis would show that he did commit the crime. B.H. was supposed to have known information that only the offender would have known—specifically, the child's sexual assault and that her underwear was placed in her mouth. When asked at first, he said he did not know if or how she was assaulted. He then said the assault took place on the couch and her underwear was placed in her mouth. But the specific questions asked of him were not recorded, so it is unknown whether the police mentioned the couch and underwear to him at some prior point.

A neighbor who knew that the children were alone the day they were killed was not extensively questioned because the detectives believed that B.H. committed the crime. Moreover, B.H. (in his first statement) lied to the police about being in a fight, failed the polygraph (even though the polygrapher said the results should not be relied on given B.H.'s lack of sleep), and gave times (regarding his whereabouts and when phone calls were made) different from the times supplied by other individuals. B.H. also said he ate hotdogs and did not immediately call the police when the children were discovered missing, behavior the detectives believed was inconsistent with how an innocent person in his position should have behaved.

In truthful confessions, there are frequently false statements; in false confessions, the offenders' statements are often accurate in details because many times they are getting the details (inadvertently) from the police. It is not uncommon for individuals not to know exactly when they carried out certain activities. Because B.H.'s timeline was different from those of others does not mean B.H. was lying; it is equally possible that the other individuals were incorrect in their times. B.H. said he did not call the police because the children's mother told him that she would call. His eating hotdogs during the time the children were missing was interpreted by the detectives to be an indication of his callousness.

According to various records, B.H. was in a number of institutions as a child and adolescent, in addition to having lived in foster care. While serving his sentence for the crime for 23 years, B.H. always proclaimed his innocence and had a number of DNA tests done, which were inconclusive. Finally, an advanced analysis of DNA was carried out, and it was determined that B.H.'s DNA was not at the crime scene. Instead, his neighbor's DNA was at the scene, including on cigarette butts as well as on the victims' bodies. When the police went to arrest the offender, he was already in prison for a number of rapes, which were committed in a manner similar to the way the children were killed. He was interviewed by the police and revealed his sexual arousal to the 8-year-old female victim. Unfortunately, this man died in the county jail just prior to his trial, so many of the questions that were raised in the initial case were not fully resolved.

This seems to have been a case of a coerced-compliant false confession. However, the defendant's attorney believed that during the interrogation itself B.H. may have come to believe that he actually did carry out the murders. His doing so would possibly indicate a coerced-internalized false confession. This case is interesting because both types of false confession seem to be present.

Case 2.8: Spontaneous-Voluntary False Confession

A 29-year-old woman stayed at a welfare hotel with a 32-year-old male. The male paid the rent, and she had sex with him as her contribution. They got into an argument, which resulted in the female fatally stabbing the male. Following the homicide, she left the hotel and, after a few days, checked into an alcohol rehabilitation program in another town.

The victim's body was found by his homeless brother, who came to visit periodically. He called the police and spontaneously confessed to them that it was he who killed his brother as well as the woman who also resided there. He said that he stabbed his brother about nine times and reported being the victim of physical and mental cruelty by his brother. He also said that he stabbed the woman four times and discarded her body in a nearby dumpster. When the authorities searched the dumpster, they did not find the remains of a female's body.

As the investigation proceeded, police eventually located the woman, arrested her, and took her to the county jail. They said to her, "There's your co-defendant," the victim's brother. At this point, the woman told the police she had no co-defendant and that she killed the man herself during an argument.

When the police confronted the brother with the fact that the woman was alive and said she acted alone, he told the police he concocted the entire confession because "I was telling you what you wanted to hear." It was later determined that the victim's brother lied to the police in order to get a place to stay, as the weather was turning colder and he was tired of being homeless. This false confession indicates that individuals have many motives for falsely confessing, and many cases do not neatly fit into one classification category or another, as confession cases—like all criminal cases—are complicated, with often unique sets of facts and circumstances.

2.5 Crime Scene Behavioral Analysis

A forensic examination is not simply an evaluation of an individual for the presence or absence of a mental illness. Forensic assessments must include an examination of the behavioral evidence in the case, which is often much more relevant than any type of mental disorder. For instance, a defendant can have any type of mental illness, including a psychotic-level diagnosis, and still be able to plan, execute, and cover up a crime.

Staging: Crime scene staging—altering the crime scene to redirect the investigation— is a common way some criminal defendants behave. Schlesinger, Gardenier, Jarvis, and Sheehan-Cook (2014) carried out what was at the time the most comprehensive empirical study of crime scene staging in homicide. These authors examined 946 homicide crime scenes and delineated the prevalence, types, levels, and motivations for staging in domestic, nonserial sexual, serial sexual, and general felony homicides. Those individuals who staged a crime scene were found to be a relatively small group who employed a variety of methods—for example, the homicide appeared to be an accident, a burglary, an arson, a suicide, and a sexual homicide. Staging an arson was the most common method followed by staging a burglary and an accident. The ways defendants can alter a crime scene is limited only by their creativity, intelligence, physical strength, and capabilities.

Schlesinger et al.'s (2014) results indicate that different types of homicides have different staging rates, based primarily on the relationship the offender had to the victim. For example, 19% of domestic homicides were staged, while only 6% of nonserial sexual homicides and 5% of general felony homicides were staged. An unexpected, but important, finding was that serial sexual homicide offenders did not stage any of their 195 crime scenes studied. The serial sexual murderers appeared more concerned with posing the victim to gain sexual gratification than with staging the scene in order to elude law enforcement. The researchers also evaluated the crime scenes to determine whether the staging involved a minimal amount of effort, moderate effort, or an elaborate attempt with many elements of the scene altered. The results indicated that the levels of staging were evenly distributed.

Domestic homicide offenders had the largest percentage of staged crime scenes. Here, the verbal staging was the primary method; the offender killed the victim, disposed of the body, and then filed a false police report that the victim was missing. The researchers concluded that domestic homicide offenders staged the scene because they correctly viewed themselves as a logical suspect. In cases of nonserial sexual homicides and general felony homicides, where the scene was staged with no documented prior relationship between the offender and victim, it was found that there may have been a relationship that was unknown and undocumented. In four of the eight cases, an arrest was made because a witness had raised the possibility in the offender's mind that they may have been seen together; this possibility motivated the offender to stage the crime scene.

Undoing: Another form of crime scene behavior that is poorly understood is undoing. Here, offenders try to symbolically reverse a homicide based on feelings of guilt or remorse for what they have just done. Douglas, Burgess, Burgess, and Ressler (2013) describe a case of undoing.

> A son stabbed his mother to death during a fierce argument. After calming down, the son was hit by the full impact of his actions. First, he changed the victim's bloody shirt, then placed her body on the couch with the head on a pillow; he covered her with a blanket and folded her hands over her chest so she appeared to be sleeping peacefully. (p. 251)

Several other authors (e.g., Schröer and Puschel, 2007; Chancellor and Grahan, 2014; Litzcke, Horn, and Schinke, 2015) report cases of what appeared to be undoing at a crime scene.

Russell, Schlesinger, Leon, and Holdren (2018) carried out an extensive empirical study of undoing. Their examination of 975 homicide crime scenes disclosed 11 cases (1.13%) of undoing behavior. These authors looked at the frequency of various methods of undoing such using blankets to cover the victim's body (55%), positioning the body (55%), using a bed or couch (42%), washing the body (36%), using pillows (36%), and removing clothing and adding other types of adornments (27%). An unexpected finding was that 10 of the 11 offenders were male, and all victims were female. It had been speculated by the researchers before the study that women would be more likely to engage in undoing behavior, possibly because they might be more sensitive. However, as the findings indicate, men can experience just as much guilt or remorse as women. Ten of the twelve victims were family members or relationship intimates, a finding that supports the notion that the motivation for engaging in undoing is to compensate for guilt or remorse for having committed the murder of someone with whom the offender had been close.

Case 2.9: Staged Homicide

A 20-year-old male with superior intelligence—but without any motivation for doing schoolwork—was unable to attract a girlfriend although he desperately wanted to. He was a likable individual who weighed over 300 pounds. T.H. was friends with many female classmates, but none of the young women wanted to have any romantic involvement with him. The defendant graduated from high school, began community college, but stopped going to classes after about a month.

The defendant's father, a well-respected and popular police officer, often bragged (in his son's presence) that when he died, T.H. would inherit close to a million dollars, based on his police pension, life insurance, home, cars, and possessions. The offender exchanged many e-mails and text messages with a female friend who wanted to move out of her parents' home but could not afford to do so. In one text, T.H. wrote, "If my plan works, I'll have enough money to buy a damn mansion."

Twelve days after that text message, hoping he would have close to a million dollars and his female friend could move in with him, he shot his father in the middle of the night with the father's service revolver. The defendant staged the crime scene by shooting himself superficially in his arm, shooting a hole in the wall, making the rear door appear as if it had been broken into, and then calling 911. He told the operator an intruder came to the house, "we tussled," and he managed to take his father's gun away from the intruder who fled, unharmed, through the rear door.

There was no evidence anyone left through the rear door, as there were no footprints in the fresh snow; neighbors heard nothing other than the gunshots; and an examination of T.H.'s wound indicated that it was self-inflicted. After a brief interview with the police, he admitted to killing his father. At trial, he unsuccessfully raised a defense that the motive for killing his father was abuse, for which there was absolutely no evidence at all.

Case 2.10: Undoing

A 23-year-old single female had a 5-year-old son; she found it difficult to care for the child because of financial problems, time commitments and, most of all, an inability to get a boyfriend to marry her. Most young men her age, whom she dated, said they did not want to marry a woman who already had a 5-year-old.

About a week before the homicide, L.M. got her son a special haircut that he wanted and a new set of clothing that depicted a cartoon figure popular at the time. She had the child sleep in his new clothing and, in the middle of the night, killed him by smothering him. She then placed the pillowcase with the body and wrapped him in his blanket, along with a balloon, highlighting the cartoon figure. L.M. drove the victim's body several miles away to a swamp she had familiarity with because she had previously worked in a building close to the area. After disposing of the body, she left the area and was next seen at about 7 o'clock that night at a carnival she had planned to attend.

While at the carnival, her 14-year-old niece and the niece's friend—both of whom had babysat for the 5-year-old—approached L.M. and asked where her son was. L.M. told them that she had turned her back at the carnival, and he was gone. The offender then gave about ten different versions to the authorities as to what has happened to her son. After a prolonged search, the body was found, but L.M. never admitted guilt and the case went cold for about 20 years.

When the cold case was re-examined, it was determined that the blanket with distinct markings the child was wrapped in and that was found in the swamp was never shown—at that time—to the two adolescents who babysat for the child. The blanket, when recovered, was shown only to L.M. who said she never saw it before. The former babysitters, now in their 30s, became visibly upset when they saw the blanket (with distinct markings) because they knew it well. The child could not have been abducted from the carnival because the offender would have to have then gone to the mother's home, stolen the blanket, and wrapped the child in it in order to leave both the body and the blanket in the swamp.

When the investigators went to a distant state to which the mother had moved and told her where they were from, L.M.'s first response was "Are you here to arrest me?" There was no physical evidence (such as DNA) because the body was in the swamp for about year before it was recovered, and it was greatly decomposed. Nevertheless, the behavioral evidence, in this case, including undoing behavior, was persuasive. The mother's dressing the child in the clothes that he wanted, getting him a special haircut, placing a balloon with his body wrapped in a blanket are all examples of her attempt to symbolically reverse what she had done.

2.6 Application of Findings to Legal Standards

Although forensic practitioners today have much more training than in the past (Roesch, Zapf, Golding, and Skeem, 1999), much of this training, as described in various books on the topic, is on the laws and legal standards that practitioners need to know. Laws and legal standards are obviously necessary, but the basics of a forensic assessment—and how it differs from a clinical assessment—are rarely stressed. And if the forensic assessment is touched upon, the emphasis is on various specialized forensic tests.

Forensic assessment should be a three-step process: (1) a detailed review of the facts of the case as derived from the investigation, not from what the defendant self-reports; (2) an evaluation of the psychopathology or any disorder that the defendant may have; and (3) both these findings should then be applied to a legal standard (such as competency to waive *Miranda* rights, competency to stand trial, or various state-of-mind defenses such as insanity, diminished capacity, passion-provocation, voluntary intoxication, and the like). That criminal defendants lie and distort is well known; however, it is surprising how often forensic evaluators rely primarily (often only) on what the defendant told them, without looking at what actually occurred by examining the details of the legal discovery. When Heilbrun, Rosenfeld, Warren, and Collins (1994) asked forensic practitioners whether they used and relied on corroborative information, in addition to their own clinical evaluation, the majority said that they did. But an examination of their reports did not indicate how this information was integrated, if at all. Because litigants have an obvious motive to lie or distort, forensic practitioners cannot conduct assessments as they would a clinical evaluation of patients who come to their private offices or are in a hospital or mental health center. Case after case is found in which forensic practitioners reach conclusions based solely on what defendants have told them, even though these contradict the undisputed facts of the case (as indicated in Case 2.2).

One common example of an assessment of legal insanity, using the M'Naghten Rule, is that offenders must not have known, or appreciated, that their behavior was wrong. Many evaluators conclude that the defendants did not know what they were doing was wrong because the defendants told them they did not know what they were doing was wrong at the time. However, leaving the crime scene, staging the crime scene, or lying about various behaviors all indicate consciousness of guilt and an awareness of the wrongfulness of defendants' behavior.

The Place of Sexual Murder in the Classification of Crime

3

Sexual murder cannot be understood in isolation from other types of crimes and homicides. Thus, a broad appreciation of crime theory and classification of offenders is necessary to fully grasp this or any other type of criminal behavior. Theories and classification systems of crime developed slowly over the course of many years, as did various laws to govern such conduct (Garland, 1990). For example, in early tribal cultures, normative behaviors became ritualized and primitive punishments were assigned to unacceptable actions. Later on, biblical laws developed and specified various crimes, along with accompanying retribution. In medieval society, crime was equated with evil. As human behavior was supposed to be guided by free will, a criminal act was a free choice by an evil person. As society developed further, governments—rather than unorganized groups—enacted laws and carried out punishments.

During the 19th and the early 20th century, various scientific theories of crime began to be expounded. These theories can be generally divided into three groups: biological, psychological, and sociological.

3.1 Theories of Crime

3.1.1 Biological Theories

Early theories: Among the biological theories of the 19th century, the most prominent was the "criminal activism" doctrine of Cesare Lombroso (1876/1911). Lombroso believed that certain hereditary and constitutional characteristics prevented a criminal from advancing as far along the evolutionary scale as a normal person was able to do. Lombroso even believed that the skulls and brains of criminals resembled those of primitive and prehistoric man. According to this theory, an individual was born a criminal and had no choice but to remain one. This point of view was widely acclaimed at the end of the 1890s, but by the beginning of the 20th century, it had lost its popularity. Goring (1913), for example, was unable to find any of the anatomical differences between criminal and noncriminal groups that were proposed by Lombroso.

Another popular biological theory of criminal behavior was advanced by Sheldon (1940), who was influenced by the constitutional theories of the German psychiatrist Ernest Kretschmer (1925). Sheldon believed, for instance, that delinquent boys could be easily identified since they were better physically developed than nondelinquent boys, a result of their biology, he maintained, rather than their environment. Toward the middle of the 20th century, Bachet (1951) resurrected some of Lombroso's notions, but he believed that Lombroso paid too much attention to external anatomical characteristics. Bachet thought that the true differences between the criminal and the noncriminal population could be detected through measurements of their internal brain functions—assessments made possible by the newly developed electroencephalogram (EEG). Bachet studied EEG differences in prison and nonprison populations and concluded that abnormal brain functioning—greater in criminals than in noncriminals—accounted for criminal behavior.

Contemporary theories: There has been a great deal of contemporary research and thinking regarding the biological underpinnings of criminal behavior including murder. Some (e.g., Rowe, 2002 and Raine, 2014) have argued that certain people are predisposed to commit crime based on various biological markers. Palmer and Thornhill (2000) and Rowe (2002) have advanced an evolutionary perspective. Raine (2002) noted that genetic factors play a role based on twin and adoption studies; he has also summarized physiological under-arousal (e.g., EEG and cardiovascular) and brain imaging studies as important new research as well.

3.1.2 Psychological Theories

Psychoanalytic theory: Prominent among the psychological theories of criminal behavior is Freud's notion that unconscious guilt is the cause of crime: "It is a fact that large groups of criminals long for punishment. Their superego demands it and so saves itself the necessity for inflicting the punishment itself" (Freud, 1928, p. 178). Freud believed that the sense of guilt derives from the Oedipus complex and is a result of the two great criminal intentions of the male—killing his father and having sexual relations with his mother. Freud (1916) commented that criminal acts are performed

> precisely because they are forbidden. … Paradoxical as it may sound, I must maintain that the sense of guilt was present prior to the transgression, that it did not arise from this, but contrariwise—the transgression from the sense of guilt. These persons we might justifiably describe as criminals from a sense of guilt. (p. 342)

Glover (1960) argued that Freud's seminal thinking on unconscious guilt as the cause of crime would alone be sufficient to revolutionize the whole system of penology. A slightly different point of view was advanced by Woddis (1957), who connected violent and non-violent criminal acts to states of depression. Woddis generally supported Freud's theory of crime as he believed that criminals bring retribution on themselves as a result of guilt and other negative feelings caused by depression.

Psychopathic personality: Psychopathic personality is perhaps the most widely known concept connecting a psychological disorder to criminal behavior. It was first described by the 19th-century alienists. Pinel (1806) reported individuals with no outward signs of psychosis, who nevertheless behaved with "moral depravity." Pritchard (1835) elaborated on the concept, which he called "moral insanity" or "moral imbecility." He questioned why some prisoners—without any mental illness or intellectual disability—repetitively committed crimes. Krafft-Ebing (1886) also reported cases of individuals who lacked moral judgment and ethics. Koch (1888) coined the term "constitutional psychopathic inferiority," which he believed described born criminals. Such individuals, from childhood throughout adulthood, repetitively committed crimes, did not change, and incarceration and punishment had no impact on them.

Kraepelin (1913) discussed psychopathic personality in the early days of the 20th century. Kahn (1931) also discussed psychopathic personality, focusing on inadequate social skills and impulsivity; he believed such individuals were unable to contain their impulsive drives because of genetics. Partridge (1928) believed that psychopathic personality was a result of lack of socialization; he preferred the term *sociopath*, earlier referred to by Birnbaum (1914). These authors believed that social learning and defective early environmental influences resulted in repetitive criminal conduct. Revitch (1950) considered emotional immaturity with an "inability to form deep feelings such as lasting friendships, love or for that matter, lasting deep hatred" (p. 3) to be the basic characteristics of the psychopath.

In his landmark book with an iconic title, *The Mask of Sanity*, Cleckley (1941) described what had since become the hallmark feature of psychopathic personality: individuals who appear normal but have a severe psychological disturbance that involves a lack of interpersonal bonding.

Cleckley believed that the deficit in interpersonal connectedness is so significant that it is at the level of a psychosis—not a psychosis with overt symptoms such as hallucinations and delusions, but rather a disruption of the personality structure. He listed 16 traits found in a psychopath including superficial charm, good intelligence, absence of nervousness, unreliability, insincerity, lack of remorse or shame, and failure to learn from experience. Cleckley noted that this level of disturbance is "masked" and is unable to be easily detected by observation, even with extended interaction with such an individual. Accordingly, Cleckley concluded that the diagnosis of psychopathy is difficult to make and can be made only by examiners who know exactly what they are looking for and spending extended time with the subject.

In the early 1980s, Hare (1980) introduced the *Psychopathy Checklist* (*PCL*) and later the *Psychopathy Checklist-Revised* (*PCL-R*) (*1991*), based largely on Cleckley's initial work, which listed and described traits of psychopathic disturbance. Hare's checklists provide a numerical assessment of the extent of psychopathy in an individual, and this assessment made empirical research much easier than it had been. But as Litwack and Schlesinger (1999) point out, the derived numbers of the *PCL-R* are nothing more than subjective clinical impressions used to rate an individual on traits and characteristics.

> An evaluator must make a clinical judgment regarding the extent to which the evaluee manifests such traits as superficial charm, a grandiose sense of self-worth, a lack of remorse or empathy, and conning or being manipulative. That is, obtaining a *PCL-R* score, even from file data, is not simply a mechanical operation. (pp. 188–189)

Table 3.1 summarizes the viewpoints, some of which have become classic, of various theorists who have offered their perspectives on the psychological makeup of individuals who habitually find themselves in difficulty with the law.

The research on psychopathic personality has been voluminous. Moreover, psychopathy has been used to predict future violence and potential for rehabilitation, as well as to make decisions about civil commitment, juvenile transfer, and other serious legal and criminal justice determinations.

But notwithstanding the fact that psychopathy has been referred to in the mental health literature extensively for almost 200 years, it has never been established as an official diagnosis in any of the five editions of the *Diagnostic and Statistical Manual*. The *DSM* has referred to various forms of personality disturbance related either directly or indirectly to criminal behavior but has never labeled such behavior as psychopathy. In fact, the closest *DSM* diagnosis to psychopathy is an antisocial personality disorder, which encompasses traits and behaviors different from those conceptualized by Cleckley and others. Table 3.2

Table 3.1   **Various Views of Psychopathic Personality/Criminal Conduct**

Author	Year	Conception of Disorder
Pinel Prichard	1806	No outward signs of psychosis, but behave with "moral depravity."
Koch	1888	Constitutional psychopathic inferiority; born criminals.
Kraepelin	1913	Constitutional psychopathic state includes sex offenders plus anxious and despondent individuals. Psychopathic personality includes born criminals, murderers, liars, and swindlers.
Partridge	1928	Sociopathy; the problem is lack of socialization.
Cleckley	1941	Underlying disturbance involves lack of emotional bonding to others which extends to the level of a psychosis. The psychosis is "masked," and the outward facade appears normal.
Fenichel	1945	Impulse neurosis; psychopaths release tension the way an infant does.
Karpman	1948	Anethopathy (primary psychopathy); true psychopathic state, which is inborn.
Revitch	1950	Condition marked by emotional immaturity and superficiality.
Yochelson & Samenow	1976	Thinking patterns differentiate criminals and noncriminals; extremely difficult to change.
Schlesinger	1980	Differentiates psychopathic, sociopathic, and antisocial personality disorders.
Hare	1980	Developed a test to assess psychopathy in an objective manner.

Table 3.2   **Psychopathy and the *DSM***

Pre-*DSM*—1927–1951	Reference to psychopathic personality and constitutional psychopathic state.
DSM-I—1952	Sociopathic personality disturbance, antisocial reaction; dissocial reaction.
DSM-II—1968	Antisocial personality disorder.
DSM-III—1980	Antisocial personality disorder with specific enumerated criteria.
DSM-5—2013	Antisocial personality disorder; conduct disorder (for children and adolescents); adult antisocial behavior.

lists the different views of the *DSM* regarding a psychological disturbance and criminal behavior.

There is no legitimate reason why psychopathic personality should not be included in the next edition of the *Diagnostic and Statistical Manual*. The reasons for noninclusion, such as the difficulty of operationally defining traits such as superficial charm, insincerity, and shallow emotions, have always been unclear. Schlesinger (1980) noted that distinctions among psychopathic, sociopathic, and antisocial personality disorders are legitimate and not just an academic argument. It is difficult to understand why all three personality disorders cannot become official diagnoses (Schlesinger, 2018). Inclusion in the *DSM* would, at least, encourage further research and enhance our understanding of criminal behavior and the various types of individuals who engage in this conduct.

3.1.3 Sociological Theories

Social theories of crime have been advanced by sociologists or criminologists who argue that various societal factors such as broken homes, poverty, social role, or the influence of others are responsible for the commission of crimes. The most widely known among the social theories was put forth by Sutherland (1937, 1949) and Sutherland and Cressey (1939). According to this theory, known as "differential association," individuals learn criminal behavior by interacting with others in intimate personal groups. They learn techniques of committing crimes (which are sometimes complicated and sometimes simple), as well as specific rationalizations and attitudes regarding criminal behavior. An individual who commits a crime has, therefore, acquired attitudes in favor of law violation that outweigh attitudes and beliefs in favor of acting in accordance with the law.

The concept of differential association, although perhaps the most prominent socio-logical explanation of criminal behavior, is not without its critics. The theory has been criticized for lacking clarity and precision, and for failing to account for certain forms of criminality, including sexually motivated crimes such as sexual murder or crimes that are a result of a mental disorder. It has also been faulted for ignoring personality vari-ables and for being unable to predict with accuracy (Gibbons, 1968). In fact, there is now a voluminous literature composed of criticisms and defenses of the theory. Nevertheless, Sutherland's concept has played a dominant role in criminological theory since its concep-tion over a half a century ago and is still widely regarded.

Merton's (1938) strain theory is another early sociological theory. This theory finds that people who fail to achieve society's expectations in terms of success by socially approved methods resort to crime.

More contemporary sociological theories of crime involve "broken windows" theory. This view, which argues that visible signs of neighborhood decay encourage further crime, also has its supporters and critics (Harcourt, 1998). Some sociologists support a social net-work theory of crime (Papachristos, 2009), while others argue for an integrated approach (Lee and Choi, 2014).

3.2 Classification of Homicide

Although crime theory is helpful for an understanding of antisocial conduct as a whole, the first and most basic step in understanding any form of human behavior, including criminal behavior, is classification. Without classification, naturally occurring events would seem random, unrelated, and chaotic. Classification is certainly the approach that medicine has taken since Hypocrites' initial grouping of diseases. Similarly, psychiatry has always valued classification of symptoms and behaviors, especially since *DSM-III* (pub-lished in 1980) which first listed specific criteria of disorders. However, complex phenom-ena such as human behavior, criminal behavior, and homicide are difficult to classify. Rigid boundaries cannot be established, and there are often many borderline cases, especially as one deviates from the nuclear condition.

Over the past 70 years, many researchers have attempted to develop a system of clas-sification for the different types of homicide. Brancale (1955) proposed a simple classifica-tion of homicide into two basic groups: administrative and psychiatric. In the psychiatric group, he placed offenders who are neurotic, psychotic, and mentally deficient. All oth-ers—a much larger number—would be placed in the administrative group. The psychiatric offenders would be treated in a specialized setting, whereas the others would be handled in correctional facilities.

Bromberg (1961) also divided murderers into two general categories: the normal and the psychopathic. A "normal murder" might occur when, for example, a man finds his wife in bed with a paramour and kills one or both of them. Bromberg explained this type of "triangle murder" as a "reaction to extreme humiliation in a sensitive individual" (p. 30); the stronger the unconscious feelings of inadequacy in the perpetrator, the more vicious the attack will be. Under the heading of psychopathic murderers (or more accurately murderers with psychopathology), Bromberg included a wide range of offenders with various levels of disturbance, including the sex and lust killer, the thrill killer, the rapist who murders, and the alcoholic who kills. Psychopathic murderers are generally unstable, unpredictable, impulsive, and without conscience; they frequently describe their crime with an emotionally flat attitude. Such homicides are rarely premeditated but instead follow an impulse.

Also using a two-pronged system, Megargee (1966) classified individuals who commit acts of violence, including murder, as either undercontrolled or overcontrolled. The undercontrolled person commonly responds with violence when frustrated or provoked. The overcontrolled person displays moral rigidity, often proclaims antiviolence sentiments, and is a proponent of law and order; at the same time, he builds up an underlying (and unrecognized) rage that results in an unanticipated explosion.

Tanay's (1969, 1972) classification system includes three types of homicide: ego-syntonic, ego-dystonic (dissociative), and psychotic. The ego-syntonic homicide is, in essence, a goal-directed, purposeful act; the psychotic homicide is the result of an overt psychosis, such as a response to hallucinations or delusions; the dissociative or ego-dystonic homicide is carried out in an altered state of consciousness, against the recognized wishes of the perpetrator. In a later publication, Tanay (1978) further describes the person who commits (dissociative) ego-dystonic homicides as having an "aggressophobic personality." This disorder is characterized by rigidity, moral preoccupation, and a high degree of inner conflict regarding the subject's own aggressive strivings. He represses angry impulses to such an extent that he does not conceive of a gun as a dangerous instrument, and he may even deny that he has ever had an aggressive fantasy. These aggressophobic personalities have such an overdeveloped superego that they are afraid of their own anger and have little ability to express hostility on any level. Because of these characteristics, the aggressophobe is prone toward a sudden loss of control, resulting in an explosive ego-dystonic homicide.

Halleck (1971) classifies criminal behavior, including homicide, into adaptive and maladaptive groups. The adaptive murder is committed for some self-serving and logical, albeit socially unacceptable, purpose—for instance, to obtain money or to eliminate someone who might interfere with a plan. The maladaptive homicide is illogical, basically not purposeful, and is caused by some type of psychopathology, such as an overt psychosis, intoxication, or pronounced internal conflicts.

Other classification systems have been proposed by Guttmacher (1960) and Wille (1974). Guttmacher differentiated six types of murderers: (1) average murderers, free from prominent psychopathology; (2) individuals angry at the world because of their own mistreatment in earlier years; (3) alcoholics who kill their wives out of fear of rejection; (4) murderers who kill to avenge a prior intimate partner's rejection; (5) schizophrenics who respond to hallucinations and delusions; and (6) sadists who kill to achieve sexual gratification. Wille (1974) grouped murderers into ten different types: (1) depressives, (2) psychotics, (3) organics, (4) psychopaths, (5) passive–aggressive individuals, (6) alcoholics, (7) hysterical personalities, (8) child murderers, (9) mentally retarded individuals, and (10) those who kill for sexual gratification.

Two methods of classification were derived from empirical research. Simon (1977) studied 30 murderers and classified them into three general groups. Type A homicides are impulsive and occur usually while the offender is under the influence of alcohol; type B homicides are victim-induced, typically stemming from rejection by a former intimate partner; and type AB murders are committed by sadistic individuals who probably cannot be rehabilitated. In their research on adolescent homicidal offenders, Miller and Looney (1974) developed a classification system that is focused on prediction. The groupings here are based on the degree of "dehumanization" of the victim by the perpetrator. Thus, the classification includes (1) offenders who are at high risk for repetition because they have totally and permanently dehumanized their victim; (2) offenders who are at high risk for repetition because of partial and transient dehumanization; and (3) individuals who have a low risk to commit a future homicide because the degree of dehumanization, although transient and partial, required consensual validation by peers.

Still another system of homicide classification, utilizing a law enforcement perspective based on crime scene characteristics, was offered by Douglas, Burgess, Burgess, and Ressler (1992; 2013). These authors differentiate 43 different types of homicide, including criminal enterprise homicide, personal cause homicide, sexual homicide, and group cause homicide. Personal cause homicides would include domestic murders, homicides triggered by arguments, or revenge killings. Included in group cause homicides are cult murders, murders of hostages, and paramilitary homicides. Within each category, the authors list crime scene and forensic findings, victim characteristics, and investigative considerations. Douglas, Ressler, Burgess, and Hartman (1986) also describe the distinguishing features of mass murder (killing multiple individuals at one time in one place), spree murder (killing multiple persons at different locations, with no cooling-off period between murders), and serial murder (killing multiple victims, with a cooling-off period between events). Recently Safarik and Ramsland (2020) differentiated types of spree killing also from a law enforcement perspective.

Although the various classification schemes cited above are different in overall approach, purpose, and extent of differentiation, there is a common denominator among many of them: those that include (1) a large group of homicidal offenders with no overt psychopathology or disturbance and (2) a smaller group of offenders with overt psychopathology (see Table 3.3). For example, Brancale's administrative grouping is similar to Tanay's ego-syntonic group; Bromberg's normal (triangle) offenders; Halleck's adaptive murderers; and Guttmacher's average, angry, sadistic, and avenging individuals. Those with a more overt disturbance would include Brancale's psychiatric group, Guttmacher's schizophrenics and alcoholics, Tanay's ego-dystonic and psychotic groups, Bromberg's psychopathic category, and Halleck's maladaptive murderers.

Table 3.3 **Systems of Homicide Classification: Common Groupings**

Author	Year	Term Reflecting Absence of Overt Disturbance	Term Reflecting Overt Disturbance
Brancale	1955	Administrative	Psychiatric
Bromberg	1961	Normal (triangle)	Psychopathic
Megargee	1966	Overcontrolled	Undercontrolled
Tanay	1969	Ego-syntonic	Ego-dystonic (dissociative) and psychotic
Halleck	1971	Adaptive	Maladaptive
Guttmacher	1960	Average, angry, sadistic, and avenging	Alcoholics and schizophrenics
Wille	1974	Psychopaths, passive–aggressive hysterical, mentally retarded, who kill for sexual gratification	Depressives, psychotics, organics, alcoholics, those

The legal system's method of classification of crime attempts to assess an offender's level of intent; the more intent, the more criminal responsibility, the greater the punishment. However, since the various legal definitions of homicide deal with motivational factors, both the prosecution and the defense may stress different aspects of the same set of facts. The prosecution may emphasize logical behavior and explain away irrational acts. In many cases, however, what may seem to be premeditation is actually a compelling irrational need with reasons obscure even to the offender. Moreover, different examiners will often stress and emphasize different aspects of the same symptoms and behavior (Perr, 1975). Shah (1972) illustrates the many other levels of motivation in homicide by recounting a conversation between a scholar and a mullah. The scholar, believing totally in logic and in cause and effect, regards murder as an uncomplicated event. However, he was taken aback when the mullah pointed to a group of people passing in the street; they were taking a man to be hanged for committing a murder. "Is that because someone gave him a silver piece and enabled him to buy the knife with which he committed the murder," the mullah asks, "or is it because someone saw him do it, or because nobody stopped him?" (p. 112).

Psychiatric diagnoses per se cannot be used as a sole common denominator in the classification of crime or homicide, since crimes committed under the influence of delusions and the occasional violence resulting from organic and toxic-confusional states are primarily relevant. Psychoanalytic penetration into various nonconscious levels is frequently too theoretical and esoteric. On the other hand, the legal method, although appropriate for assigning moral responsibility and extent of punishment, is not always helpful in understanding all types of criminal behavior or the varying levels of motivation and dynamics of a homicide.

In an attempt to develop a method to classify crime, in general, and homicide, in particular, Revitch and Schlesinger developed a system of classification based on an analysis of the motivational dynamics of the antisocial act itself (Revitch, 1977; Revitch and Schlesinger, 1978, 1981, 1989). The remainder of this chapter—following a discussion of organic, toxic, and paranoid homicides—describes the motivational spectrum, in order to place sexual murder within the overall classification of crime and homicide.

3.3 Organic, Toxic, and Paranoid Homicides

The motivational spectrum does not include homicides that are largely a direct result of a primary psychiatric/neurological condition, such as an organic disorder, a toxic state, or psychotic symptoms. These homicides form a group of their own and are therefore discussed separately here.

3.3.1 Organic Disorders

The organic disorders represent a wide range of conditions, including various types of brain impairment and brain injury. Epilepsy is frequently cited as a cause of sudden, often unprovoked, attacks of violence and aggression. However, epileptics are no more violent than the general population. The most common characteristics of a psychomotor seizure are staring, smacking of the lips, various stereotyped movements, and automatisms. When an epileptic does commit a homicide, the murder usually has nothing to do with his epilepsy. An example is the case of Jack Ruby who killed President Kennedy's assassin Lee

Harvey Oswald. Ruby's attorney attempted to explain his client's action as a result of epilepsy; however, the experts involved in this case determined that Ruby's epilepsy had nothing to do with the murder (Causey and Dempsey, 2000).

Lewis (1975) believes that the notion of epileptic violence is a myth and denies that psychomotor seizures can prompt any coordinated or unprovoked aggressive act. Mark and Ervin (1970) disagree and have presented a number of cases in which violence seemed to be perpetrated as a direct result of a seizure. More recently, other forms of seizures such as partial seizures with complex symptomatology have been held accountable for outbursts of violence, including homicide (Delgado-Escueta, Mattson, and King, 1981). However, these cases are rare and often questionable; a close examination frequently reveals a psychogenic element involved at some level.

Gunn and Bonn (1971) found more epileptics among prisoners than in the general population. That finding in itself, however, does not prove that there is a causal connection between epilepsy and crime or violence, especially since the offenses committed by the epileptics were no more violent than offenses committed by nonepileptics. Moreover, as most of the prison population comes from economically deprived environments, which include poor prenatal and postnatal care, exposure to various toxins, and an increase in head injuries, the high number of epileptics among prisoners may well be a socially determined phenomenon. There are occasional cases of murder committed in ictal and postictal states, but most crimes committed by epileptics are not connected, at least directly, to their epilepsy.

Some investigators also have found a relationship between brain injuries or brain disease and violence (Bowman and Blau, 1949; Mark and Southgate, 1971). Mark and Southgate cite the case of a 27-year-old male who held a number of people at gunpoint, threatened to commit mass murder and suicide, and wound up killing one individual and wounding another. Eleven years before the incident, the subject had sustained a head injury that resulted in a left hemiparesis. Prior to the head injury, however, this man had abused alcohol, shown a fascination with firearms, and threatened to shoot his family and himself. Just before the incident, he had lost his job and was drinking heavily. Thus, a state of emotional distress in combination with alcohol, and his history of aggressive fantasies and violent behavior prior to the injury, leads one to suspect a strong contribution of psychogenic factors.

Chronic traumatic encephalopathy (CTE)—a neurodegenerative disease caused by repeated head injury—has received a great deal of attention recently since it has been found in athletes, primarily football players (Omalu, Dekosky, Minster, and Kamboh, 2005; McKee, Stein, Nowjnski, 2013). Aaron Hernandez, who won a multimillion-dollar football contract was convicted of a murder and suspected of several others. He committed suicide in prison and was found to have had CTE on autopsy. The brain damage may have weakened inhibitory controls, as he seemed more interested in associating with low-level drug users and criminals than professional athletes.

Not only brain injury but also brain infection has been cited as a cause of violence and homicide. Bachet (1951), for example, presented the concept of "criminogenic encephalosis." He found major behavioral changes, characterized by violence and antisocial conduct or an increase in preexisting behavior, following exposure to viral encephalitis. This condition was found mostly in male adolescents but was also encountered in adults of both sexes. One of his cases was a 24-year-old female who engaged in violent outbursts, thefts, and attempted murder of her friend, following recovery from encephalitis.

Various types of brain tumors have also been linked to acts of violence and homicide (Relkin, Plum, Mattis, Eidelberg, and Tranel, 1996). Mark and Ervin (1970) reported the case of an individual whose frequent eruptions of homicidal violence (including one murder) stopped after a tumor in the limbic system was removed. Perhaps the most-publicized case connecting homicide with a brain tumor is that of Charles Whitman (Lavergne, 1998). During a 90-minute period atop a tower at the University of Texas, Whitman shot and killed 12 people and wounded 31. Prior to the campus shooting, he had murdered his wife and his mother. After Whitman was killed by the police, a pathologist discovered a brain tumor at autopsy. Although it was widely believed that the tumor had caused Whitman's violent behavior, he also displayed a number of psychological features that could, to a large extent, have accounted for the mass murder: his history of violence and brutality, his preoccupation with firearms and his skill as a marine sharpshooter, his history of depression, his periodic outbursts of hostility, and his long-held fantasies of committing mass murder.

Thus, in many instances, epilepsy, encephalopathies, brain injuries, brain tumors, and other organic conditions (Dinniss, 1999; Raine, Phil, Stoddard, Bihrle, and Buchsbaum, 1998) may just serve to weaken inhibitory controls and indirectly contribute to violence and homicide. It is certainly possible that, if not for the organicity, the murder might not have occurred. However, it is equally likely that the organicity alone, without the contribution of psychogenic factors, might not have resulted in homicide (Blake, Pincus, and Buckner, 1996; Volavka, 1995).

3.3.2 Toxic States

The most common substance associated with homicide is alcohol (Auerhahn and Parker, 1999; Martin, 1992; Yarvis, 1990). Wolfgang's (1958) findings that 54% of homicidal offenders and 53% of the victims were under the influence of alcohol at the time of the offense basically still holds true (*UCR*). The general view (Fagan, 1990; Parker and Rebhun, 1995) is that alcohol acts as a disinhibitor and under certain circumstances—a combination of setting, personality factors, and absence of social controls—can lead to homicide. In very rare cases, people who are prone to pathological (or idiosyncratic) intoxication (Pandina, 1996) may drink a very small quantity of alcohol and become extremely violent. This condition has been questioned since its inception over a hundred years ago, but such cases have consistently been reported. In these rare cases, the unusually violent reactions to alcohol have been thought to be similar to an allergic reaction (Urschel and Woody, 1994).

Some drugs such as cocaine, amphetamines, inhalants, and phencyclidine (PCP or Angel Dust) can act to increase violence, as illustrated by the case of a 37-year-old who, while under the influence of PCP, assaulted a 60-year-old police officer. He was only deterred by a good samaritan who hit the offender over the head with a bat. He stopped his aggression when the police arrived and pointed their guns at him. Recently, several man-made drugs such as synthetic cathinones ("Bath Salts"), MDMA ("Molly or Ecstasy"), and synthetic marijuana ("Spice, K2") have been noted to weaken controls, stimulate psychotic symptoms, and contribute to bizarre violence and murder.

Other drugs such as heroin can actually decrease aggressive behavior. For the vast majority of users, marijuana does not precipitate violence. However, this substance is often connected to homicide since many offenders have regularly used the drug (Spunt, Brownstein, Goldstein, Fendrich, and Liberty, 1995), and in some rare cases, marijuana has been directly responsible for violence (Abel, 1977). The same connection has also been found between cocaine and violence (Goldstein, Brownstein, and Ryan, 1992) and between anabolic steroids and violence (Pope, 1988). Reich and Hepps (1972) report the case of a homicide committed under the influence of lysergic acid diethylamide (LSD). In this instance, as well as in most other cases where murder is connected to psychedelics, the substance did not merely act as a disinhibitor but induced a psychosis which precipitated the offense. Here, the individual was a chronic LSD user who developed psychotic delusions to which he responded. A similar case was reported by Klepfisz and Racy (1973), wherein a 22-year-old student, without any history of violence, killed his girlfriend during a psychotic period precipitated by the ingestion of LSD.

3.3.3 Paranoid Disorders and Homicide

The entire array of paranoid disorders has a much more complex relationship to violence and homicide than the organic and toxic conditions. The various paranoid illnesses can be viewed on a spectrum. On one end are cases of pure paranoia which blends almost imperceptibly into normal personality; on the opposite end of the scale are the more disorganized forms of paranoid schizophrenia. The conclusion of Swanson, Bohnert, and Smith (1970) that paranoid delusions, as well as delusional jealousy, are major causes of homicide still holds true (Palermo et al., 1997; Silva, Harry, Leong, and Weinstock, 1996). Lanzkron (1963) studied 150 mental patients charged with murder. He found that 37.3% had paranoid delusions and 20% displayed delusional jealousy and delusions of infidelity. The prevalence of paranoia among homicidal offenders has held up not only over time (Wilcox, 1985) but cross-culturally as well (Benezech, 1984). Revitch (1979) found that most patients who kill their physicians (often urologists because of the sexual aspects of urological disorders) are paranoiacs. In addition, many mass murderers (Hempel, Meloy, and Richards, 1999) have strong paranoid proclivities, as do many political assassins (Lewis, 1987).

The classic example of a homicidal act motivated directly by delusions of persecution was the murder committed by Daniel M'Naghten, from which the legal test of insanity, the M'Naghten Rule, arose. M'Naghten, a Scotsman, believed that he was being persecuted and followed by members of the ruling political party in England, and he requested protection from the provost of Glasgow. In an attempt to assassinate his persecutor (the prime minister of England), M'Naghten accidentally killed the press secretary. As a result of this 1843 case, the English Court established the M'Naghten Rule (having to do with a defendant's ability to know the nature and quality of his acts and to distinguish between right and wrong), which has since served as the standard for insanity in most of the English-speaking countries of the world.

The following case typifies a homicide that was a direct result of paranoid delusions.

Case 3.1: Disorganized Paranoid Psychosis and Matricide

A 22-year-old male was evaluated to determine his state of mind at the time of the homicide. He was charged with murdering his 50-year-old mother by bludgeoning her with his fists and a door. The victim, who had been repeatedly struck in the head and neck area, died of multiple skull fractures.

For 6 years prior to the murder, AA had had numerous consultations with psychiatrists and was hospitalized several times; there were four separate hospitalizations during the year immediately preceding the homicide. On one occasion, AA's father pleaded with the judge to keep his son in an institution, since the father recognized—as did most of the neighbors—the potential for severe violence. Unfortunately, the court-appointed psychiatrist who evaluated AA believed that he could be easily managed on an outpatient basis.

AA slowly developed paranoid delusions where he believed that his mother was a Communist who was plotting to kill him and also was plotting with other Communists to take over the world. He became convinced that the "real purpose" of his mother's European trip was to attend secret meetings to put her plan into action. In order to protect the world, he decided that the only course of action was to kill his mother. According to police reports, the victim was found dead at home. The crime scene was described as follows: "There was blood on the walls … broken furniture … broken windows … blood in the bathroom. A broken and bent door of the medicine cabinet was also noted." When AA was arrested that evening while riding his bicycle a few blocks away from the scene of the murder, he was "soaked with blood." He stated, "I hit her with anything I could get my hands on. I hit her with furniture. I wanted to kill her as fast as I could. I am glad she is dead."

When evaluated in the county jail, AA was extremely agitated and questioned the examiner in great detail about his credentials and identity and the purpose of his visit. He inspected all notes and refused to sit down, pacing in the examination room. After about 20 minutes, AA made a fist and refused to continue the examination because "I am as sane as you are. They're trying to make me a mental case and I am not."

About 1 month later, AA was much more cooperative but still paranoid. He was unable to concentrate and stated that noises and telephones bothered him. His conversation was bizarre. He stared into space for long periods of time, repeating one or two words. He said,

> I can't think. How can a dead man think? I am dead. People are conspiring. I am the center of everyone's conversation. I am the nucleus. They say things like "It's only a disease." And they talk about me. People don't act the way they should. Everyone's out to make a buck and they want to destroy me. The secret society is doing it. They want to get rich and start a world war.

He explained that he heard voices telling him that he should kill her, and so he did.

This as is an excellent example of a homicide that was a direct result of a paranoid psychosis. Unlike Daniel M'Naghten, whose overall personality seemed intact (except for his delusions), AA appeared bizarre, decompensated, and disorganized. The murder and the crime scene itself reflected the extent of his disorganization. Although family members, neighbors, and friends recognized the potential for extreme violence, the court, following the advice of the court-appointed psychiatrist, did not listen. AA was found not guilty by reason of insanity (in accordance with the M'Naghten Rule) and placed in a psychiatric facility.

In the following case, a 19-year-old man killed a child, also as a direct result of paranoid delusions. However, in this case, the offender was not as overtly disorganized as in Case 3.1. Family members, friends, and schoolmates viewed him as very odd, but they had no idea of the extent of his bizarre delusions which led to the act.

Case 3.2: Encapsulated Delusions and Murder of a Young Girl

A 19-year-old male killed an 11-year-old girl by throwing her in the back of a garbage truck when the garbage men were not looking. The motivation for the homicide was revealed in a letter that he wrote 2 days after the murder.

The haircut I got changed me completely. It gave me a new personality. Then the devil possessed me. I went to Toronto to see my cousins. I was so attractive that they got mad if I didn't look at my girl cousin. I was like a prince. I started to communicate by looking straight at people's eyes, which took a lot out of me. It made me more feminine. I was free so I wanted to set people free. They had a record player so I communicated with music, which took a lot out of me again. My cousin said that he would like to show me Toronto. While riding in his car, I told him that I never had sex with a girl. That took a lot out of me, also. I was feminine because I gave too much too fast. I was becoming a homosexual. I was becoming very blind because of a need for sex.

I came home. My father noticed I was becoming gay. I went back home to my mother. There were ESP people downstairs. While I drew pictures, I played the radio to communicate with the people downstairs. They got angry because I was communicating by sound waves like the serpent. The whole town didn't like me. The ESP people told my father to bring me to New York City to the Hare Krishna place to cure me. It did not work. I went to live with my father.

Everyone was out one day when I started to communicate with car sounds. Then that night I made my heart to physically drop from sound waves. In the morning, my homosexuality was gone and I was like a dead man because in the daytime I thought that whatever I ate would not come out; instead it would stay in me and the poison would kill me.

The next morning I started following garbage trucks because I knew that the more the heart beats, the smaller it gets and it would get smaller and smaller until infinitely small and I could physically live forever. The pain I would bear would be outstanding. I thought I would freeze a thousand times more than I can and boil like the latter. I went to my mother's house the next morning.

I thought if I threw someone in a garbage truck I could be saved. I saw a little girl just standing in front of her house. I got to talk to her, grabbed her, and threw her in the garbage truck when the guys weren't looking. Then I got caught and was sent to the hospital. I thought worms and insects would eat me. I also thought I would be the devil himself and I would be locked up in a room forever. I thought I was going to be a suffering thing. I thought if electricity was in me, I wouldn't be hurting people. If I did not kill the girl, my mother would have been killed. Everyone in the world was quarantined and they used to say the devil may care. I hope I didn't lose my soul. Everything was made for me. Once the sun obeyed me. I thought I was here to be blessed on. Thank God everything is all right now, Thank God.

This individual was viewed by others as withdrawn and strange, but no one recognized the depth and complexity of his delusions or the potential violence that could flow directly from them. His thinking did not appear especially disorganized when he discussed topics unrelated to his delusional ideas. He was found not guilty by reason of insanity.

In many instances the relationship between paranoia and homicide is indirect and more complex than in the preceding cases. Such an indirect relationship often exists in cases of delusional jealousy, a condition first described by Revitch (1954) under the name "conjugal paranoia." The symptomatology in delusional jealousy consists basically of accusations of infidelity; destructive, hostile, and aggressive attitudes toward the partner; and feelings of insecurity and dependency. These accusations reflect a break with reality so that there is actually an encapsulated psychosis. Thus, delusional jealousy is far more extreme than pathological jealousy (Morenz and Lane, 2007), which is a more common condition. At times, the paranoid accusations may have some basis in reality, but the truth is distorted and "evidence" is frequently fabricated. It is sometimes difficult to diagnose delusional jealousy because the subject's personality appears to be intact, he is able to work, and his performance during the examination is convincing. He is able to mislead not only his own family members and friends but also many mental health professionals as well. Thus, his (or her) partner often is incorrectly considered mentally disturbed as the partner appears agitated, whereas the paranoiac maintains a cool and calm demeanor and is viewed as normal.

The following case exemplifies a homicide associated with delusional jealousy.

Case 3.3: Delusional Jealousy and Homicide

A 73-year-old male killed his wife under these circumstances: a year prior to the homicide, while attending a church picnic, BB observed a young man, who looked about 35 years old, kissing his 68-year-old wife.

> I said, "Hey, what's going on." My wife told me, "Be quiet, he is a priest." I said, "You better go to confession." My wife said, "He is a priest, you can't talk to him like that." I told him he needs absolution before he says mass. Word, thought, and deed. If the thought is there, that's evil. It's the same as the act. He turned around and gave me a dirty look. He walked away with another male friend. They both had sports shirts on.

After this incident, BB slowly developed an idea that his wife was having a sexual relationship with the parish priest.

> She was always going to church and she was so clever on hiding it. I asked her what was going on, and she said that I was crazy. She refused to talk to me, so I let it go. I felt I had to really start to understand this. I hid all of this from our children. I tried to present a good marital image.

As time went on, the delusion became fixed when BB found "incontrovertible evidence" to support his belief.

> She'd go out at 8:30 p.m. and come home at 12:30 in the morning. She said she went to play bingo at the church, but I could smell cigarettes and cigars on her. She'd come home with a certain cigar odor.

Finally, the children, all of whom were adults and well situated with their own families, became aware of BB's ideation. They spoke to their father many times, but he remained unconvinced. He spent hours in the basement of his home crying, "How could she do this after almost 50 years of marriage?"

On one occasion, BB confronted his wife before they went to church.

> I asked her what was in the bag that she was carrying. She wouldn't show me. I said to her, "It is probably a present for the con artist you are going to. A whoremaster." I broke down and cried like a baby.

The following day, BB went to the parish monsignor in order to explain the situation and enlist his help. The monsignor said that he would look into the matter and that BB should come back the following week. When BB returned, the monsignor said that there was no substance to BB's allegations. He explained that Mrs. B attended church functions regularly along with her daughters. He described the parish priest as friendly, well liked, and not involved with his wife as BB had thought. This did not satisfy BB, because a delusion—which does not stem from reality—cannot be dissipated by facts of reality. Thus, BB incorporated the monsignor into his delusional ideas and concluded that he was covering up the affair to avoid embarrassment to the church. In addition, BB reasoned that his wife's 83-year-old lady friend was also "in on it," covering up the affair as well.

After several more weeks of brooding and thinking about his wife's behavior, BB attempted to contact the bishop, as he had had no success at the parish level. He made numerous phone calls but was unable to arrange a meeting with the bishop. He therefore became very despondent. "Through my whole life I did everything right. I followed the Church to the letter, and this is how I'm treated. The priest has an affair with my wife, and the monsignor and the bishop won't help me." That afternoon, while watching a TV talk show whose topic was infidelity, BB called the show's producer. The show's representatives were very interested in this case, as it involved themes of older woman, younger man, sex, and the clergy. BB became agitated following the conversation. His wife returned home at around 6 o'clock and went into the bathroom. From the closet, BB took the gun he had for many years and shot his wife in the stomach when she came out. He then called the police and explained what happened.

When interviewed in the county jail 1 month later, BB was adamant that his wife was having an affair. He spoke about "clues" that supported his assertions of his wife's unfaithfulness. For example, he stated that his wife "used to wear cotton underwear. She changed her underwear to pink silk or satin underwear. What did it mean? I saw this on TV." He also had found a box of candy that he believed was a gift from the priest. "Also there was a pillow and blanket in the back of her car. I think it was there for a quickie in the back seat. That's what I presume. I checked the car for other tell-tale signs."

A thorough investigation by the prosecutor's office, as well as his defense attorney's investigator, revealed that there was absolutely no evidence that Mrs. B was unfaithful. When she went to the church functions, she was always accompanied by one of her daughters. One daughter said,

> My father had a one-track mind that my mother was running around. He went crazy. My mother was calling me up crying, stating "He accuses me of having a boyfriend." She said, "He is sobbing like a baby in the basement." She was crying several times to me on the phone. "He is accusing me of having a boyfriend, the priest." She was so upset about all of these accusations.

Both prosecution and defense experts agreed that BB suffered from a delusional disorder (jealous type). In addition, the defendant had no insight into his delusional beliefs. He continued to remain adamant that his wife was unfaithful and involved with the priest or another "high church official." When gently challenged that he might have misinterpreted or imagined his wife's actions, BB became irritated, animated, and excited, emotions typical of a paranoiac and atypical of someone who simply has significant jealousy.

Although BB was psychotic, this case is different from the M'Naghten case, and from Cases 3.1 and 3.2, since here the homicide was not a direct result of his delusions. BB did not believe that his wife was going to harm him, nor did he believe that killing her was a command from God or a way to save himself from dying. BB killed his wife out of anger and humiliation, emotions that were a result of his psychosis. Accordingly, he was not totally absolved of criminal responsibility. However, the degree of intent was reduced, as a result of his illness, from first degree murder to manslaughter.

Case 3.4: Delusional Jealousy vs. Persecutory Delusions

A 47-year-old female, married to a physician, had a long history of multiple contacts with the police as a direct result of her disturbed behavior, specifically leaving her home because she did not feel it was safe. D.T. was hospitalized multiple times, and some admissions were for several months. Typically, D.T. would leave her home and sleep in her car in various parking lots, dressed inappropriately in cold weather. She stayed away for extended periods of time, hiding, because "she did not feel safe at home." Once, she lived in her car for 7 days during February. Questioned by the police when they made several welfare checks, D.T. told them there were no arguments between her and her husband and no domestic violence, but she thought that in some way being at home was unsafe. At one point, she went to a police station to see if they could help her with housing because she no longer wanted to live at home. In fact, she inquired about homeless shelters in the area. During this period of time, she was under the care of a local psychiatrist.

About 7 weeks before the homicide, D.T. went to the police station and told an officer that something could happen to her in the future, that her husband "could do something" to her, and she was concerned. About 10 days or so before the homicide, she went to an Army Navy store and purchased a can of pepper spray. Three days later, D.T. came back to the same store and bought a large hunting knife, which she kept in a satchel in her closet during the day and under her bed at night.

On the day of the homicide, her delusional belief that her husband and her husband's family were plotting to harm her "in some way" intensified. She took a marble vase and hit her mother-in-law on the head multiple times, killing her as a result of massive blunt-force trauma. D.T. fled the crime scene, gave a false name at a hotel where she stayed for several days, and was found wandering at a bus terminal. She told the authorities she had lost her wallet and had no credentials. When interviewed by the police, she said,

> I can't stay in that house anymore, the marriage is over, I don't trust my husband. He can do anything to me. I didn't want anyone to find me. She [the mother-in-law] was up to something. I had a feeling, it's hard to explain.

A defense expert evaluated D.T. and believed she had a delusional disorder, jealous type. Upon further analysis, it became obvious that delusional jealousy was not the underlying problem, but rather delusions of persecution. D.T. did not leave her home and live in her car multiple times prior to the homicide, and buy pepper spray and a large hunting knife because she was jealous, she did it because she felt unsafe and believed her husband's family was going to harm her. Any jealous thoughts and beliefs, while present, were secondary to a more basic persecutory delusion. It was not that her husband was going to divorce her, the delusional belief that ultimately led to the homicide was that her husband and mother-in-law were going to get rid of her, and she believed she was not safe. D.T.'s delusional belief fluctuated—as do all symptoms—in intensity and became stronger and more intolerable just before the homicide. "I was really scared. It is possible they [her husband and mother-in-law] were in it together .... [The mother-in-law] perhaps was planning to kill me." D.T. was found legally insane, and even while at the hospital, she still felt unsafe. She believed that her husband could poison her hospital food in some way and that "he could get to me."

This case presents a problem not only in diagnosis but in clinical management as well. Individuals who have encapsulated delusions—particularly delusional jealousy as well as a persecutory type of delusion—are extremely difficult to treat. The delusions are so encapsulated that they are often intractable, even with medication (which, however, can possibly reduce the intensity of the delusion). Psychotherapy is of minimal value because a delusion does not stem from facts of reality; therefore, it cannot be dissipated by facts of reality. Moreover, these types of delusions are often missed diagnostically in both their incipient and residual stages. And such delusions are extremely dangerous—especially a delusion of persecution—because individuals act out in self-protective ways which can easily result in violence.

Although it is not uncommon for individuals with a psychotic disorder to commit homicide, in some cases, such as the following, the killing is not at all directly connected to the psychosis.

Case 3.5: Paranoid Psychosis, Arson, and Murder of Four Women

A 27-year-old male (CC) with a well-documented history of paranoid schizophrenia gave a detailed statement to the police explaining how and why he had set fire to his mother's home and therefore caused the deaths of four women. He explained that he had set his alarm for 3 o'clock in the morning, so that "while everyone was asleep I could do what I planned." He poured gasoline into two bottles, placed both bottles in the oven, turned on the broiler, and set the temperature to 550 degrees. "I knew the broiler was on because of the pilot light. I knew when the oven heated up, the bottles would melt, and the gasoline would start a fire." He was aware that four relatives besides his mother were sleeping in the house, but "I didn't care, I just wanted to hurt my mother." He hoped that eventually everyone would get out all right, "but I was so mad at my mother [that] I just didn't care."

CC admitted that in his initial statement he had lied to the police about various details of the offense and the reason he had gasoline on his clothes when arrested. "I lied because I was scared and wanted to cover my tracks. I'm sorry for what happened and knew what I did was wrong. I was angry and I didn't care. I wasn't thinking about anything else."

The argument with his mother that precipitated the arson occurred about 1 week before the offense. CC felt that his mother made fun of him because of his inability to hold a job or keep a girlfriend. His mother (the only survivor) explained her comments in a much different light, stating that she was trying to offer counsel and guidance in order to prevent him from making irrational decisions.

CC stated that he had intended to burn down the house so that

> my mother would lose the house. She made fun of me, so I wanted to take away from her something that she was proud of. I didn't want to hurt or kill anybody. I was so angry. She worked hard for the house. She told me I was nothing. I felt real bad, and I had an idea to burn down her house. My mother teased me and said I was garbage.

When he was asked whether he had heard voices directing him to set the fire (as he had told a previous examiner), CC stated,

> I didn't hear voices. I am sorry I lied part of the way, but I've been covering my tracks. A guy in the jail told me, "Whatever you do, lie." I am gonna be honest with you; I was hurt and destroyed. She said I was nothing and I'd never make nothing of myself. Every car I got

always broke down. She wants me to better myself, but every time I try to better myself, nothing would satisfy her. To be truthful, it was anger. Voices may have played a part in it, but it was really anger.

This offender had a clear history of paranoid schizophrenia with auditory hallucinations and delusions. When he was initially arrested, he gave a very clear statement explaining his motivation for the arson: anger at his mother. He never mentioned anything remotely connected to hearing voices. He denied, upon careful questioning, that voices played a direct role in the arson and subsequent homicides.

His primary motivation, then, was anger toward his mother; his mental illness played a secondary, and important, role since it was largely responsible for the extreme level of anger that he displayed. If he did hear command hallucinations (as he told a defense psychiatrist, but later recanted), they were consistent with his intentions and may simply have given a concrete utterance to his own wishes. The defendant pleaded guilty to aggravated manslaughter and was sentenced to a correctional facility, where he will likely be treated within the structure of the prison system.

3.4 Motivational Spectrum in the Classification of Homicide

Revitch and Schlesinger (Revitch, 1977; Revitch and Schlesinger, 1978, 1981, 1989) developed a classification system of crime and homicide based on the "motivational spectrum" of the antisocial act itself. At one end of the motivational spectrum are external or sociogenic factors that stimulate the homicide. At the extreme opposite end of the spectrum are offenses motivated by internal or psychogenic factors. From the external or exogenous end of the scale to the endogenous end, offenses are divided into (1) environmental, (2) situational, (3) impulsive, (4) catathymic, and (5) compulsive categories. External, environmental, or sociogenic factors play less and less of a role as one approaches the extreme end of the scale occupied by the compulsive offenses, which are determined almost entirely by internal psychogenic sources. This classification system is not intended to be rigid, as borderline cases with characteristics belonging to adjoining areas are inevitable. The motivational spectrum is illustrated graphically in Figure 3.1.

3.4.1 Social and Environmentally Stimulated Homicides

The sociological study of homicide is chiefly concerned with the relationship of murder to other societal variables, including culture, religion, race, age, region, and socioeconomic status. As all behavior takes place within the context of society and is more or less influenced by it, such determinants have to be taken into account when one is trying to understand specific types of conduct, such as crime and homicide.

For instance, Wolfgang's (1958) comprehensive study of 588 homicides in Philadelphia between 1948 and 1952 detailed numerous social and environmental factors associated with murder, and most of these relationships are relevant today. Merton (1957) specifically pointed to social breakdown and feelings of "anomie" as major contributors to crime and homicide. Other theorists have investigated the relationship between crime and economic depression (Gibbons, 1968), and also, paradoxically, the increase in crimes and homicides sometimes noted in periods of economic prosperity (Cohen and Felson, 1979).

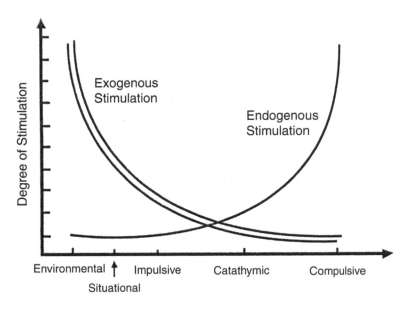

Figure 3.1 The motivational spectrum.

Still others, beginning with LeBon (1910), have emphasized the role of society as a restraining force. LeBon believed that the social environment not only stimulates homicide but also keeps homicide in check. He theorized that the need to kill is primitive, an ancestral residue always ready to appear unless vigorously repressed; thus, only severe societal punishment will keep murder and crime in abeyance.

In keeping with LeBon's theory, numerous historical examples demonstrate an increase in crime, violence, and murder when society is unable to impose restraints and discipline. One such example is the biblical account of a group rape and murder of the victim. "In those days there was no King in Israel; every man did that which was right in his own eyes" (Judges 21:25). In fact, a reading of the Book of Judges gives the impression that crime, violence, and murder were rampant in the loosely organized tribal society of Israel in the 11th and 12th centuries B.C. The Thirty Years War (1618–1648) was marked by a complete absence of discipline among the mercenaries. Officers were corrupt, and troops frequently committed acts of vandalism, robbery, and homicide of innocent civilians. Wedgewood (1957), describing these conditions, speaks of soldiers

> having fine sport firing at the feet of passers-by through low set windows of the cellars. It was sport to shoot prisoners tied in long rows one behind the other, and lay wagers on the number of people that one charge of shot would penetrate. (p. 228)

Social disorganization also was rampant during the various epidemics of plague which fostered bizarre behavior, disruption of interpersonal bonds, dehumanization, violent crime, and murder.

In his seminal work on group psychology, Freud (1921) supported LeBon's concept that a group is not just a collection of individuals but has dynamics of its own. Individual characteristics are dissolved in the anonymity of a group, repression is discarded, and unconscious urges dominate behavior. Thus, suggestibility, contagion, and a feeling of power are the main features. This account of group dynamics helps to explain gang behavior, where individuals commit homicide only within the security of a group because individual responsibility becomes dissolved in the group (Kogan and Wallach, 1964). Arendt (1966), Lifton (1986), and others have linked various Nazi atrocities directly to general societal and subgroup influences. In fact, psychological evaluations of Nazi leaders (Gilbert, 1947) have demonstrated that their conduct was the result not of personal psychopathology but, rather, of social, environmental, and group influences.

In the same vein, Gault (1971) described several episodes of murder perpetrated by U.S. soldiers during the Vietnam War. Here, many ordinary men, without overt disturbance or a particular predisposition toward violence, became engaged in slaughter because of the general social atmosphere of war, which fostered dehumanization of the enemy, dilution of responsibility through groups, and the pressure to act. One veteran stated, "You become a hunter. We'd bomb the village and take turns going down for clean-up. Whoever is alive, you kill." Another described an incident where he and his friends drove jeeps and ran over civilians, including women and children. "We would run them over. Run them off sides of cliffs. I must have killed hundreds of them. At the time it was fun. Everyone did it. But now it bothers me."

Of course, pathological individuals with a need for violence—assassins or would-be assassins, terrorists, or cult members—also are influenced by the social context and social climate, which may release, give meaning to, and direct the aggressive act. The social environment of the late 1960s, along with the social pressure found in the cult itself, influenced many of the members of the infamous Manson family (Bugliosi and Gentry, 1975). Many of the middle-class women who were involved in these cult murders overidentified with Manson, a rather charismatic leader. Their irrational acts seemed at that time consistent with the goals of their cult. There is even some experimental research (Milgram, 1963; Zimbardo, 1973) demonstrating that ordinary people can easily be made to engage in all sorts of potentially aggressive behavior if the context or environment condones it. A lot of gang related murder—which is easy to understand—is stimulated by social, environmental, and personal motives. An example is a 26-year-old male, with a long arrest record and gang affiliation, killed a rival gang member in retaliation for "disrespectful" acts toward his group.

Homicides committed by amateur, semiprofessional, and professional contract killers are other examples of subculturally stimulated murder. Schlesinger (2001c) reported the case of an individual who claimed to have killed over 100 people for profit. This case also illustrates the distinction between a contract murderer (who kills multiple people for money) and a serial murderer (who kills multiple people for sexual gratification, rather than profit).

Case 3.5: Professional Contract Murder

A 52-year-old male described a professional career as a contract murderer that spanned over 30 years. He used traditional methods of killing such as shooting, choking, and knifing, but he became most noted for his proficiency in cyanide poisoning. The murders were carefully planned and his techniques were methodical and disciplined, often involving elaborate staging to throw off law enforcement.

DD was apprehended not for contract murder but for killing several close associates who he believed could implicate him in a number of other crimes. His history was replete with instances of childhood abuse, family disruption, and the adoption of a criminal lifestyle where antisocial behavior—including murder—was condoned. This offender had been married for more than 25 years, raised several children, and provided his family with a traditional middle-class upbringing, much different from his own experiences.

Extensive psychological evaluation found no indications of mental illness, except for antisocial personality disorder. Antisocial personality, however, does not explain DD's numerous homicides; in fact, most individuals with antisocial personality disorder never commit a murder (Revitch and Schlesinger, 1981; Tanay, 1969).

Acquired subcultural values played a dominant role in DD's decision to pursue a career as a contract killer. Personality traits involving a need for order, control, and hypervigilance helped DD in his methodical approach and subsequent thwarting of law enforcement. He also had a good capacity to rationalize his actions and encapsulate his emotions; he demonstrated superior practical and social judgment as well. Thus, multiple factors in his social background and personality contributed to this unique criminal career.

Interestingly, DD did express a feeling of "power and control" during several of the murders. Some individuals may therefore consider him a "serial" murderer because this feeling has been reported by many sexual murderers. It could be argued that these murders were perhaps sexually stimulating or erotized at an unconscious level. However, whatever inner gratification DD achieved from the killings was not even close to the main motivation for his crimes, which was simply profit.

Case 3.6: Amateur Contract Murder

A physician had his license suspended in the 1980s for insurance fraud. After about 25 years, he once again came to the attention of an insurance fraud task force, which utilized a cooperating witness. The cooperating witness—a former patient of Dr. A.—brought various individuals to the medical practice in order to get prescriptions for narcotics. The fake patients were paid just to get the prescription and fill it. The pills were sold on the street, and Dr. A. received several thousand dollars per month for his part in the scheme.

At one meeting between Dr. A. and the cooperating witness, the doctor asked him whether he would be able to kill a woman with whom the doctor had a relationship and to whom he owed $250,000. The cooperating witness said that he would, and the insurance task force then turned the entire investigation over to the homicide unit. In numerous recorded meetings between the cooperating witness and Dr. A., the offender wanted to know all the details of the planned murder, which would benefit him as he would not have to pay the target the money he owed her. Dr. A. was curious as to whether the targeted victim would be dead before or after being placed in a wood chipper. Dr. A. thought it was a good idea for her to be killed and then placed in a wood chipper. Dr. A. also wanted to have the cooperating witness kill a former business partner to whom he also owed money.

After obtaining enough evidence, the authorities arrested Dr. A. While in the county jail, he met another inmate and asked him whether he would kill his wife, who had several hundred thousand dollars of life insurance and who he believed would leave him when she found out about his prior affair. The inmate then contacted the prosecutor's office, and he also became a cooperating witness.

At the time of sentencing, Dr. A. told the court he was "a new man" and that the targeted victims would not have to worry. Individuals such as Dr. A who hire amateurs to kill somebody do so because they have no contacts or means to hire a more professional or experienced assassin.

A contemporary example of the impact of subcultural environmental factors on behavior is the case of three adolescent boys who killed a female classmate. After becoming obsessed with a "death-metal" band's music—which included lyrics of sacrificial killing, necrophilia, and mass murder—the boys stalked, abducted, and killed a 15-year-old girl in a ritualistic fashion under an altar they had constructed. They said they wanted to mimic the lyrics of the music they admired. Following the girl's murder, the three offenders engaged in various necrophilic acts with the body for over a week. None of the teens had a history of significant psychological disturbance or violence. In this case the murder, as well as the necrophilic acts, were not (primarily) sexually motivated, but were stimulated by their cult-like adherence to the death-metal music and its message.

3.4.2 Situational Homicides

Situational homicides are murders that occur when a particular set of circumstances, present at a particular time, gives rise to powerful feelings of stress, especially in susceptible people. These murders, including domestic homicides, many felony homicides, and murders during arguments, may be premeditated or spontaneous acts. However, a common element in all situational murders—even those with clear premeditation—is stress stemming from external or internal sources (Schlesinger and Revitch, 1980). Stressful feelings such as despair, helplessness, depression, fear, or anger can trigger such murders under the right circumstances, especially when the stress is intense and chronic. All types of personalities may commit situational murders; however, inadequate or immature individuals and those raised in a subculture of violence are most vulnerable to engage in such acts (Steadman, 1982).

A review of the *UCR* over the years reveals that about 60% of all murders are basically of a situational nature and occur under stressful circumstances such as arguments, often within the context of another felony. For example, many murders that occur during armed robberies are due to the tremendous stress the offender feels while committing the crime (MacDonald, 1975). The overall recidivism rate for situational murders is rather low; consequently, the recidivism rate for murder in general is low since most murders are of this category.

Theodore Dreiser in his novel *An American Tragedy* describes a situational homicide with clear premeditation. The murder was committed by an individual raised in a background of poverty and insignificance. He met a rich young woman who fell in love with him; at the same time, a factory worker he had dated became pregnant. Thus, his prospects for a rich future appeared bleak. Then, after reading a newspaper account of a canoe accident in which a young woman drowned, he decided to kill the pregnant girlfriend and stage the event to make it appear that the homicide was an accident. Even after successful completion of the murder, he consoled himself with the fantasy that the victim's death was purely accidental.

Other situational murders include accidental homicides with a background of stress, as well as murders induced by anticipation of violence. Orenstein and Weisstein (1958) reported a case of an individual who complained to the police that another person had been threatening him. When the complainant noticed the other person with hands in his pockets, he shot and killed him under the impression that the victim had a gun. Domestic violence, in general, and child abuse and child murder, in particular, have always been thought to be a result, to a large extent, of prolonged stress (Gil, 1970; Gelles, 1973). Some individuals kill simply as a result of anger and jealousy. For example, a 25-year-old male who lacked any type of accomplishment killed his long-term girlfriend after she left him for another man who was a successful young attorney. He planned the murder by researching methods to kill on the internet.

The following case of a domestic homicide, triggered by an angry quarrel over money, is instructive. Here, the offender attempted to stage the crime scene so that it would appear to be a sexual murder—behavior not uncommon in this type of crime.

Case 3.7: Domestic Homicide Staged as a Sexual Murder

A 58-year-old male (EE) described the events leading up to the killing of his wife, as follows. For the past 2 years he had been unemployed after being laid off from a lucrative computer job that he had held for many years. His wife continued to work as an administrative assistant. This was the second marriage for both of them, and they had no children together. Several weeks prior to the homicide, EE became increasingly angry at his wife "because she would not come home right after work. It hurt me. She went to her secretary's house without me. I wasn't invited." Four days before the killing, he overheard Mrs. E telling her (adult) son

> that she was with another person. It could have been a man, it could have been a woman. She once went to Maine by herself, but I believe she wasn't alone. She could have been with a man or a woman.

Two days before the homicide, Mrs. E "came home late, tired and irritable. She didn't want to talk. She changed her sex habits and didn't want sex. I thought she was involved with another woman. Maybe she was a lesbian." When asked why he thought that his wife was a lesbian, EE stated,

> She always went with divorced women and did it everywhere we lived. Her personality changed. She wasn't interested in me or the house. She had a look of hatred. I wanted to discuss the problems with our budget. I needed data and I wanted to talk, but she wouldn't contribute money from her raise. We got into an argument, then I went to work on my computer. Twenty minutes later I talked to her and she was more receptive.
>
> The next day I called her at work and she was impersonal and nasty. I was nervous and couldn't settle down. I was depressed. I continued to work on my budget at the computer. My wife called to say that she wouldn't be home. I was disappointed and discouraged because I hoped we could talk about the budget. I tried working on the computer but I couldn't, so I went to lay down and went to sleep.
>
> When she came home, I got up and we got into another argument. I pointed my finger at her, and she grabbed my finger and my arm. I said, "Let go." She was angry. The look on her face was a hateful look. She wanted me to stop gesturing with my finger. This bothered her and she wouldn't let go. We were on the floor before I knew it. She said, "That does it," and went to a drawer for a French cook's knife. I said, "We can't solve our money problems with a knife."
>
> I then went into another room to get something to protect myself. I didn't dare turn around. I grabbed a magazine and threw it at her. It didn't hit her. I reached for something else and there was a hammer. I told her to put the knife away. I tried to strike at the knife. I hit the blade. I had to hit her hand to knock it out. She screamed louder. I said, "That does it," and hit her hand again, and she moved. I hit her forehead. She was hysterical and I was frightened to death. I raised my hand again. I saw the image of the big muscle in my neck being cut open.

EE denied memory for most subsequent events, but the evidence indicated that he put the hammer and knife in a bag and disposed of them. "I don't know why. I think I took 'em in a car some place and dropped them off." He next wrapped his wife's body in a tarpaulin. "I don't remember covering the body up. I think, looking back at it, I probably put her under the tarp to protect her against flies and insects. I loved her."

Her body was eventually found in a wooded area. Her trousers and underpants had been pulled down below her hips, and her shirt and bra had been pulled up to her neck, exposing her breasts. Mrs. E's clothing was drenched in blood, but there was little or no blood on the ground directly beneath her, indicating that the body had been moved. According to the autopsy, the victim died as a result of 23 blows to the head by a hammer, causing multiple skull fractures and injury to her brain.

When asked why the body was moved into the woods about 100 yards from his home, EE said, "That was my place to meditate. I loved her still." When asked why her blouse was pulled up and her pants pulled down, he stated, "I think I wanted to see if somebody had intercourse that night. I think that's why. I wanted to see her breasts. If it was a lesbian, it would show some redness from fondling or from another girl's mouth."

When Mrs. E failed to show up for work the next morning, co-workers became concerned since she was usually very punctual. Her supervisor telephoned her home and spoke with EE who said he had been working on his computer until 2:30 a.m. and did not know whether or not his wife had returned home.

> He then related that his tarpaulin, used to cover his lawn mower, was missing, and expressed the hope that no one had killed and raped his wife, wrapped her up in a tarpaulin, and dumped her by the side of the road—or words to that effect.

The homicide itself was unplanned and occurred in a state of rage, within the context of marital strife and a bizarre belief that his wife might have been having a lesbian relationship with her secretary. EE's behavior following the homicide indicates that he had tried to make the crime appear to be a sexual murder—a common attempt to redirect an investigation away from oneself. However, he quickly abandoned this approach the next day and led police directly to the body.

Although this was not a sexually motivated murder, there is a sexual element noted throughout. Not only did he have a strange belief that his wife was a lesbian, but his figure drawings of people with exposed genitalia reveal a sexual preoccupation (see Figure 3.2). In addition, EE got into a dispute with his attorneys, claiming "They told me if I did not plead guilty to a lesser charge, I will be sentenced to state prison where I would be forced to become the homosexual wife of some hardened criminal." EE had no prior psychological or psychiatric history. His intelligence fell within the superior range (full-scale IQ = 125); compulsive personality traits, characterized by a need for order and control, were found.

Situational homicides are relatively common and, in most cases, quite straightforward with obvious and clear motives. An example is the case of a 28-year-old who killed his friend over jealousy that he was not part of a three-way sexual encounter; or the case of a 27-year-old who strangled and stabbed to death a neighbor who resisted having a sexual encounter with him. Some situational murders, however, are exceptionally complex, so that all levels of motivation often remain elusive. The following case of a 20-year-old male who sadistically murdered his 1-year-old daughter is an example.

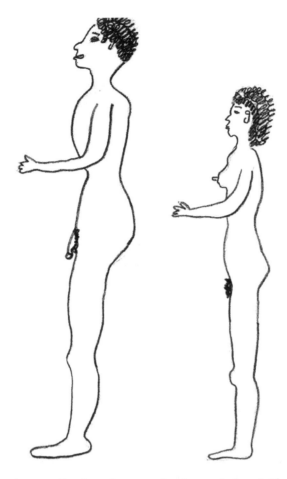

Figure 3.2 Drawings by an offender who staged a domestic homicide to appear as a sexual murder. His sexual conflicts are revealed by his sketches involving exposed genitalia.

Case 3.8: Sadistic Murder of a Child, with Unclear Motivation

The 20-year-old offender was immediately apprehended after torturing and finally sadistically killing his 1-year-old daughter. He initially gave an untruthful statement to the police but then recanted "to get it off my chest so the truth could be known." What follows is the verbatim account of FF's description of the murder of his daughter.

Carol had a cold. She refused to take the bottle of cough medicine, so I forced it into her mouth and squeezed the bottle real hard to make her try to drink it. She started crying again, so I slapped her across the face twice on each side. I punched her hard on her forehead and then, after that, I punched her two times hard in the back of her head. I stumbled on a pillow and dropped Carol on the floor accidentally. She landed on her back. She cried for a second and then started crying again. This is around 5 o'clock. I picked her up, cradled her, and punched her hard with my fist, twice on each side of her face. Then I put her on the floor. She was bleeding out of her nose, so I laid her on the floor behind the couch.

While I was eating, I took a piece of cheese and stuffed it in Carol's mouth. She chewed on it and ate it. I got up and walked across to the bathroom and got a green can of aerosol spray that's for underarm deodorant. I sat next to Carol and sprayed the rest of the can in her mouth by holding it down for three seconds at first, and then fifteen seconds later on. She started choking and coughing and sticking her tongue through her lips like she was getting a taste of it.

After that I took a piece of chicken and a piece of cheese, wrapped it together, and stuck it in her mouth, but she wouldn't take it. I pushed it down her throat with my index finger. She started choking again. I turned her over and slapped her on the back to burp her. She stopped coughing, so I put her on the couch. She was still crying, so I got angry. I grabbed her by the wrist and pulled her up off the couch real hard and I heard a bone in her arm snap. I dislocated her arm at the shoulder. I threw her down on the wooden table in the corner of the family room between the two lounge chairs. Carol landed head first on the table. She fell on the floor and I just left her there.

I was watching TV and I picked Carol up again and I started bending her hands back one at a time to break them. I heard each one pop. Then I took her to the bathroom. I took her clothes off. She was crying loud so I grabbed the green scouring brush that has a sponge on one side and a rough scouring brush on the other. I scrubbed her vagina back and forth real hard with the brush side, and it made a bad bruise on her. I did it on purpose because I was mad that she was crying. I then got a tube of ointment from the top of my mother's dresser and went back to the bathroom with it. I squeezed some on my index finger and rubbed it around and swiped it inside of Carol's vagina. I put a new diaper on her and brought her back downstairs.

I covered her mouth and nose with my hand to try to quiet her. Then I picked her up by the neck and threw her across the room and she landed on her stomach behind the couch. She was still crying, so I picked her up by her leg, over my head, and dropped her on the floor on her back. This time she still kept crying.

Then I decided to go to my metal tool box and take out a pair of red-handled needle-nose pliers. I used the needle-nose pliers to beat Carol over the hands and to squeeze each of her hands to make her cry. I kept doing that for a half an hour on and off, squeezing and letting go, squeezing and letting go. She cried the whole time, and it caused my mother to wake up and walk downstairs to the family room. She asked what was going on. I told my mother nothing was wrong, and she walked back upstairs.

Carol fell back asleep on the couch and I leaned over and suffocated her by holding my hand over her mouth and nose. I let go after about two minutes. I thought I killed her by then because her eyes were closed, so I let go. She was still breathing and trying to catch her breath. I watched TV for another fifteen minutes. Then I leaned over and placed my hand over Carol's nose and mouth and placed more pressure than the first time. That's when her eyes opened and she was trying to push my hands away from her nose and mouth. She was squirming. I held my hands there much longer than the first time because I didn't want to make the same mistake. I didn't want to release my hands too soon.

After Carol died, I carried her upstairs to my bedroom, wrapped her in a blanket, and placed her on the floor next to my bed. I then put her in my bed. She slept next to me all night.

When asked how Carol received the bite marks all over her body, the offender responded,

I bit her all over her body while I was beating her when she was still alive. I bit her on her cheeks, her stomach, her chest, her arms, her foot, both her hands, her back, the back of her ear, and her neck. I scratched her with my fingernails on her nose and pinched her with my fingers on her thigh. This all happened while I was beating her through the night while she was still alive.

I was worried that I would get blamed for this because doctors could see bruises all over her. So I changed her clothes and got my mother's powder and make-up. I used it to cover over the bruises that I gave to Carol, so nobody would be able to tell. I hoped that nobody would notice them and that way, when she goes back home to her mother, her mother would think she was still alive.

This individual had low average intelligence and no history of any type of diagnosed psychological disturbance. He denied engaging in sadistic fantasies, and there was no evidence, after a thorough investigation, that FF had displayed any prior inclination to be sadistic. Crepault and Couture (1980) found that over 60% of "normal" men have had some type of sadistic fantasy but do not act out. Since sadism is not primarily about inflicting pain but, rather, having total control over another person with pain just one expression of that control (Schlesinger, 2000a), evidently, a situation where a person has total control over someone else can, in some cases, trigger sadistic behavior typical of what Krafft-Ebing (1886) referred to as "outbreaks of sadism." We know, for example, that some individuals who have complete control over others (such as Nazi guards, prison guards, and nursing home attendants, as well as some supervisors) often exhibit sadistic behavior at different levels of intensity.

Sadistic acts can vary greatly from cases where the dynamics are overt and obvious to cases where the dynamics are much more subtle. In many cases of homicide that seem largely situational, the offender also engages in gratuitous sadistic behavior. One example is the case of a 24-year-old man who killed the parents of his teenage girlfriend because they objected to the relationship. Following the murder itself, the offender mutilated the victims' bodies and cut out their eyes. In another case, a woman (with the help of her boyfriend) killed her aunt and uncle in order to steal their money. The girl took a knife and made numerous stab wounds over the victims' faces. She could not explain why she had mutilated their faces because she always got along well with both of them.

In the case of FF, sadistic behavior emerged spontaneously, given the context of total control over the victim. Perhaps extended therapeutic involvement with FF might eventually provide further understanding of all levels of motivation of his behavior. He was sentenced to life imprisonment and spared the death penalty primarily because of his age.

Case 3.9: Murder Following Previous Sexual Abuse

A 39-year-old male killed his former scout leader who had sexually abused him 30 years previously. When he was between 8 and 2 years old, he was sexually abused repetitively, including one episode of anal rape. For many years, he made an adequate adjustment coping with severe trauma which went untreated. But for about 10 years before the homicide, he was unable to sustain employment and went home to live with his mother.

F.C. had a number of stressful situations, in addition to the sexual abuse. For example, a friend of F.C. committed suicide, which he believed was a result of being sexually abused by the same scoutmaster. The defendant's grandmother was raped and murdered, and a female friend was also threatened with rape. About a year before the homicide, F.C. lost $50,000 in some type of business transaction; he did everything right legally, but was unable to gain any compensation from the swindler because he went bankrupt. For years, F.C. viewed himself as weak and damaged in some way.

The defendant's level of stress increased significantly the night of the homicide, and he disclosed to a friend for the first time what had happened to him. Both men went to the home of the individual who F.C. said abused him and the defendant killed him with multiple stab wounds, just about decapitating him. This was a complex case legally as well as psychologically. F.C. was found guilty of passion-provocation manslaughter, served several years in prison, and subsequently devoted himself to helping other victims of abuse.

3.4.3 Impulsive Offenders Who Commit Homicide

The word *impulse* is derived from the Latin verb *impulsus*, which essentially means to "push, drive, urge, stimulate, or force." In a psychological context, impulse is defined as an unexpected urge motivated by conscious or unconscious feelings over which the person has little or no control (Freedman, Kaplan, and Sadock, 1972). Impulsive offenders who commit homicide are distinguished mainly by their lack of direction, randomness of actions, and unpredictability. These individuals are passive, easily led, and overinfluenced by circumstances; their personality structures are loose and poorly integrated. They cannot see life in perspective but, instead, view it on an immediate basis. The offenses they commit, whether homicides or some other crimes, are generally poorly structured and only partially, if at all, premeditated.

Impulsive offenders differ from situational offenders mainly by the number of antisocial acts in their background. Whereas a situational homicide is often a one-time event, the impulsive offender has a history of multiple criminal events with homicide being just one in a series. Impulsive offenders are often recruited into semiprofessional crime, but they lack the purposefulness and know-how of the professional. Impulsive offenders often have a disorganized family life; sometimes they even have developmental handicaps such as attention deficit disorder, learning disabilities, physical maladies, or speech problems. As a result of their background, they have acquired strong feelings of inadequacy and feel especially inferior in the competitive world. These feelings of inadequacy bring about feelings of hostility which result in chronic anger and a vague need for revenge. Offenders discharge their tension by action, as they are largely unable to modulate their emotions.

Impulsive offenders merge with antisocial personality disorder to some extent, as these offenders usually manifest more personality or characterological disturbance than do other offenders. The concept of impulsive offender, however, cuts across all personality diagnoses. Impulsive offenders do not, in our view, suffer from an impulse disorder per se, although some of them may fall into this category. Mainly, they are not driven to commit the offense but are simply reacting to circumstances. In the prison population, nonhomicidal offenders are usually less reliable, less integrated, and more disturbed than offenders serving time for homicide. That is because most prisoners have a lifestyle with multiple prior antisocial acts similar to the lifestyle of impulsive offenders, whereas most murderers commit situational, one-time events. Table 3.4 lists characteristics of impulsive offenders who commit homicide.

The following case is an example of an impulsive offender who killed a woman. A detailed account of the crime and the crime scene, provided by the offender's 15-year-old girlfriend, provides a graphic description of the thinking and behavior patterns of individuals who commit a sudden, unplanned, and unexpected act of violence with grave consequences.

Case 3.10: Impulsive Offender Who Killed a Woman

A 20-year-old male lived with his mother until 6 months prior to the homicide. He had learning problems, was teased in school ("Kids called me retard"), and eventually dropped out in the tenth grade. His biological father left the family as a result of marital strife, but

Table 3.4 **Characteristics of Impulsive Offenders Who Commit Homicide**

- History of multiple antisocial acts.
- Offenses are poorly structured, committed without planning.
- Frequent involvement in amateurish and semiprofessional crime.
- Lifestyle characterized by lack of direction, random actions, and unpredictability.
- Offenders are passive, easily led, and overreact to environmental circumstances.
- Personality is loosely integrated, with strong feelings of inadequacy.
- Frequent history of developmental disabilities (e.g., ADHD, learning and speech problems, and minor physical handicaps).
- Chronic feelings of hostility and anger, and a nonspecific need for revenge.
- May not have impulse control disorder per se.

the offender believed that he left "because I had a growth and he couldn't take it," referring to a nonmalignant tumor on his neck, which was hardly noticeable but bothered him greatly. His mother remarried, and her husband inflicted cruel physical and emotional punishment on GG, beating him with a hose and making him kneel on rice. As an adolescent, GG was involved in repetitive minor antisocial acts, including theft of radios, public intoxication, marijuana possession, minor assaults, school behavior problems, and one or two violation of probation offenses.

GG's mother was unable to tolerate his conduct, lack of steady employment, and general lack of direction. She asked a friend of hers, a 35-year-old divorced woman, if GG could live with her for a period of time. GG moved in and stayed with her for several months.

The offender became involved with what was known as the "party line," a predecessor of the present-day computer chat room. Individuals could dial a 900 telephone number and talk to strangers. On the party line, GG met a 15-year-old female (A) who lived about 70 miles away. After extended conversations, they decided to meet. He showed up at her home, but after 1 or 2 days of "hanging out," A was unable to get rid of him. Her parents, as well as the school vice-principal, talked to GG. Out of desperation, A's father called the police, who threatened to have him arrested if he returned to their town.

But the following week, after again talking to GG on the party line, A agreed to meet with him "for one last time" before finally terminating the relationship. Without telling her parents where she was going, she took a train to his residence. Later, A provided a vivid description of the unplanned murder of the 35-year-old woman (B) whom GG had been living with.

> G started yelling at B. I got up from my seat to look, and they were arguing about something, I don't know what. They were fighting a lot. I heard a thump, and they were doing a lot of yelling. I heard him yelling, saying how she was a problem. The next thing I heard was B screaming. She was screaming hysterically. I heard a banging noise. Screaming and banging was going on.
>
> G came downstairs. He was crying and told me that he had just killed B. He said to me that she was just another problem and he had to take care of her. He was screaming at me. "You gotta come with me. You gotta help me clean this up. I can't leave her there."
>
> B's bedroom door was half open and half closed. I walked into the room. She was lying on the floor. She was covered with sheets from the bed. The rug was covered in blood. The walls had blood all over them. On the floor, there was a knife and there was some kind of stick. G was full of blood. He had a green surf shirt on. It was full of blood. His white socks were full of blood, too. His hands had blood all over them. He was nervous, huffing and puffing, out

of breath. He told me, "Don't tell anybody. This is not happening. I did this for us. She would have been a problem."

He brought her out of the room. I could see he was dragging her by four belts he tied around the sheets. I didn't see her face until later. When I did, her face was a mess. I saw her arms. They were all bloody. He was still mad because I was screaming. Then he started to drag her down the stairs. While she was in the hallway, she bled onto the rug. He had a hard time getting her downstairs. She was very heavy and he was screaming. Her body kept falling on the stairs. Her body was rolled up and just lying there. He said her car keys were on the counter and told me to get them.

He couldn't carry her because she was heavy and he wanted me to help him. He said, "Never mind, never mind." He then took the body and jammed her in the trunk of her car. I felt really sick. I might have blacked out because I remember some things and some things I don't. I looked in the house; there was blood on the floor. G got steel wool, dish detergent, and bleach. There was a sponge in the sink, but there was nothing really to clean up this mess. Everything was covered in blood. On the floor were blood stains. The phone was ripped out of the wall and covered with blood. Her white sneakers were full of blood. B's nightgown was white; it was short, ripped in half, and full of blood.

He told me to go downstairs to get bleach and steel wool to clean the walls. The blood was not coming off the walls, and he started yelling at me again to help him. I was standing there hysterical. He went from the walls to the rug with the bleach, trying to get the blood stains out. It didn't work and it made the room stink. It made the blood stains black. There was no way he was going to get this out of the rugs. The rugs were wet, so wet with blood. There were spots of blood where she was lying. He was getting nuts. He was getting crazy. He kept screaming, "Just don't touch nothing."

He was rolling the rug as he cut it out, and he told me to help him. He cut the rug in sections. He went down, grabbed the rugs, and went down to the lake. He threw the rugs into the water, but the rugs just sat on top of the water. They wouldn't sink. He started going crazy. "What am I going to do? I gotta get rid of these rugs." Then he went into the water, stepped on them to make them sink. Finally they sank and we came back to the condo. He was drenched in blood and soaking wet.

Underneath the padding from the bed there was blood on the wood floor. He said to me, "We gotta get her outa the trunk and gotta get far away from here." He swept the floor and tried to get the blood stains up from the floor. As he put more bleach on it, it made the blood stains more visible. By this time, it was almost morning and you could see the sun shining on the floor, making the blood stains stand out.

I don't remember how we left the condo, whether it was in the front or the back. He kept saying "We have to get rid of her." In the trunk of the car I could see her face and arms. She was full of blood and still bleeding. I could see bruises, and her face and body were just broken. She was a mess. She wouldn't move.

He got her out of the trunk of the car and she fell on the road, and everything that she was wrapped in fell off of her. She was completely nude on the roadway. Finally, he threw her into the lake also.

We walked back to the condo and went through the back door. That's when G painted the walls in B's room. It took him about three hours to paint them. As he was painting the walls, the blood kept seeping through, and he was going nuts because he couldn't get rid of the blood. He would put another coat of paint on and the dark spots of blood would still come through.

After this, I took a shower and he made me go to the food store with him to buy hair dye. He said my red hair stood out too much and he wanted me to dye it blonde. It changed my hair color to brown. He took B's car and was driving south on our way to Florida. We were gonna stop to get a room but then G realized "I can't let you go in alone, because I can't trust you." We went to get a room. We were going to use B's credit card, but the lady said we needed a driver's license. So we went back to the car and then we just drove off. G started to drive faster and faster and the cops started to follow us. Finally the police pulled over and I jumped outta the car. It was over.

When GG was interviewed in the county jail, he gave a very different account of the events. He said that A was pregnant (which was untrue), and it was A's idea to kill B. He said,

I did it because of her. A and B got into an argument, a sexual argument. B was a lesbian and came on to A. A said if I don't do something about it, she would do something. A said she didn't want her around. If she wasn't around, we could stay in the condo. So I got a knife, went to B's room, and stabbed her in the back and I hit her with a billy club. I stabbed her three more times so that she'd die.

When asked if he had any remorse, he said, "I feel bad. I feel stupid because I did something like that for a girl. I deserve to be here. I'd rather be executed than do life in prison."

Psychological test findings revealed a great deal about the psychodynamics of this offender. His figure drawings are shown in Figure 3.3. The house, tree, and drawing of a member of the opposite sex are bland and empty and reflect serious depression and

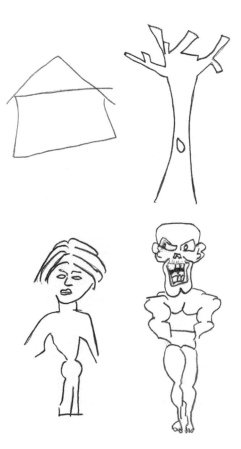

Figure 3.3 Drawings by an impulsive offender who killed a woman. His sketches of a house, tree, and member of the opposite sex are bland and empty, indicating deep depression and inadequacy. His drawing of a male reflects how this young man would like others to perceive him.

inadequacy. The drawing of a male shows a person of massive strength, the opposite of how he truly feels about himself but probably how he would like others to see him.

His TAT stories were filled with themes of inadequacy and deep depression, including the following. Card 1: "This boy is depressed. He feels he can't do anything. He is useless. He has no friends." Card 3BM: "This is a guy crying. He shot himself. He was depressed. He killed himself because it's the only way he can deal with his grief. He shoots himself in the head." Card 14: "This person is lonely. He is thinking of suicide. He doesn't have a normal life. People keep rejecting him. He is not liked." Card 18GF:

> A woman strangling another woman. She wanted her money. He gets rid of the body. Puts it in the car, drives it off a cliff, and makes it look like an accident. The police thinks it's an accident. It bothers him, so he kills himself.

The following story (to Card 13MF) is most revealing of his inner thoughts:

> This is a guy who had a prostitute and then killed her. Maybe something happened in his past. Women used to reject him or treat him like dirt and tease him. He figured he'd get back. He did it to a prostitute because they are easy to get away with. The police won't try as hard with a prostitute. He hates woman. Women teased him. He feels good while he is doing it. Some kind of revenge. He feels like he is getting back at the world.

Expressions of self-deprecation, inadequacy, and self-loathing poured out of this offender. The day before his capital murder trial was to begin, GG stabbed himself in the eye with a pen, which resulted in his death. He was found in his cell, lying on his back with a pen sticking out of his left eye.

3.4.4 Catathymic and Compulsive Homicides

There are essentially four types of sexual homicide (1) a compulsive-repetitive homicide, where an offender seeks out a victim to kill because killing itself is sexually arousing and part of the offender's sexual arousal pattern; (2) a catathymic homicide, where the murder occurs suddenly as a result of breakthrough of underlying sexual conflicts or, the offender develops a fixed idea that murdering the victim will resolve an internal conflict; (3) a murder to cover up a sex crime, as when an offender rapes a victim and then kills her so he is not identified and arrested; and (4) a sex-related homicide, where there is a sexual element to the murder but it is hard to understand the exact motivational dynamics, as when a man kills another man, steals his money, and then cuts off his penis. Murder to cover up a sex crime is fairly straightforward; however, in sex-related homicides the exact dynamics motivating the sexual component often remains unclear.

A catathymic homicide, beginning with Wertham's (1937) conception of "catathymic crisis," involves an individual with underlying emotionally charged conflicts, who develops a fixed idea (a "root like fixation") that he must kill the future victim, and he does so after a protracted period of rumination. Catathymic homicides may also be sudden acts of violence, similarly induced by underlying conflicts that erupt with a trigger. In both forms, the chronic and the acute, a superficially integrated individual who is secretly struggling with feelings of inadequacy, particularly sexual inadequacy, resorts to violence when the potential victim challenges his sense of integrity, adequacy, or sexual competence. Thus, the violent act serves the purpose of freeing one's self from the source of threat to psychological stability.

The compulsive homicides are at the extreme endogenous end of the motivational spectrum and are determined entirely by internal psychogenic sources, with little environmental influence. The urge to commit the act is powerful, and the offender may experience inner discomfort and anxiety if he attempts to resist action. Compulsive homicides have a strong potential for repetition and are frequently committed in a similar and ritualistic manner. These murders have a different underlying basis of sexual motivation; rather than sexual conflicts, there is a fusion of sex and aggression so that the violent act itself is eroticized. In some cases, the compulsion breaks through spontaneously when a victim of opportunity emerges. In other cases, the murder is planned out in such a thoughtful manner that the offender is not easily apprehended. Thus, he may kill multiple individuals in serial fashion.

In the following chapters, catathymic and compulsive homicides will be explored in depth. It is hoped that these two different types of sexual murders will be better understood by viewing them within the overall spectrum of crime and (nonsexual) homicide.

3.5 Sexual Murder in Context

Crime theory, crime categorization, and the various classification systems of homicide provide a necessary context in which to understand sexual murder. In this chapter, an attempt was made to draw distinctions between killings that are not sexually motivated and those that are. Therefore, several of the case examples chosen are of men who killed women as a result of psychosis or with motivation that was not directly sexual but, instead, was environmentally, situationally, or impulsively induced. In contrast, catathymic and compulsive murders (discussed in the following chapters) are sexually motivated murders. We believe that the motivational spectrum is of practical help in placing the homicidal act in context.

The concept of the motivational spectrum—seen within the context of the offender's personality, inner resources, and empathic capacity—is also of help in prognostication. At times the question arises as to what do we evaluate, the offender or the criminal act? In essence, we must first evaluate the act itself, but this merges with the evaluation of the offender. Situational offenders have the best prognosis as most situational homicides are one-time events. The prognosis for homicides that are a result of environmental factors is influenced by the offender's value system, opportunities, associations, and level of maturity. Impulsive offenders who commit a murder may continue to engage in antisocial activities, but those activities may not necessarily be homicidal or severely aggressive. Compulsive offenders who commit a violent act or homicide will almost always repeat the offense after they are released from incarceration. These offenders who kill because of an inner need to kill are clearly the most dangerous. Catathymic offenses are often limited to a single episode. However, if the offender's underlying (sexual) conflicts that fueled the murder are not resolved, another catathymic murder, following years of incarceration, has been known to occur.

Catathymia and Catathymic Crisis
Contributions of Hans W. Maier and Fredric Wertham

4

The term *catathymia* is derived from the Greek *kata* ("according to") and *thymos* ("spirits or temper"). Feyerabend's (1969) Greek dictionary gives various translations, the most appropriate of which is "in accordance with emotions." *Catathymia* (*Katathymie*) was first used by Hans W. Maier (1912) as a psychodynamic explanation for the development of the content of delusions. The concept later became used, notably by Fredric Wertham, as an explanation for extreme acts of violence, including homicide and some types of sexual homicide. This chapter provides an in-depth analysis of Maier's seminal papers (published in 1912 and 1923), which have never been translated or fully reviewed, as well as a discussion of Wertham's writings on "the catathymic crisis."

4.1 Hans W. Maier: The Concept of Catathymia

After studying medicine at Zurich, Strassburg, and Vienna, Hans Maier joined the staff of the well-known Burghölzli Hospital in 1905. Burghölzli, founded in Switzerland in the mid-19th century, was the first mental hospital to accept psychoanalysis as a modality of treatment. Therapeutic work programs, as well as the concept of the halfway house, were introduced there. Nearby, the first residential treatment center in the field of child psychiatry was established in 1920. In fact, the entire child guidance movement, in an indirect way, was influenced by the hospital and the intellectual climate it created (Mora, 1975) (see Figure 4.1).

Many well-known psychiatrists were affiliated with Burghölzli. Eugen Bleuler, during his tenure there (1898–1927), coined the term *schizophrenia* and wrote his classic text *Dementia Praecox or the Group of Schizophrenias* (1st ed., 1911/2nd ed., 1951). Carl Jung worked at Burghölzli under Bleuler from 1900 to 1909. While working at the hospital, Hermann Rorschach published his classic *Psychodiagnostik* (1st ed., 1921/2nd ed., 1947), a fusion of psychoanalysis, clinical psychiatry, and applied psychology, which laid the foundation for his well-known inkblot test. Around the same time, three other prominent Swiss psychiatrists who trained at Burghölzli left Switzerland and established themselves permanently in the United States. August Hoch became active in the New York State psychiatric system; Emil Oberholzer helped to introduce the Rorschach in the United States; and Adolf Meyer exercised a great influence on the entire American psychiatric field.

Maier had a multifaceted career, succeeding Bleuler as the medical director of Burghölzli and also working as a teacher and researcher. He tried to combine theory and practice in order to confront and alleviate social problems. Thus, he was especially interested in forensic psychiatry, child psychiatry, and community mental health and frequently gave lectures on these subjects to lawyers and members of the police department. The following sample of topics he routinely lectured on gives some indication of the diversity of

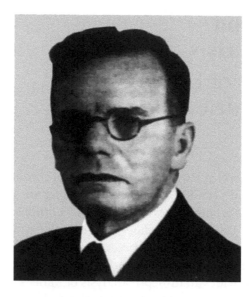

Figure 4.1 Hans Wolfgang Maier, MD (1882–1945).

his interests: (1) the attitude of psychiatrists toward criminals, (2) changes needed in the criminal code, (3) challenges facing the juvenile court, (4) psychiatric thoughts on abortion, (5) guidelines on raising children, (6) psychiatric problems in youth, (7) principles of psychiatry applied in schools, including corporal punishment, (8) development of mental health centers, (9) prevention of crime, (10) the fundamentals of psychiatry as an aid to police, (11) sterilization of criminals as a means of mental hygiene, and (12) development of laws prohibiting inheritance by criminals and the mentally ill. His influence on legal thought in Switzerland was substantial; he even helped write some of the country's criminal codes. Maier also studied the effects of encephalitis and various infections on mental functioning, and he explored the possible relationship of accidents and military service to the development of schizophrenia.

Maier had a particular interest in substance abuse, and in 1926, wrote *Der Kokainismus* (*Cocaine Addiction*), which is considered a classic. In the mid-1980s, there was an extensive cocaine epidemic in the United States, and a great deal of research was begun on the evaluation and treatment of cocaine users. In 1987, Maier's book was translated into English, as this text had already examined all the major areas of cocaine addiction some 60 years earlier. A review of the topics covered in *Cocaine Addiction* reveals the depth of Maier's understanding of the problem: physiological actions of cocaine; cocaine-related illnesses; the effects of cocaine, including disturbances of perception, cognition, emotion, and motivation; and various symptom pictures in cocaine intoxication, cocaine psychosis, and cocaine-related psychiatric problems. Maier also provided numerous clinical histories of cocaine addicts with additional chapters on differential diagnosis, prognosis for acute intoxication vs. the chronic abuser, anatomical alterations, and an outline for a program of treatment. The book ends with Maier's view of the legal steps needed to control cocaine addiction.

But most relevant for the present book is Maier's pioneering work on the development of the content of delusions (for which he received a professorship and ultimately was appointed chairman of the department of psychiatry at Zurich). In 1912, Maier published his dissertation research, "On the Subject of Catathymic Delusions and Paranoia."

A detailed look at Maier's paper illuminates his use of the concept of catathymia to explain how underlying, emotionally laden conflicts can result in such a change in thinking that delusions develop.

Maier begins his treatise by defining catathymia and attempting to show how it relates to cases of (what we would call today) pure paranoia or delusional disorder. In an effort to understand why individuals develop specific delusional content in the way they do, he searched for unconscious connections that determine the makeup of psychotic ideas. The stream of associations, he believed, "can go in a wrong direction through the predominance of a relatively strong affectivity" (p. 556). The delusional content is therefore greatly influenced by emotionally charged unconscious "complexes" such as a wish, a fear, or an ambivalent ambition. Delusions that grow out of these underlying conflicts are catathymic delusions and are to be differentiated from delusions that do not stem from complexes such as those with an organic base. But even in mental illnesses that are primarily organic in origin such as manic–depressive psychosis, catathymic delusions can still occur secondarily, as long as the delusional ideas have a causal connection to an underlying complex. In contrast, delusions that are not a result of complexes, as in substance abuse, are not catathymic. Maier presents as an example an individual who became delusional as a result of bromine intoxication. Here, the delusions were not the consequence of any complexes but occurred solely because of the effects of the substance and are therefore not catathymic.

The tenacity of the emotions connected to the underlying complex in catathymic delusions is an important consideration. As the delusion is (partially) caused by the emotional conflicts that are closely connected to the individual's life experiences, it is not easily dissipated. The content of the catathymic delusion is especially shaped by the individual's emotional attitude (*Affecteinstellungen*) toward his underlying conflicts.

In an attempt to further clarify the meaning of catathymic delusions, Maier presents several clinical conditions with illustrative cases: (1) paranoia, (2) mental retardation, (3) "utter nonsense," (4) manic–depressive psychosis, (5) *pseudologia fantastica* (pathological lying), and (6) organic and intoxication disorders.

Paranoia, in Maier's view, is the quintessential disorder in which catathymic delusions occur. The first case he presents is of a highly intelligent woman who had a successful academic career but several unhappy marriages. She developed paranoia of a persecutory type but showed no other signs or symptoms that would indicate schizophrenia. The catathymic content of her delusional system was obvious, and it formed the groundwork for her successful treatment. In another case, an individual's strong wish for financial security could not be fulfilled because he developed a physical handicap; this conflict became the center of his catathymic delusional system, which was more intractable than the first case. Finally, Maier describes the case of a severely ill individual who had "gigantic ideas of persecution" that grew from underlying conflicts and rendered him extremely dangerous, difficult to control, and resistant to treatment. The same underlying mechanism is operative in both paranoia and paranoid schizophrenia, but treatment for paranoid schizophrenia is clearly more difficult.

Maier also presents several cases of mentally retarded individuals who developed catathymic symptoms. One such woman had a childhood sexual relationship with her father and became pregnant. An innocent man was accused of assaulting her and was sent to jail for some time before her father was eventually arrested. All this produced major internal conflicts in her. She hated her father as a woman, but loved him as a daughter. Simultaneously, she felt jealousy, anger, and pity toward her mother. She also believed that members of the community who knew of her circumstances were scornful of her. These emotional conflicts were too overwhelming for her limited intellectual capacity. "Her psychological balance is destroyed and the groundwork for catathymic delusions and hallucinations is created" (p. 582). In this and similar cases, Maier looks for unconscious connections between emotion-laden memories from childhood and the content of the developed delusion.

Under the heading "Utter Nonsense," Maier describes the case of a man who published brochures and books devoted to subjects such as natural living and healing, attacks on the government, and various sexual and philosophical topics. He earned a great deal of money from his speeches and publications, which afforded him a comfortable lifestyle. He organized a "life society" and promised his followers health if they adhered to his system. This man was eventually institutionalized at Burghölzli for 7 years. Maier noted that his mood was always euphoric, with a flight of ideas, and he diagnosed him as a chronic sub-manic, a category of manic–depressive psychosis.

Maier was struck by the content of this patient's "utter nonsense" ideas. According to Maier, this man's delusions were a direct result of his manic illness and therefore were not catathymic. Since his beliefs were not caused by any consistent, underlying, emotionally charged conflicts or trauma, his condition would not be considered catathymia but, instead, should be called "emotional psychosis." In another case, a manic–depressive who had many delusions of grandeur and ideas of persecution also had no apparent inner conflicts to account for his delusions; Maier therefore concluded that the symptomatology was solely due to mania.

The next case reported is a woman who had engaged in repetitive pathological lying (*pseudologia fantastica*) since childhood. She was intelligent, but she lied continuously, stating, for example, that she would inherit a million dollars, including diamond and gold mines in South Africa. The lies became more and more bizarre, manifesting delusions of grandeur and persecution. She stole money, served time in prison, and continued to lie to the authorities and to her doctors. Eventually, the *pseudologia fantastica* developed into paranoia. Because of time constraints, Maier was unable to specify the underlying complex of ideas that would definitely indicate catathymia, but he believed it was present. In some cases, catathymically determined symptoms can be uncovered only by in-depth analysis of the patient.

Delusions caused by an organic disorder or intoxication are not rooted in a complex and therefore should not be considered catathymic. However, an organic disease can trigger catathymic delusions in a predisposed individual. In addition, underlying complexes involving a fear or a wish can result in catathymic delusions in an individual who has an independent organic illness such as epilepsy. In alcoholic psychosis, catathymic delusions may play a role but usually only a secondary role. In Korsakoff's syndrome, catathymic symptoms usually are not found, but there are cases of delirium tremens where catathymic delusional ideas do occasionally occur.

Maier concluded his lengthy paper by emphasizing his central point: catathymic symptoms are a result of emotionally charged complexes, usually a desire, a fear, or an ambivalent tendency. If the underlying complex is not present, the symptom is not catathymic. Maier also offered several additional observations about catathymic symptoms. Because catathymic manifestations concern only one selection of ideas, the catathymic delusion can be encapsulated while the rest of the patient's psychological functioning remains intact, as in pure paranoia. In such cases, however, catathymia can also lead to catathymic syndromes in which one idea-complex is so strongly emotionally charged that logic in several other areas is overcome. In normal individuals, the equilibrium between logic and emotion can be disturbed but the effect is usually not of long duration. The healthy individual can generally correct the error in his thinking as soon as the emotion subsides. A predisposition to catathymic symptoms does exist in cases where an excess of emotion destroys the balance between emotion and logic. This kind of imbalance could occur in cases of low intelligence (especially if there is a severe trauma); in different types of schizophrenia; and in cases of hysteria where the emotions are especially strong and the catathymic symptoms are especially persistent.

Several years later, Maier (1923) published a second paper that clarified his view on the psychogenic development of symptoms. Again, he asserted that a psychologically determined symptom can be considered catathymic in origin only when it reflects an underlying emotional conflict representing a wish, a fear, or an ambivalent tendency. Catathymic symptoms exist only where "the balance between logic and affectivity is displaced" (p. 193).

As examples of psychogenic symptoms that are not catathymically induced, Maier pointed to patients who developed psychological sequelae of encephalitis. Several of these encephalitic patients suffered sleep disturbances that were purely psychogenic in origin but did not offer any secondary gain for the patients. Other types of psychogenic symptoms in postencephalitic patients such as abnormal breathing rhythms also had no organic basis. In another case, a 25-year-old woman developed a psychogenic tic which quickly disappeared with hypnosis and suggestion but returned the next day. After a year of psychotherapy ("as thorough an analysis as possible," p. 195), no catathymic genesis could be established. Slowly, the tic appeared less and less frequently so that the patient was able to resume work; eventually she terminated treatment after the symptom subsided completely.

Maier believed that such examples of sequelae of organic illnesses are purely psychogenic but are not catathymic. "Thus, there is a mechanism present where an organically damaged pathway no longer functions correctly due to psychological influences and without any emotionally charged complexes being at work" (p. 197). Maier referred to this type of psychogenic symptom as "athymic."* In athymic psychogenic symptom formation, emotion plays no role at all; rather, a previously organic symptom continues to function psychologically on its own.

Maier also described two other patients who developed noncatathymic psychogenic symptoms: a paralyzed individual who in an angry outburst suddenly broke the furniture in a room because one chair was misplaced, and a senile individual who set fire to the house because the door did not open immediately. In these instances, "an emotion is caused psychogenically and carries the entire personality along with it in such a way that all inhibitions and other considerations are eliminated" (p. 198) and "the emotion [by itself] leads to psychogenic symptoms, and the intellect plays no role at all" (p. 198). Maier referred to this psychogenic symptom mechanism as "synthymic."

Table 4.1 lists the three psychogenic mechanisms differentiated by Maier (1923). In short, the catathymic is a result of emotion as well as intellect. In the athymic, emotion plays no role, but an organically caused symptom continues to function psychogenically. In the synthymic, an emotion suddenly takes control of the entire personality; the intellect plays no role. In Maier's view, cases of catathymic symptom formation are best treated

---

* Maier's use of *athymic* is not to be confused with Hypocrites' term for melancholia, which was also called *athymia*.

Table 4.1   Three Types of Psychogenic Mechanisms as Described by Maier (1923)

Name	Process	Symptom	Treatment
Catathymic	Caused by affect as well as intellect.	Various neurotic symptoms; paranoia and hysteria.	Psychoanalysis and psychoanalytic therapy.
Athymic	Emotion plays no role; an organic symptom continues to function on its own.	Various psychogenic symptoms that are vestiges of an organic illness.	Education, suggestion, and hypnosis.
Synthymic	Intellect plays no role; an emotion suddenly takes control of entire personality.	Various stages of agitation and aggression.	Education, suggestion, and hypnosis.

with psychoanalysis, psychoanalytic therapy, and other "in-depth methods." The athymic and synthymic symptom formations should be treated through education, suggestion, or hypnosis; psychoanalysis would have little effect on these mechanisms because there is no underlying complex to be analyzed.

4.2 Catathymic Crisis

Fredric Wertham studied at the universities of Erlangen and Munich, obtaining his medical degree from the University of Würzburg in 1921 and continuing his studies in Paris and Vienna. He then joined the Kraepelin Clinic in Munich. The distinguished psychiatrist Emil Kraepelin, who developed the standard system for classifying mental disorders, was Wertham's first significant mentor (Reibman, 1990) (see Figure 4.2).

Wertham left Europe to accept a position with Adolf Meyer at Worcester State Hospital in Massachusetts. He later followed Meyer to the Phipps Psychiatric Clinic at Johns Hopkins University, where he stayed for 7 years. While at the Phipps Clinic,

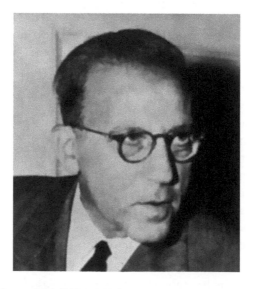

Figure 4.2 Fredric Wertham, MD (1895–1981).

Wertham wrote his first book, *The Brain as an Organ: Its Postmortem Study and Interpretation* (1934). He left Johns Hopkins to become affiliated with Bellevue Hospital in New York. Founded in 1736, Bellevue is the oldest public hospital in the United States. Bellevue was also home to several individuals who would later become key figures in the mental health field. For example, David Wechsler—who developed the Wechsler–Bellevue Intelligence Scale—and Lauretta Bender, known mostly for developing the popular Bender–Gestalt, were also at Bellevue Hospital at around that time period (Oshinsky, 2017). At Bellevue, Wertham organized the nation's first court clinic (that is still operative), which conducted psychiatric screenings on every convicted felon. He also founded the Lafargue Clinic in Harlem, a low-cost mental health center to treat inner-city patients, who otherwise would not be able to receive such services. In 1947, Wertham began a treatment center for sex offenders as well.

In addition to his work on violence and murder, for which he is best known, Wertham was a social critic and an advocate for social justice and human rights. He testified in several desegregation cases, explaining the harmful effects of segregation on children. His testimony was subsequently used in the landmark school desegregation case *Brown v. Board of Education* (1951; decided by the U.S. Supreme Court in 1954 and 1955). Wertham also testified at the Julius and Ethel Rosenberg spy trial in 1951 and was a psychiatric consultant to Estes Kefauver's Senate subcommittee for the study of organized crime.

In the 1950s, the American people faced two major fears: the threat of communism and the increase in juvenile delinquency. Wertham's book *Seduction of the Innocent* (1954) was the culmination of a 7-year research study on the effects of violence-filled comic books on children. He attempted to show a connection between the rise in juvenile delinquency and what he believed to be the injurious influence of comic books in promoting a culture that encouraged antisocial acting out. Wertham was vigorously maligned, investigated, and harassed by members of the comic book industry for years. The degree of animosity felt toward Wertham is illustrated by Catherine Yronwode's column in *The Comic Buyer's Guide* (1983):

> Probably the single individual most responsible for causing comic books to be so reviled in America is our good friend and nemesis, Dr. Fredric Wertham. ... We hate him, despise him ... he and he alone virtually brought about the collapse of the comic book industry during the 1950s. (p. 12)

Wertham's book *The Circle of Guilt* (1956) was also a study of juvenile delinquency and the role that the media plays in creating and distorting various social and psychological problems of teenagers. In this book Wertham attempted to expose the failures and hypocrisies of the legal system and the social service establishment, which did not adequately serve those whom they were intended to help.

In *A Sign for Cain: An Exploration of Human Violence* (1966), Wertham again argued that aggression is not innate but, instead, is created and perpetuated by the mass media and a culture that seems to legitimize violence. As he stated in an earlier book,

> It is always ... negative factors in [the] social medium where the growth of the personality takes place that lead to murderous acts of violence. The murderer can never kill without a transformation of values which may come from his innermost mind, but is always derived ultimately from social prejudgments and prejudices. (Wertham, 1949, p. 253)

Wertham's most lasting contribution to understanding violence, and particularly mur-der, was his concept of catathymic crisis. In his seminal paper "The Catathymic Crisis: A Clinical Entity" (1937), Wertham sought to explain the behavior of individuals who have committed severely violent acts—murder, arson, self-castration, infanticide, or suicide—for which there was no obvious motivation. Wertham's syndrome was summarized in the first (1937) and the last (1978) paper he wrote on the topic.

Individuals who commit out-of-character violent acts which they are not able to explain adequately intrigued Wertham. Why would a girl who was not psychotic or men-tally deficient become jealous of a friend and pour lye on her eyes while she slept, causing her to become blind? How does thinking about severe violence become translated into action? Wertham immediately dismissed the simplistic and incorrect notion that criminal behavior is a result of a mental disorder or a psychopathic personality; he intended to delve much deeper into the motives, dynamics, and hidden factors that result in such antisocial conduct.

In attempting to develop an explanation for such acts of violence, Wertham relied on the concept of catathymia introduced by Maier 25 years earlier. As noted in the first part of this chapter, Maier did not use the concept of catathymia as an explanation for violent or criminal behavior. Instead, he used it to explain how underlying emotionally charged conflicts result in such a pronounced change in thinking that an idea reaches a delusional proportion. Wertham borrowed Maier's concept and defined catathymic crisis as "the transformation of the stream of thought as the result of certain complexes of ideas that are charged with a strong affect—usually a wish, a fear, or an ambivalent striving" (Wertham, 1937, p. 975). Catathymic symptoms are caused by "one latent idea that takes on a rutlike fixation"; catathymic thinking develops when "the balance between logic and affectivity is disturbed" (p. 976).

> The patient acquires the idea that he must carry out a violent act against others or against himself. The idea does not arise in an obsessive form. It appears as a definite plan, accompa-nied by a tremendous urge to act it out. The plan itself meets such resistance in the mind of the patient that he is likely to hesitate and delay. The violent act usually has some symbolic significance over and above its obvious meaning. ... The thinking of the patient may have an almost delusional character in its rigidity and inaccessibility to logical reasoning. (p. 976)

Wertham argued that catathymic crisis is a clinical entity and should be considered only after other diagnostic possibilities are ruled out. For example, the syndrome excludes impulsive or explosive acts of violence associated with psychiatric disorders such as schizophrenia.

After committing a violent act such as murder (or after attempting suicide), many indi-viduals actually improve. The next day in the hospital or jail, the patient often appears calm and no longer wants to commit the act of violence that was all-consuming just hours previously. Jameison (1936) also noted that "certain patients after failure to commit sui-cide abruptly become much better mentally. The depression seems to lift; they are cheerful and agreeable, and temporarily (occasionally permanently) all the various fears and ten-sion disappear" (p. 9). Following the criminal act, Wertham believed, there is a superficial appearance of normality. During this period, a marked inner adjustment can take place, which could lead to a complete shift in the person's attitude; as a result, the individual might develop insight and reestablish an inner equilibrium that could be lasting. Thus,

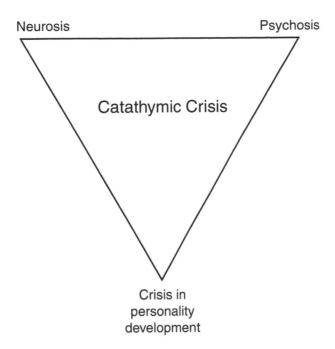

Figure 4.3 Diagrammatic representation of catathymic crisis. (Adapted from Wertham, F., *Archives of Neurology and Psychiatry, 37,* 1937.)

the violent act enables the personality to safeguard itself and thereby prevent more serious forms of regression such as psychosis. Wertham (1937) envisioned the catathymic crisis as lying within a triangle, "the outer points of which are a neurosis, a crisis in personality development, and a psychosis" (p. 977), as illustrated in Figure 4.3.

In 1978, Wertham summarized the five stages of the catathymic crisis:

1. An initial thinking disorder that follows an original precipitating (or traumatic) circumstance.
2. Crystallization of a plan, when the idea of a violent act emerges into consciousness. The violent act is seen as the only way out. Emotional tension becomes extreme and thinking becomes more and more egocentric.
3. Extreme emotional tension culminating in a crisis in which a violent act against one's self or others is attempted or carried out.
4. Superficial normality, beginning with a period of lifting of tension and calmness immediately after the violent act. This period is of varying length, usually several months.
5. Insight and recovery, with the reestablishment of an inner equilibrium.

A full clinical example of the catathymic crisis appears in Wertham's *Dark Legend: A Study in Murder* (1941) in which is detailed the case of Gino, a 17-year-old male with average intelligence and an absence of significant mental disturbance, who murdered his promiscuous mother. The work was acclaimed by literary giants of the time, including Thomas Mann and Arthur Miller; however, since the focus was matricide, many people denounced it. In England, its publication was delayed because it was considered obscene, suitable for distribution only to physicians and mental health professionals (Reibman, 1990).

Gino became enraged at his mother's sexually promiscuous conduct following his father's death. He was preoccupied not only with his mother's sexual indiscretions but with sexual activities of women in general.

> Prostitutes are bad girls. I will destroy them—kill them, that's all. If I would be in charge, I would kill every one of them. They shouldn't do that. It is the women who spoil the men. They do it to make money and because they like it. (Wertham, 1941, p. 101)

Gino slowly developed an idea to kill his mother, and he could not put this idea out of his mind. "I tried not to think of it. I tried to read. To play. But nobody would play with me. I had to think about it" (p. 105). He had recurrent thoughts of "making her realize how bad she was, and then finally shoot her" (p. 106). One afternoon, while he was chopping ice with an ice pick,

> In my mind, just like a vision, I would see my mother being kissed and intercoursed. I had no idea how to kill my mother. Then it came to my mind how to do it. … Cutting the ice gave me the idea of what I could do to her. From that day I couldn't stand it no more. (p. 107)

He described the murder to Wertham:

> My mother was in bed, turned to the right with her shoulders toward me, facing out into the room. … I went to the kitchen and took off my shoes, and I prayed to God again to help me do it. … I went to the kitchen. I took the knife and I came back. … I was standing there with the knife in my hand. I was so nervous. … But my hand was steady, though. I put my head through the curtain. I saw my mother … "You dishonored my family." … Then I stabbed her two, three times in the neck and chest. She said "You are going crazy." I said, "I am not crazy." I did not look at her face. When I was stabbing her, I don't know how, but the knife slipped through my hand and stuck me.
>
> Then it came to my mind to cut the whole head off, not to make her live anymore. That's why I stabbed her in the neck. She was not dead yet. I put my arm up to do it, and then I found they were holding my arm—Mario and my cousin. I gave my cousin a punch in the jaw to stop holding me. Everybody was awake. The baby was crying, my sister was crying, Mario was hollering, my cousin was hollering.

Gino then ran out of the apartment and yelled to a few passersby, "Call the cops. I killed my mother." As he was laughing at the time, people did not believe him.

Following his quick arrest, Gino was taken to the prison hospital because of his hand injury. He explained that he "felt fine" and that his injured hand did not even hurt.

> I was laughing and talking. I never slept so well. I was glad I did it. I did what I thought was right. I will never be sorry. Nothing bothers me now. I am sorry I didn't do it a long time ago. I don't believe in forgiving. … I can forgive anybody who would give me a slap, but not one who dishonors my family. … I don't forgive. They said I am crazy, but I am not crazy. They told me they might have to send me to the electric chair, but that doesn't make any difference to me. … I'm glad, I'm glad, I'm glad. I was always happy since the day I killed her. I was glad I had done it. For 5 years it had been growing on me. For a month I knew I had to do it. I did not think about the electric chair. I did not worry about it.

According to Wertham, Gino's belief that all women are bad "had an almost delusional character. But this abnormal trend was isolated and none of the essential signs of schizophrenia were present" (p. 128). "Gino was guided only by one idea or one complex of ideas. It originated years before the actual onset of what might conceivably have been regarded as the phase similar to a depressive psychosis" (p. 130). Gino was under "a terrific and mounting tension. This tension was the result of a conflict within him; a conflict between his wish to kill his mother and a counter action of restraining forces" (p. 133). Gino said, "If any of my sisters did the same as my mother, I would tear them apart. I would kill my wife if she did anything like that. The wives and mothers wouldn't do it then, if that was done" (p. 137). Wertham concluded that Gino's conflict—to kill or not to kill—seemed rooted in the "battle between two social taboos," but "behind the facade of family honor lay a deeper, more primitive impulse" that he himself was unaware of (p. 154).

How are thoughts of murder translated into action? Many individuals have criminal, perverse sexual, or suicidal ideas in one form or another, but few put these ideas into action. "An obsessive idea can reach consciousness but it … cannot make the body obey it" (p. 194). Wertham reasoned that Gino did not understand why he was planning violence. "He was conscious only of the wrong reasons he had made up for its justification. In other words, the full control of the forces of his personality could not be applied to an impulse which, when he became aware of it, was already a descendant of highly complicated, latent, and repressed ideas" (p. 196). Thus, Wertham became convinced that Gino's matricidal impulse "stemmed from a deeply submerged, unconscious conflict" that he had harbored for some time before the murder of his mother (p. 217).

> The murder was like a self-operation. Gino acted like a man who cuts off his arm to escape blood poisoning. By the cruel deed he eradicated his own mother complex. This was shown by his changed attitude towards women in general [after the matricide]. He now wanted to marry and correct his idea that all women are bad. (p. 219)
>
> Gino's hatred against women was therefore not something basic but only due to his fixation on the mother image. The bad experiences that had influenced him were only those with one woman, his mother. In this woman, he killed all [bad] women. If this were not so, he would have continued to hate women in general. (p. 220)

Instead, he changed his opinion of women and understood that he was wrong when he condemned them all. This change in sentiment "shows that the disorder was very localized and very well circumscribed" and also "explains … why, after he gained insight, he thought of marriage, but not of suicide. He wanted to get married to replace the mother. He had no desire for self-punishment" (p. 220).

Thus, Wertham reasoned, Gino's matricidal act was a catathymic crisis. "The thought processes lost their plasticity and became more and more rigid along definite lines as the result of repressed ungratified wishes, unallayed fears, or any unresolved feeling" (p. 224).

> Catathymic crisis is a circumscribed mental disorder, psychologically determined, non-hereditary, without physical manifestations, and not necessarily occurring in a psychopathic constitution. A central manifestation consists in the development of the idea that a violent act—against another person or against one's self—is the only solution to a profound emotional conflict whose real nature remains below the threshold of the consciousness of the patient. A violent climax is reached as a direct result of the inner tension. There is usually no provocation at all, or provocation which is utterly insufficient. (p. 225)

The catathymic crisis develops as follows:

> An injurious life experience precipitates an unbearable and seemingly unsolvable inner situation, leading to persistent and increasing emotional tension. The individual's hold on the outer situation is entirely responsible for his inner tension. His thinking becomes more and more self-centered. With apparent suddenness, a crystallization point is reached in the idea that some violent act against another or against himself is "the only way out." After a prolonged inner struggle leading finally to extreme emotional tension, this violent act is carried out or attempted. It is followed immediately by an almost complete removal of the preceding emotional tension, [but] the patient does not gain insight at this time. There follows a superficially normal period of varying length. During this period the complex determined train of thought of the patient makes him still see the need for the violent act in a wrong light. Finally, an inner equilibrium is re-established, which leads to insight. It then becomes clear to the patient that the outer situation with which he was faced after the initial traumatic experience does not sufficiently account for the violent act committed, and that this act satisfied a deep inner need he had not been aware of. He realizes that the motives for the violent act with which he had credited himself were not the real driving power. (p. 227)

Wertham explained the five stages of the catathymic crisis as they specifically relate to Gino's life:

- *Stage 1*: Following the precipitating circumstances, mainly his father's death, his mother's misconduct and his own physical deprivations, an inner situation arose with which he could not cope.
- *Stage 2*: The latent complex of ideas at the base of this inner situation developed into a chronic irritant because it was fraught with such strong emotion and because it had never found unreserved expression in feeling. One day the plan of matricide came to him, and henceforth he could not give the idea up.
- *Stage 3*: After doubts and delays, his preoccupation with his plan finally became so acute that it excluded everything else from his mind.
- *Stage 4*: Then he committed the murder. The phase following his violent act has a superficial appearance of normalcy, but it is obvious that his satisfaction with the matricide still rested on a delusional basis.
- *Stage 5*: During this phase, a profound inner adjustment was initiated, which finally led to a complete shift in his attitude. Eventually an inner equilibrium was reestablished which was lasting and which in psychological structure was a continuation of that existing before the original precipitating circumstances (pp. 229, 230).

Wertham believed that Gino's act of murder averted a more serious form of psychological regression. Thus, "the matricide was an expression of Gino's struggle to safeguard the core of his personality. ... The violent act was a defense" (p. 230). After a period of treatment, Wertham contended Gino would gain complete insight, recover fully, and never again constitute a danger to himself or others. Wertham testified in court that the young man was insane at the time of the murder. Gino was subsequently committed to a psychiatric hospital and discharged 9 years later. In accordance with Wertham's predictions, Gino eventually married, led a productive life, and experienced no subsequent difficulties of this type.

In *Show of Violence* (1949), Wertham discussed a number of cases where he was directly involved in the offender's evaluation as well as in subsequent criminal court proceedings. One of these offenders, Robert Irwin, a 28-year-old male, killed three people, two by strangulation and one by multiple stab wounds made with an ice pick. Before committing these murders, Robert was a patient at Bellevue Hospital, admitted for attempted self-castration. Prior to this hospitalization, Robert had asked three doctors to amputate his penis; when all of them refused, he decided to do it himself. Wertham first saw Robert at Bellevue.

> On the one hand, he was almost ashamed and very secretive about [the attempt at castration]. He didn't want any of the other patients to know what he had done. On the other hand, he was insistent that what he had attempted was the right thing for him, and he insisted on having the doctors complete it. At that point, he was adamant. If the doctors in the hospital [would] not do it there and then, he declared emphatically, he would get somebody else to do it as soon as he left the hospital. (p. 107)

Robert wanted to be castrated in order to "bottle up sexual energy for higher purposes" (p. 122). After some psychotherapy with Wertham, the patient was transferred to a state hospital for long-term treatment and was eventually discharged.

Robert was raised in an atmosphere of religious fervor, fanaticism, and fear. His mother was a college graduate, and his extended family members were businessmen, judges, and individuals of considerable wealth. Robert's father was a schoolteacher, a lawyer, and later a minister in several churches. However, his father abandoned the family, and his mother was forced to raise the children by herself under very strained financial circumstances. Much later his mother also abandoned her son and placed him in a juvenile home.

Robert had a very conflicted relationship with his mother and developed major sexual conflicts in this regard. His mother

> used to bathe in front of the children, nude from the waist up. He remembers seeing his mother when he was about nine and admiring her beautiful breasts. "They were neither too large nor too small." The beauty of women's breasts played a considerable role in his later life. (p. 113)

Themes of mother, religion, and sex were woven into Robert's consciousness in a disturbed manner. As he told Wertham,

> There is another thing that made me hate my mother. I was the only one of her kids that ever paid any attention to her, or even realized what she was going through. One day I was helping her to do the washing, and somebody came over to me and congratulated me on helping my mother, and my mother laughed and said, "Yes, he is just like a regular girl," and it made me so mad, I just saw blood. I was seven or eight then. (p. 116)

Wertham concluded that Robert's fixation on his mother was at the root of many of his problems. In describing a sexual encounter with a prostitute, Robert stated, "She treated me in a motherly way." He also became attached to several older married women and had relations with some of them; afterward he felt ashamed: "We were like mother and son. We liked each other and quarreled a lot" (p. 118).

Wertham concluded that his patient did not suffer from schizophrenia; rather, Robert's fixed idea and attempt to castrate himself pointed to a diagnosis of catathymic crisis.

Although Robert improved with psychotherapy, Wertham believed he was not cured and remained a danger both to himself and others.

> I expressed my conclusion that he was in a greatly improved stage of disease, but that the pattern of violence was still latent—violence either against himself or against others. I added that these cases could recover if they were given prolonged sympathetic and active psychoanalytic psychotherapy, and said I was convinced that if they did get it, they could be returned to the stage of recovery and normality. (p. 128)

However, by the time of his discharge, Robert still had not achieved substantial insight, and the catathymic dynamic continued.

Eventually, Robert's idea of castrating himself transferred to the idea of killing a female acquaintance named Ethel. The thought came to him while he was walking by himself, feeling lonely and desperate. For a period of time, he ruminated and brooded, "and then I made up my mind to kill Ethel and to go to the chair for it" (p. 133). He purchased an ice pick and went to Ethel's house to kill her, but she was not there. He talked calmly for an hour or so with Ethel's mother. Then, since Ethel still had not arrived, he decided to kill her mother.

> I hit her a terrific blow with my fist and knocked her down. ... I grabbed her by the neck. ... I continued choking her, and in the struggle she kicked me and scratched me something terrible. I continued to choke her for about 20 minutes before I was sure she was lifeless. (p. 135)

Hearing the commotion, Ethel's sister came out of an adjoining room. Robert quickly hit her, grabbed her by the throat, carried her to her bedroom, and put her on her bed. He did not kill this victim immediately but kept her there for about 2 hours.

> First, all she said was "Who are you?" I supposed she thought I was going to rape her. She said, "Please don't touch me. I just had an operation and the doctor said if I have intercourse I could die." (p. 136)

Robert denied that he had any sexual thoughts at this time. He was simply afraid that she recognized him as an acquaintance of her sister:

> When she said "Bob, I know you are going to get in trouble for this," I clamped down on her and choked her till she was lifeless. I turned on the lights and ripped off her chemise, leaving her on top of the bed, her mother's body lying beneath. At that moment, she was the most repulsive thing I ever knew. (p. 136)

Robert then got his ice pick and went into an adjoining room where a boarder was staying. While he slept, Robert stabbed him in the temple "as far in as it could go. ... I wanted to put him out of his misery, so I stabbed him a number of other blows about his head" (p. 137).

Ethel, the initial object of Robert's homicidal plan, never returned home. He went through the various drawers in the house looking for pictures of Ethel but could not find any. He finally took two photos of her sister and then took a small alarm clock and put it in his pocket. He said later that he had no remorse for the killings, but was ashamed of the stealing. "To kill is one thing. But to be a sneak thief ..." (p. 137).

Following the murders, Robert felt "as calm as I've been in my life before" (p. 138). He stayed in New York for a week, then traveled to Philadelphia, Washington, and later Cleveland. While reading a newspaper, he saw his mother's obituary, which triggered an immediate urge to turn himself in. Wertham explained, "Now he could never go home to his mother after having made something of himself. So he might as well give himself up and die now" (p. 138). He traveled to Chicago and then surrendered.

Wertham found a parallel between the first violent act of self-emasculation and the subsequent violent acts against others. Following the self-castration attempt, the impulse to destroy transferred itself to another person. Eventually Robert came to believe that "the only way out was murder," an idea that was closely related to prior suicide thoughts and his attempt at self-castration.

> The impulse to murder Ethel had an even closer psychological relationship to his attempt at self-emasculation 4½ years before. As he saw it, either act of violence would have put him "under pressure" and forced him—provided he were not electrocuted—to use all his energies on self-perfection. ... "You know yourself that without sex life, if you have no other purpose, no other goal, there is no life." (p. 176)

Thus, said Wertham, "sexlessness would have solved his innermost conflict between his inability, on the one hand, to love a woman normally and his inability to renounce the desire for a normal love relationship with a woman, on the other" (p. 177).

> Symbolically the two overt violent acts are the expression of the components of the ambivalent feelings towards his mother's image: self-castration as punishment activated by guilt feelings arising from his libidinal fixation on her; murder as an expression of his hostility against her. (p. 181)

Since Robert was not cured by psychotherapy, the critical stages of the catathymic process could easily recur. Wertham explained Robert's stages of the catathymic crisis as follows:

- *Stage 1*: In an attempt to cope with the trauma of his mother's conduct, at age 17, Robert developed a bizarre idea that you have to "visualize things first."
- *Stage 2*: At age 23, after reading Schopenhauer and trying to visualize his ideas, he planned to cut off his penis.
- *Stage 3*: The next year, his preoccupation with self-castration and accompanying tension became overwhelming and all-absorbing.
- *Stage 4*: After the actual attempt at self-emasculation, his tension was immediately relieved, and he felt as calm as he ever had been. He gained partial insight but went no further.
- *Stage 3 (recurred)*: Five years later, the tension became overwhelming, along with emergence of the violent idea to kill Ethel.
- *Stage 4 (recurred)*: Following the homicides, the extreme tension was completely relieved and he felt perfectly calm. While he was a fugitive, he made a fairly good social adjustment.
- *Stage 5*: This stage had not yet been reached because complete insight had not taken place.

Robert was found guilty and sent to prison, but was immediately transferred to a psychiatric hospital. Over the years, Wertham kept in touch with Robert's treating physicians who, he believed, confirmed his diagnosis of catathymic crisis.

4.3 Comment

Catathymic crisis has had a long and notable history in the forensic psychiatric/psychological literature. Maier conceived of the concept of catathymia as a way of explaining delusional thinking. Although Maier did make contributions to the field of forensic psychiatry, he did not apply his concept to cases of violence or homicide but, instead, restricted it to cases of psychotic ideation, especially cases of pure paranoia where fixed ideas are implanted in an otherwise normal personality.

Wertham borrowed Maier's concept 25 years later and used it to explain extremely violent acts that he could not otherwise understand. Such acts, he believed, are a result of a change in thinking—of adopting an idea with a rootlike fixation—whereby the individual believes the only solution to his inner conflict is through violence. The two cases summarized in this chapter are Wertham's most complete examples of catathymic crisis. In both cases, an underlying basis of sexual conflict was directly related to the homicides. Gino's internal conflict was ignited by his mother's sexual behavior, which upset his psychic homeostasis and eventually resulted in matricide. Robert's sexual disturbance was more diffuse. He, like Gino, had conflicts initiated by a sexually seductive (and abandoning) mother which expanded into an enormous disturbance regarding women in general. His attempt at self-castration was the result of a catathymic crisis. Although Robert received some treatment, it was not fully effective, and the catathymic dynamic remained operative. He finally committed three (sexual) murders, a result of the same process that earlier had led to the attempt at castration.

Although the catathymic crisis has been recognized as a clinical entity for almost a century, its usefulness as a model for understanding acts of extreme violence, especially when there is an underlying sexual component, has been undervalued. Perhaps because of the syndrome's complexity, or perhaps because the process is psychodynamic—and not merely an explanation of behavior as a consequence of a traditional *DSM* psychiatric diagnosis—it has not had the level of clinical study it warrants. In addition, the process is not often found in its pure form, as initially described and presented by Wertham. It is very clear, however, that many sexual murders cannot be fully understood without reliance on the early work of Hans W. Maier, Fredric Wertham, and the catathymic crisis.

Acute Catathymic Homicides

5

Since Maier's (1912) initial conception of catathymia, devised to explain the development of the content of delusions, the term has been used mostly, but not exclusively (Sedman, 1966), to describe various forms of violent behavior. Wertham (1937) was the first to borrow Maier's notion to explain severe aggression that stems from a process similar to a delusion. The homicidal ideas that Wertham's subjects developed were not exactly delusional, but Wertham considered them quasi-delusional in that they were fixed, rootlike, and inaccessible to reason. However, not all authors have used the theory of catathymia to explain violence that is preceded by a protracted period of obsessional rumination. Some have used the term to explain sudden unplanned acts of extreme violence. This chapter discusses acute catathymic homicides: sexual murders involving a sudden loss of control when an underlying conflict is triggered by an external circumstance.

5.1 Varying Views of Catathymia and Sudden Violence

5.1.1 A Subtype of Episodic Dyscontrol

Menninger and Mayman (1956) viewed personality disintegration as a series of stages of adaptation to life's stresses. Their notion is based on Freud's (1923) concept of the protective function of the ego. With increasingly greater degrees of failure in adaptation come correspondingly lower levels of functioning. Their "first order" of adaptation is the experience of anxiety. If anxiety becomes too intense, neurotic defenses are formed, which constitute a "second order" of adaptation. The "third order" of adaptation is episodic dyscontrol. This explosive outburst of violence represents a failure of the higher order stages to prevent disintegration. It is also a concomitant attempt to prevent a (lower) "fourth order" of adaptation, which is psychosis, or a "fifth order," suicide, which represents a person's total inability to adapt to life's stress.

Menninger and Mayman (1956) divided episodic dyscontrol into two general types: dyscontrol with organized (consciously rationalized) patterns of aggressive behavior and dyscontrol with disorganized (unjustified or unexplained) patterns of aggressive behavior. One type of disorganized aggressive dyscontrol involves attacks of assaultive violence, which the authors referred to as catathymic. These explosions are like "the sudden unstructured release of great quantities of energy characteristic of a convulsion, ... an outburst of primitive, disorganized violence like an enormous temper tantrum or an aborted suicide" (p. 160).

Thus, Menninger and Mayman's catathymia is a subtype of a larger episodic dyscontrol syndrome. In many of these catathymic explosions, the offender had no explanation at all for the crimes. Sometimes the individual may rationalize the act by presenting a convincing story, but this explanation "usually has little to do with the real motivation of the murder" (p. 161). The authors found that many of these catathymic outbursts contained elements of sexuality within the motivational dynamics.

The view of catathymia as a subtype of episodic dyscontrol was elaborated further by Satten, Menninger, and Mayman (1960), who presented four cases in which an explosive homicide was triggered by an individual whom the perpetrator had just met. After killing the strangers, the offenders were puzzled about their actions. The following are summaries of their cases:

- *Case A, Thomas*: A 31-year-old military officer suddenly grabbed a 9-year-old female, choked her, and held her head under water long after she was dead. Thomas was unable to explain what happened. He could not recall the beginning of the attack but "suddenly discovered" himself strangling the child.
- *Case B, Adams*: A 13-year-old boy refused to make change for a 23-year-old corporal. The soldier, who felt the boy was making fun of him, struck the youngster. Adams denied any recollection of the homicide and insisted he had no intention of killing the victim. He had no explanation when he "found out" that the boy's body had been severely mutilated.
- *Case C, Mason*: Following an argument with a friend, a 20-year-old truck driver picked up a 14-year-old boy. When the boy refused Mason's sexual advances and kept "nagging" the offender to take him home, he struck the boy and choked him. Mason denied any intent to kill, and he described "finding" the victim dead.
- *Case D, Elliot*: A 43-year-old male reported being teased by a prostitute who attempted to seduce him and take his money. Elliot described a dissociative-like state during which he struck and killed the woman with a tire iron, then mutilated and dismembered the body.

Following an extensive evaluation of each case, the authors concluded that the offenders were predisposed to kill because of strong conflicts they were secretly trying to resolve, such as incestuous feelings, self-hatred, or strong ambivalence. They

> unconsciously perceived [the victim] as a key figure in some past traumatic configuration. [The] … mere presence of [the victim] add[ed] a stress to the unstable balance of forces, which result[ed] in a sudden extreme discharge of violence, similar to the explosion that takes place when a percussion cap ignites a charge of dynamite. (p. 52)

Thus, the victims, often strangers, triggered in the offenders a repressed conflict that rushed to the surface, which was unable to be contained defensively and resulted in the violent outburst. The victims lost their real meaning and assumed "an identity in the unconscious traumatic configuration" of the offenders (p. 52).

Satten et al. (1960) found a number of common characteristics in the four offenders: severe weakening of impulses, blurring of boundaries between reality and fantasy, periods of what seemed to be altered states of consciousness, blunted and shallow emotional reactions to the homicides, and violent and primitive fantasy lives (elicited by interviewing and psychological testing). The subjects' inner lives were often of a bizarre, violent, and primitive nature. Several of the men reported repetitive dreams of violently killing, mutilating, burning, or destroying others. Their TAT stories were filled with primitive homicidal hostility, often rationalized on the basis of the victims' provoking their acts.

The authors raised the issue of possible organic component as a factor in these cases. Two of the men had ambiguous EEG findings, and one reported a history of childhood seizures. One offender had a more definite EEG abnormality and reported having had a head injury as a child. Satten et al. postulated that had they done more extensive neurological evaluations, some underlying physiological factor might have been detected.

The researchers also spent a great deal of time attempting to understand the unconscious motivational dynamics that may have induced the sudden murders. They concluded that for Thomas, the victim represented his dead sister, with whom he had had a conflictual incestuous relationship. The authors believed that Adams' victim symbolized his own hated self-image. In the case of Mason, Satten and colleagues were unable to delineate any further unconscious conflicts that the victim may have triggered beyond the overt homosexual component. Elliot's victim seemingly released an unresolved conflict regarding his deceased girlfriend, for whom his feelings were intense but quite ambivalent.

Finally, the authors found it significant that three of the four murderers conveyed a fear of losing control to either legal officials or psychiatrists prior to the homicides. Unfortunately, all of the warnings either were disregarded entirely or were not taken seriously.

5.1.2 The Role of Inadequacy

Lamberti, Blackman, and Weiss (1958) conducted a descriptive study of 13 sudden murderers in order to gain insight into the profile and motivations of such offenders. Typical of their sample was a 22-year-old who killed a 30-year-old woman (the cousin of his first wife) in a rather brutal fashion. He carried the remains in a laundry bag in the trunk of his car for several weeks before dumping the body in a creek. Following the homicide, and when evaluated, his affect was flat and bland even when discussing disturbing topics. The authors found underlying conflicts involving inadequacy and extreme dependence on and fear of women to be central in understanding this person's dynamics.

Surprisingly, Lamberti et al. found that their subjects' families of origin were overtly cohesive, in that they were intact and included both parents. However, further observations revealed that the fathers were generally hostile, rejecting, or indifferent, while the mothers were overprotective. Only in one case was the mother warm or accepting. In fact, only 1 out of the 13 offenders made a complete break from home; the researchers believed this demonstrated the subjects' closeness and abnormal emotional ties to their mothers. The offenders also evidenced ambivalent feelings and bad attitudes toward authority and a concomitant feeling of not being wanted, loved, recognized, or appreciated. Most also showed a fear of failure and defeat, with accompanying resentment toward successful people. But, most importantly, all offenders expressed "marked feelings of sexual inadequacy" (p. 9), a finding that was confirmed in a follow-up study (Blackman, Lum, and Vanderpearl, 1974) and supported by McCarthy (1978).

These sudden murders and assaults were precipitated by some sort of "insult" that seemed to threaten the subjects' sense of adequacy and stability in an important relationship—for example, belittling rejection by a sexually provocative paramour, a sadistic threat by a sexual partner, or "teasing" and provocative, hostile remarks. Eleven of the 13 offenders (85%) admitted or expressed a definite sense of relief after committing the crime. The investigators concluded that some type of insult "may trigger a sudden discharge of tension into a wish fulfilling, furious, violent, hostile lashing out—the sudden murder—which may be directed against a clearly significant person or against a stranger or a passer-by" (Lamberti et al., 1958, p. 12).

In a subsequent publication, Blackman, Weiss, and Lamberti (1963) analyzed a sample of 43 sudden murderers with a focus on detection, prevention, and intervention. In addition to the traits previously reported, these researchers again stressed that underlying conflicts of inadequacy, particularly sexual inadequacy involving rejection, may have triggered the attacks. They presented several cases as illustrations:

- *Case 1*: A 34-year-old man brutally murdered and subsequently mutilated his wife when she threatened to leave him. This offender could not tolerate her threat of rejection.
- *Case 2*: A 23-year-old was unable to express anger or to assert any masculine aggressiveness in the relationship with his wife. When she announced she was leaving, he shot her several times.
- *Case 3*: A 32-year-old dishwasher discussed future plans with two waitresses who encouraged him as long as he bought them drinks. When his money was spent, the waitresses told him to get out or they would call the police. He returned to the bar and shot and killed both women.
- *Case 4*: A 52-year-old male shot his wife in the head. The offender had made a suicide threat, to which the wife replied, "Who cares? Go ahead."
- *Case 5*: A 39-year-old shot his wife following an argument in which she cast doubts about his masculinity.

Blackman et al. (1963) reported that in 21 of their sudden-murder cases (49%), the offender had been seen prior to the crime by a mental health professional who found the person stable. Because the offenders' pronounced feelings of inadequacy were not obvious to the examining professionals, the authors concluded that their subjects presented a "mask of adequacy." They stressed the need for psychiatrists, psychologists, and workers in social agencies to be aware of such masks of adequacy so that violent proclivities can be recognized and sudden murders can perhaps be prevented.

Ruotolo (1968) conducted in-depth studies of five cases of sudden murder referred for forensic assessment. Using Karen Horney's concept as a frame of reference, he found that an injury to the individual's pride was the common denominator in the genesis of the homicidal acts. The murders were triggered by "a shattering blow to the individual's pride system, triggering off enormously intense self-hate" (p. 173). He also found that the victims set off conflicts of such a magnitude "as to threaten the entire unstable neurotic structure; … the pride systems of the murderers [were] shaken to their foundations, provoking the self hate" that led to the murderous assaults (p. 174). In a follow-up paper, Ruotolo (1975) discussed the role of self-hate, emotional detachment, and a perception of the victim as symbolizing an obstacle to stability, as additional factors contributing to the homicides. Ruotolo's findings corroborated those of Blackman et al. (1963) regarding the role of underlying inadequacy as well as the work of Satten et al. (1960) regarding the role of the victim in triggering the attack.

More recently, Berkowitz (1981) described three adolescents whose sudden violent outbursts (parental shooting, vehicular homicide, and suicide attempt by jumping out a window) were a direct result of feelings of inadequacy and powerlessness. The author found that, especially in adolescents, "depression, frustrated growth, hopelessness, and repressed anger may set the stage for the unpredictable eruption of strong, occasionally violent, uncontrolled impulses" (p. 478).

5.1.3 The Role of Organicity

Gayral, Millet, Moron, and Turnin (1956) studied a spectrum of paroxysms (sudden violent outbursts), extending from quasi-voluntary acts up to true epileptic manifestations. These authors categorized such phenomena as *crises catathymiques*. This view actually revived an earlier notion of Gowers (1885), who believed in the existence of a disorder falling between pure hysteria and epilepsy. Gayral and his colleagues believed that the sudden violence of the patients they studied was a result of neither epilepsy nor hysteria but was precipitated by a combination of emotional and physiological factors. In their paper, they present a number of typical cases where the aggressive outbursts were associated with varying degrees of alteration of consciousness.

Several years later, Revitch (1958, 1964) borrowed Gayral et al.'s notion of combining organic and psychogenic factors to explain violent outbursts that present a differential diagnosis with psychomotor epilepsy. The cases he studied—many seen in a female prison population—demonstrated seemingly unprovoked explosions of rage with agitation, destructiveness, and partial amnesia for the event. Some subjects fell to the ground and thrashed about, while others cut themselves with sharp objects. One woman severely cut her breasts with a piece of glass during such an attack. After prolonged observation and in-depth interviews, including the use of hypnosis and sodium amytal, Revitch concluded that these individuals had been incorrectly diagnosed as having psychomotor epilepsy. He uncovered emotional factors and precipitating triggers which he believed better explained the behavior. Labeling such paroxysms "catathymic attacks," he discontinued anticonvulsive medication—which he viewed as unnecessary—and transferred the individuals to a less stressful environment. Long-term follow-up found a cessation of violent outbursts in almost all cases.

"While an epileptic seizure is the correlate of a cerebral discharge, catathymic attacks are emotional release phenomena connected with poor ability to control, to inhibit, and to redirect the emotional impulses into constructive activity" (Revitch, 1964, p. 669). Abnormal EEGs (found in some subjects) do not always indicate epilepsy but rather an immaturity or defect in cerebral organization that makes it impossible for the subject to withstand anger, hostility, and tension without a behavioral discharge. The overall personalities of most of Revitch's subjects were so loose and immature that internal tension was released violently with little inhibition or modulation. The function of the release is to maintain internal psychic homeostasis in patients with immature personality makeups or with weakened inhibitory controls caused by some type of defective organization of the central nervous system.

5.1.4 "Affective" Aggression

Meloy (1988, 1992) noted that sudden catathymic homicides are affective—as opposed to predatory—types of violence; in this sense, they parallel the concept of a "blitz" attack used by the FBI to describe some disorganized sexual murders (Ressler et al., 1988). Meloy (1992) delineated the acute catathymic homicide as an event marked by

> intense autonomic arousal, overwhelming anger during the violence, the perception of the victim as an imminent threat to the ego structure of the perpetrator, a time limited behavioral sequence, and a goal of threat reduction and a return to intrapsychic homeostasis. (p. 47)

He found that acute catathymic murders not only are associated with disorganized crime scenes but also include, on the part of the murderer, various personality and mood disorders, attachment pathology, moderate levels of psychopathy, autonomic hyperactivity, and a history of physical or sexual trauma (or both) (Meloy, 2000). In a recent article, Meloy (2006) discussed the empirical support for distinguishing affective from predatory forms of violence.

Catathymic homicides, in Meloy's (1992) view, are differentiated from other forms of affective violence by an "unconscious motivation for the act and the symbolic significance of the victim" (p. 47). Accordingly, the author points out that "transference distortions" which trigger the violence can be identified through a careful history taking that focuses on the offender's problems in attachment. Such distortions are precipitated by one or more traits in the victim that the offender misperceives based on his or her conflicts. Meloy finds the Rorschach and the TAT helpful in understanding the dynamics of such events.

5.1.5 Presence of Dissociation and Trauma

Additional insight into the etiology of explosive catathymic violence is provided by Dicke (1994). He described three cases involving "inexplicable, sometimes bizarre, violence suddenly acted out with explosive rage against intimates, acquaintances or even strangers" (p. 10). As these defendants had no prior criminal record, Dicke first thought they might be malingering because of "the automaticity, vagueness, or amnesia for the event" (p. 12). His offenders had unstable families, overwhelming mothers, and absent or abusive fathers. Projective-test findings showed the offenders to be very attached to their mothers as well as likely victims of emotional abuse, abandonment, or maternal sexual abuse (or some combination of these). Subjects idealized their mothers as wonderful or perfect, while at an unconscious level, as the test results indicated, they felt "a rageful life and death struggle to get dependency needs met by [the] mother without being engulfed, abused or abandoned by her" (p. 11).

Dicke (1994) believes that in many cases of sudden catathymic violence, the offender also has a concomitant dissociative disorder and/or a posttraumatic stress disorder. This view has been supported by Heide and Solomon (2006) and Muskowitz (2004). Dicke found that many of his subjects suffered trauma and developed dissociative disorders as a result. However, the offenders were unable to make a conscious connection between the early traumatic event and the catathymic explosion. Thus, Dicke essentially views the violent act as a defense against internal pain. He found hypnosis to be helpful in diagnosing cases of catathymic violence because the defendants were able to reenact or reexperience the actual trauma or abuse which laid the foundation for the catathymic dynamics. The author believes that many of these cases have viable legal defenses: "I would venture to guess that the number of dissociative defendants throughout the country who are imprisoned for catathymic acts without their lawyers having raised their mental status is very significant" (p. 12).

Kirschner and Nagel (1996) also discussed the role of dissociation in explosive catathymic violence, particularly as it relates to individuals who were adopted. These authors contend that, because of the circumstances of being adopted, adoptees have a unique form of "trauma," which often leads to rageful feelings that erupt in catathymic violence. They relied on the work of Lifton (1994), who found adoptees to have "cumulative trauma" based on their separation from their birth mothers; this trauma is compounded when they are denied knowledge of their biological parents. Kirschner and Nagel believe that rage associated with dissociation (although not specific to adoptees) is frequently found in such cases. "An eruption of catathymic violence in adoptees is always triggered by a series of perceived or actual rejections that resonates with and reactivates the dissociative primary feelings of rejection and rage" (p. 207).

The authors present an illustrative case of an adopted young man with no prior history of violence, who developed a dissociative state following rejection by his girlfriend and an ultimatum from his father that he "get a job, join the military, or move out." The offender bludgeoned his adoptive parents to death and set their bodies on fire. Kirschner and Nagel stress that "adoption pathology" is a neglected area of inquiry in similar cases of violence and homicide.

5.1.6 Overcontrolled Personalities

Megargee (1966) found that overcontrolled individuals who have rigid inhibitions and strong moral beliefs against violence explode infrequently but in extremely violent ways. Cartwright (2001) also noted that many individuals who commit "rage-type" homicides are overcontrolled and appear "apparently normal" to others. Grubin (1994) observed this personality profile in a number of murderers whose crimes were associated with sexuality. He believes such offenders bottle up their rage, remain isolated interpersonally, and then suddenly explode when triggered in some way by the victim. One of Grubin's subjects strangled his victim with a cord so tightly pulled around her neck that the ambulance crew was unable to untie it. In another case, the brutal beating of an elderly woman resulted in 16 broken ribs, a torn liver, and a ruptured heart. Grubin found that anger and overcontrol were common characteristics of such offenders, who were not any more impulsive than others. And, as noted by other investigators, these men also reported feelings of inadequacy and powerlessness. In fact, in several cases, the offenders were unable to perform sexually until after the murder. The author concluded that a sense of power derived from the assault itself "finally enabled [them] to ejaculate" (p. 627).

5.2 Revitch and Schlesinger's Catathymic Process: Acute Catathymic Homicides

Although cases of catathymic crisis reported by Wertham (1937)—which entailed a protracted period of rumination prior to the act—and the cases of sudden murder cited above—which were spontaneous and unplanned—have many differences, there are also a number of similarities among such acts. For instance, both types of homicide typically involve men killing women. The victims release underlying conflicts in the offenders, usually involving strong feelings of inadequacy, particularly sexual inadequacy. The symbolic relationship of the victim to the offender is paramount in understanding the underlying emotional conflicts and the triggers for the act. Following the homicide, after the tension is released, the offenders return to a state of psychic homeostasis, sometimes involving a feeling of relief or a flattening of emotions. Both types of offenders either turn themselves in or do not attempt to elude the authorities for long. In addition, mental health professionals see many such offenders prior to the acts but do not recognize the ominous significance of the problems the offenders are secretly struggling with. Table 5.1 provides a summary of the similarities between both types of homicides.

Such distinct similarities led Revitch and Schlesinger (1978, 1981, 1989) to conclude that both forms of homicidal violence, the sudden as well as the more protracted, stem from the same underlying psychodynamic process, but it is expressed differently in each form. Accordingly, Revitch and Schlesinger differentiated two types of catathymic homicide, the acute and the chronic. Neither type is a clinical diagnosis; rather, catathymia is a psychodynamic process, or what Meloy (1992) has been referred to as a motivational process. This process occurs along with various clinical diagnoses, which might range from different types of personality and mood disorders through the psychotic conditions (Schlesinger, 1996a,b). The chronic catathymic homicide is generally consistent with Wertham's (prolonged) catathymic crisis, while the acute catathymic homicide is sudden and unplanned.

Acute catathymic homicides should be differentiated from situational acts of violence and from common assaults committed in an explosion of anger, fear, or jealousy or under the influence of paranoid delusions, drugs, or alcohol. In some cases, however, alcohol may help release the accumulation of catathymic tension since the acute catathymic process taps a much deeper source of emotional tension. In acute catathymic homicides, superficially integrated individuals who secretly struggle with strong feelings of inadequacy, primarily sexual inadequacy, resort to violence when victims challenge their sense of integrity, adequacy, or sexual competence. The depth of the inadequacy almost always extends to the sexual area since low self-esteem by itself is not enough to stimulate the process.

5.2.1 Sexual Inadequacy

The sexual nature of acute catathymic homicides is frequently not recognized by law enforcement authorities or by many mental health professionals because of the absence of manifest expressions of genitality. Nevertheless, in almost all these cases, the underlying sexual dynamics become obvious as the offender explains, or attempts to explain, his behavior.

The following cases are illustrative of acute catathymic homicides triggered by sexual inadequacy, a motivation that was not apparent until the offender and the offense were carefully studied.

Table 5.1 Similarities between Acute and Chronic Catathymic Homicides

- Cases primarily involve men killing women.
- Victim is viewed in symbolic terms.
- Victim triggers underlying, emotionally charged conflicts.
- Conflicts center on strong feelings of inadequacy, extending to the sexual area.
- Homicide releases emotional tension.
- Following homicide, psychic homeostasis is quickly reestablished.
- Feeling of relief or flattening of emotions (or both) is common after the act.
- Offenders typically do not attempt to elude authorities for long and often tell a friend what happened or call the police themselves.
- Mental health professionals do not recognize the ominous significance of the offender's conflicts prior to the act.
- Investigators sometimes miss the underlying sexual motivation because overt manifestations of genitality are often absent.

Case 5.1: Feelings of Sexual Inadequacy Triggered by an Insult from a Woman

An 18-year-old high school senior strangled a 22-year-old female nightclub entertainer with a rubber hose after she entered the gasoline station he worked at to make a phone call. AA was a part-time attendant and was alone at the time of the homicide. When the victim entered the gas station, she asked to borrow a dime for a telephone call. After AA gave her the dime and she made her phone call, the victim pulled her dress up and invited AA to have sexual relations with her. He approached the woman and attempted intercourse but was unable to obtain an erection. The victim taunted, "Go home to your mother." AA then grabbed a piece of rubber tubing, wrapped it around the victim's neck, strangled and killed her.

He put the body in the trunk of his car, dropped it off at a local field, covered the body slightly with twigs and leaves, and went home. He slept well that night. When he woke the next morning, he thought that what had occurred was "a dream."

> I went to school as if nothing happened. At noon I picked up my girlfriend for lunch and we went shopping, and then I got ready for work. While I was working, the incident started to bother me. I thought I was dreaming. I looked in the trunk of my car and saw her eyeglasses there, and I realized that maybe I was not dreaming. I closed the gas station after work and went to the spot to see if the body was there. I thought that if they didn't find a corpse, then I was really dreaming and the whole thing had not taken place.

The police came to AA's home the next day to speak with him since he worked in the vicinity where the body had been found. He did not connect their presence with the homicide and believed, for some reason, that he was going to be questioned about a stolen car. For the next several days, he continued his usual activities as if nothing had happened. He was summoned to appear at the police station, still feeling that the homicide was a dream. However, when the detective asked whether he had killed a woman, he answered, "Yes, I did it." "I realized inside, I guess, that I would not get away with it. Inside of me I felt guilty. I felt better after I admitted doing it."

AA gave the following description of the homicide:

> It was late in the evening and the station was about to close. She took some of her clothes off and told me not to be afraid. My mind was blank. She grabbed me by the wrist and pulled me to come towards her. I pulled my hand away but she kept saying, "come on, I won't hurt you." She kissed my neck. She unbuttoned my pants. I turned around and looked at her and tried to have sex standing up. She pushed me away and said I was a little boy and told me to go back to my mother. I left, and as I was coming out of the panel room, I grabbed a rubber tubing. I got her from behind, put it around her neck. She scratched my nose and said that her husband was coming back to pick her up, and then I think she stopped moving. I guess I imagined she was dead. I pulled my car up to the front, opened the trunk, and put her in. I drove to a dirt road where people dumped things. I took her out of the trunk and her hand grabbed my pants. It scared me.

Anal intercourse (revealed by the autopsy, which found semen in the rectum) was initially denied (because of embarrassment). AA later admitted to the act and said it occurred after the homicide. The victim, once dead, was no longer threatening to AA, a common dynamic in many cases of necrophilia. When she was lifeless, he was able to obtain an erection and penetrate her. Clearly, the victim's taunting made him feel inadequate and angry, especially the victim's comment, when he was unable to effect an erection, that he should go back to his mother. In addition, the victim's aggressive approach was ego-threatening and rendered him confused and helpless by confronting him with his immaturity and inadequacy.

Psychological testing revealed average intelligence; he had a rigid personality makeup and referred to feelings of inadequacy in his TAT stories. Neither the Rorschach nor the TAT pointed to any predisposition toward or preoccupation with violence; however, they did indicate a need for control and a reliance on brittle intellectual defenses with few secondary supports. He had no history of criminal behavior prior to the murder and was well liked by friends and teachers.

In this case, memory for the event was preserved despite its explosive nature. The recollection of the incident had a dreamlike quality and was related without an emotional display, in an objective, quasi-clinical manner, typical of most of these cases. Although the event was recalled, it was perceived as ego-alien and unreal.

Case 5.2: Feelings of Inadequacy Triggered by Child's Comments

A 30-year-old male suddenly murdered a 10-year-old girl when she came to his door to sell magazine subscriptions. BB opened the door when she rang the bell. He owed her $2 for the magazines, but since he had only a $20 bill, the child told him that she would return later in the day for the money and not to be concerned. At this point, he felt angry and humiliated because he was unable to solve the problem, and "she had to tell me what to do." He forced her to go down to the basement, where he choked her, beat her, and smashed her head against the floor, inflicting serious injuries that led to her death. The autopsy of the child's body revealed extensive head injuries, laceration of the chin, hematoma of both eyes, a tear inside the upper lip, three broken teeth with bleeding inside the mouth, a bruised right knee, fractured neck, dislocation of both shoulders, fracture of the skull, contusion and hemorrhage of the brain, and evidence of a ruptured hymen and bruises throughout the vaginal wall.

Following the homicide (and vaginal necrophilia), BB wrapped the child's body in a plastic bag, covered it with a blanket, and put it in the trunk of his car. With a calm demeanor, he casually spoke with a neighbor while driving out of the driveway. BB then drove to a local field, disposed of the clothes on the way, and left the body in a garbage pile in an isolated area. He then returned home and slept well. He first denied the murder when questioned by the authorities but then admitted it following a polygraph at the police station.

BB was raised in a stable, middle-class family and lived with his mother and grandmother. As a youth, he worked as a camp counselor and was described as a gentle person, fond of animals, and "incapable of hurting even an insect." He was employed as an accountant at the time of the offense and had a master's degree in business. He had no history of any prior criminal acts. Several years earlier, he was briefly engaged to a woman but broke the commitment after he felt she might discover his "weakness and stupidity."

His intelligence fell within the superior range, and he gave no indications of violence on the Rorschach or the TAT. Even on TAT card 13MF (which usually elicits sexually aggressive content in the predisposed), he responded,

> It was the morning after a drinking party. The guy just woke up with a bad hangover and does not even recognize the girl that he was in bed with. He is trying to get it all together so he can leave, as the girl is still asleep.

His personality had some obsessive features, with dominant feelings of insecurity, inadequacy, and low self-esteem.

When interviewed under the influence of sodium amytal, BB described the homicide as follows:

> I could not solve the problem solved by the little girl. I felt embarrassed, ashamed, and angry, and felt I had to destroy her. Then after it was over, I was standing and shaking. I was sweating. I did not know what to do. I felt better when I went back to the house after disposing of the body. I slept well. It was a split feeling. It happened but it was not to me; like I was an observer of the event. I did not remember strangling the little girl, but I remember banging her head, watching myself. It was like a separate feeling. I was not upset, but, yet, I was not peaceful. I also did not want to believe that I did it. I could not convince myself of doing such a thing.

When asked why he attempted to penetrate the child sexually, he stated, "It was total domination of man over woman. A man dominates a woman through rape." He reported some vague rape fantasies while in high school, but he had never acted on them. He also developed fantasies of sexual contact with young, nonthreatening children of prepubescent age. He had fantasies about women his own age but felt they would not be receptive to his advances.

BB described tremendous self-hatred and inferiority in many aspects of his life. He despised himself for what he regarded as "inadequacies." At one point, he felt stupid because he was unable to repair a lawnmower. He also claimed he was afraid of appearing stupid to others. For example, when he had to go to an unfamiliar place, he explored the area a day ahead so he would not lose his way. The offender emphasized that because the child had so easily solved the problem of making change, he felt particularly stupid: "I hated her." Following the homicide and body disposal, he was slightly disturbed for a short time, but this feeling was replaced by a superficial calm and a degree of depersonalization, which is not uncommon in such cases.

Case 5.3: Feelings of Inadequacy Triggered by an Inability to Satisfy a Woman Sexually

A 24-year-old male (CC) was evaluated following the strangulation murder of a prostitute and the subsequent dismembering of her body. After leaving his factory job at midnight, CC went to a nightclub with his brother. He left the club at 3:00 a.m. and met a prostitute, who was obviously looking for a client, on a nearby street. CC took the prostitute back to his apartment, where his mother and two brothers were also living.

The victim came out of the bathroom, partially undressed, and got in bed with CC. She repetitively told the offender that sex had to be completed quickly because "she had to meet someone at 5:30. She constantly looked at the clock by the TV." They engaged in oral sex, and then "she got on top of me. I rolled over on her and then strangled her." But, before the strangulation, he lost an erection or "had half an erection."

In describing the homicide, CC said:

> I am watching myself do this. Looking down at myself doing this. Everything seemed hazy, like walking into a cloud. I could see myself doing it, but I couldn't stop. It was like watching a movie. Everything happened so fast, but I don't know what I was thinking about. I can't tell you what I was thinking. I was watching myself. It was like a dream.

After strangling the victim, he indicated that he sat at the edge of the bed. Then, "I put her in the bathtub, but I don't know why." He heard noises like "steam" in the room. "Then I cut her up. I got a knife out of the kitchen. It was like an impulse." When asked to explain the impulse further, he was unable to elaborate. CC remembered seeing a duffle bag in the hallway; following the dismemberment, he put the various body parts in the bag, opened the back door, and dropped the bag off the fire escape to the yard below. The offender then washed out the bathtub, put the knives in the sink, and put the sheet and blankets from the bed into the tub. When questioned further as to the dismemberment, CC said,

> I don't know. I guess I didn't want a dead body in the house because of my mother. I threw the body in the bag out the fire escape and then dragged the bag about five feet to hide it.

He next took his brother's car and drove on a major thoroughfare. He was unable to explain why he fled the scene except to say, "I just wanted to leave, but I don't know where I was going. I just drove." While driving, he hit a guardrail after falling asleep. He got out of his car when the police arrived.

> I was still trying to figure out what happened. I told the cops, "I think I killed somebody." It didn't seem real. If I turn myself in, and if it wasn't real, they'd let me go. I didn't know it was real until the second time the police came in the holding cell.

CC had a long-standing obsessional idea that "my penis is too small." In fact, he bought several devices he read about in pornographic magazines to enlarge his penis. Also of significance was his suspiciousness regarding his girlfriend. On the day of the homicide, CC had an argument with her as she had accused him of "checking on her" by driving by, calling her house and following her. He accused her of unfaithfulness.

Psychological test findings provide further insight into the dynamics of his case. The offender's intelligence fell within the low-average range, with no evidence of organicity. A number of regressive Rorschach perceptions suggest a mild borderline personality structure, illustrated by the following: "A set of lungs. Bad lungs." "A fetus and embryo cord." "A nuclear blast. The colors. The explosion. The flames." Total lack of any human (movement) perceptions on the Rorschach suggest a deficit in empathic capacity, as well as difficulty in forming reciprocal and mature interpersonal relationships. Although there was no evidence of any type of psychosis, his defenses were rather brittle. Several scale elevations on the MMPI indicated mild depression and anxiety, plus unusual thinking involving feelings of estrangement and alienation from others.

Although the offender appeared superficially intact from a clinical perspective, he was struggling with strong feelings of low self-esteem and sexual inadequacy, which were revealed particularly on the TAT. CC produced many stories demonstrating interpersonal conflicts, especially within male–female relationships. In one story, the central character revealed his view of women:

> She was messing around with someone because he wasn't satisfying her sexually, or she just wanted to go out and have some fun. She wanted to see what it was like to have two men. Girls want one-night stands. Or she did it to help him. Maybe she had sex with his boss, and this would get him a better job.

This story not only shows his fear of rejection by females due to his own sexual inadequacy, but also his view of women as untrustworthy and as using sex in a manipulative way.

The following is perhaps the most enlightening TAT story because of the reference to an inability to satisfy the victim and the expression of strong feelings of sexual inadequacy:

> He killed her. He strangled her himself. He has a sick mind. Hatred towards her or maybe he caught her the night before with somebody. He spent all his time with her and she went out and did something. He trusted her to be honest and she wasn't. He didn't totally satisfy her. He was incompetent [probably meaning impotent], or maybe premature ejaculation, or half an erection. The girl feels, "Why get mixed up with a guy like this who can't do anything for me? I'll get somebody else." He feels less than a man, not capable of satisfying her. He could commit suicide. He is on the verge of it.

The offender's drawings are shown in Figure 5.1. His sketch of a female is reasonably well done, but the rather strange male drawing reflects inadequacy, as he was unable to draw a full male figure ("I can't do it"). CC emphasized that he did not "pay for sex" but only spent money on cocaine as requested by the victim. "She just wanted to get high." The toxicology report, however, showed no substances in the victim, indicating that the offender was untruthful on this one point, perhaps because he was embarrassed to admit he paid for sex.

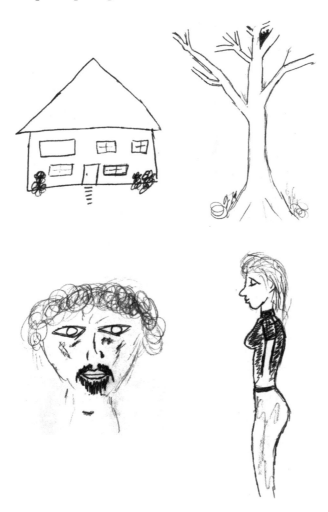

Figure 5.1 Drawings by offender who killed and dismembered a prostitute.

CC's description of the homicide is a classic expression of a depersonalized state, typical in acute catathymic murders. His history reveals sexual inadequacy, especially his persistent belief that his penis was too small. His inability to satisfy the victim, as well as the victim commenting that she had to leave and her watching the clock, triggered the explosion. The dismemberment was not an attempt to dispose of the body; he could have easily fit the body in the duffle bag without dismemberment because the victim weighed only 88 pounds. The dismemberment was thus probably a continuation of the catathymic anger which was not fully released by the strangulation. Rajs, Lundström, Broberg, Lidberg, and Lindquist (1998) reported a number of dismemberment cases with similar dynamics.

Case 5.4: Feelings of Inadequacy Triggered by
Suspicions of the Victim's Unfaithfulness

A 45-year-old male (DD) shot and killed his live-in girlfriend (B), had vaginal intercourse with the dead body, and then dismembered her in his basement. Both victim and offender were substance abusers but neither was under the influence at the time of the murder. They met in a rehabilitation program and lived together for 2 years. DD had been unemployed for several months; he had lost his clerical job because of excessive absences, a result of substance abuse. B had been employed (as a secretary) for 1 year, but lost her job as well.

The victim demanded money from DD on a continual basis. He had gone through about $30,000 of his savings (in 6 months) in order to give B money to procure cocaine. As DD's money ran out, B began to prostitute herself in order to get money for drugs. The victim and offender argued constantly about her conduct, which offended (and humiliated) him greatly. DD was unable to tolerate the thought of his girlfriend "going out on weekends doing tricks."

One afternoon, during sexual relations, the victim got dressed and said she would be back in several hours. DD assumed she was going out to earn money as a prostitute. After an argument, DD grabbed his gun and shot B at close range. Following the shooting, he had sex with her "to see who gets the last fuck." He then took the victim to his basement and dismembered the body. He cut off the arms and legs, wrapped them in bags, and deposited them in a local meadow. He took the head off and put it in a pot of boiling water (on the stove) in order to "boil it down, and remove the skin and organs." DD told the police (when eventually arrested) that he planned to keep the skull. The offender was an experienced hunter who had several deer heads mounted in his apartment. In addition, he kept the bones of several animals that he had shot. For example, he had the spinal cord of a deer (with a bullet hole in it), as well as the shoulder of another deer. He said he wanted to save the skull of the victim as another souvenir. After living with the body for about a week, he called a friend, confessed to the crime, and was subsequently arrested.

With his first wife, DD had a history of domestic violence that was also triggered by his accusations of unfaithfulness. The police were at his house several times because of arguments and fights, one of which involved breaking furniture. However, he was not arrested and had no prior criminal record. He had two children, aged 14 and 18, from whom he was estranged. The offender lived in a middle-class area, had graduated from college, and was generally respected by his neighbors. Those who knew DD never thought he was capable of homicide, necrophilia, dismemberment, or devising a plan to save the victim's skull. As in Case 5.3, the dismemberment here seems to have been a continuation of the catathymic anger, which was not fully released by the homicide. Psychological evaluation did not reveal any evidence of an underlying compulsion to kill.

5.2.2 Displaced Matricide

Conflicts regarding sexual inadequacy in acute catathymic homicides are frequently interwoven with conflicts regarding maternal images. Sometimes the offender's mother is idealized—considered pure and unsoiled by sex—or she may be perceived as rejecting, hateful, or immoral. Such ideas may be induced by the mother's infidelity to her husband or by her sexual conduct with other men. Meloy (1988, 1992) believes that maternal rage is often a result of the feelings of helplessness and dependence aroused in a male, who observes his mother's sexually promiscuous conduct. Maternal sexual promiscuity and indiscretion are more upsetting to males than to females: "A boy's perception of his mother's infidelity and sexual looseness is more traumatic than a girl's perception of the same behavior in her father" (Revitch and Schlesinger, 1989, p. 108). Perhaps cultural standards play a role in this phenomenon.

Lewis and Yarnell (1951) reported the case of a young man whose preoccupation with fire and female purity was similar to dynamics found in many cases of sexual homicide. The offender was disturbed by his mother's promiscuous sexual behavior. He hallucinated hearing his mother's voice inviting him to have sexual relations with her, and he even had a vision of flaming genitals in front of him. Following this experience, he set fire to his mother's bedroom and her clothing. These authors believed that this case could be best explained by Freud's (1910) theory of the splitting of the maternal image into "good mother" and "bad mother." In this connection, Mathis (1971) described the Madonna–prostitute syndrome, which also involves the split between good and bad images of the mother. Men with such maternal conflicts are frequently unable to obtain an erection with their wives unless the wives are sexually degraded in some manner. Only a "degraded woman" is not like the Madonna–mother and does not induce panic anxiety over the thought of an incestuous relationship. Karpman (1935) also found these oedipal preoccupations in some of his cases.

An acute catathymic homicide can be the result of a displacement of suddenly induced hostile emotions from the mother to the victim, although not all acute catathymic homicides involve such displacements. In some cases, these conflicts are masked and are not obvious until the offender is thoroughly evaluated and is willing to discuss his thoughts and feelings in an open and direct manner. Revitch (1965) noted that adolescents and preadolescents who committed unprovoked sexual attacks were particularly preoccupied with maternal sexual conduct and morality, and this conflict served as a trigger for their outbursts. The following cases are illustrative of acute catathymic homicides involving a displaced matricide.

Case 5.5: Typical Displaced Matricide

A 24-year-old male (EE) killed a 39-year-old woman, whom he had known for only several hours, by slashing her throat with a knife. Earlier in the evening, around 8:00 p.m., he had gone to a local bar.

> I hit on a chick at the bar. Some bar trash there. I talked to her. She wanted nothing to do with me, and I wasn't into her world, which was drugs. So I decided to go home. I had to go to work the next day, so the hell with it.

At around 10:00 p.m., EE ran into the victim in the parking lot of his apartment building.

I said, "What's going on?" and started bullshitting with her. I didn't think nothing of it. I said, "What are you doing tonight?" I don't remember exactly what I said. I invited her up to my apartment, and she went up there with me. She rambled on about this and that. I put the moves on her. I kissed her, and she had no objection and she proceeded down. Nothing was said; she did it herself. She didn't want intercourse. She said, "Not right now." I wouldn't force myself on her because she said no. It was just oral sex.

We stayed at my apartment for a half hour talking. I offered to go for a drive. She said, "All right," and we made small talk. She was talking about a lot of things. I thought she was dingy at the time. I pulled over one block from the boardwalk because she said she wanted to walk on the beach and look at the ocean. We got out of the car, and she mentioned it was a clear night, a nice night. A nice night. I had a hunch maybe our chemistry would work out, and she'd be in the mood if she got to know me a little better. We walked on the beach. It was about a half mile from the boardwalk. We sat down a bit. I wanted sex.

She started talking again. Then I took a change. I wasn't looking forward to sex anymore. I got tired of listening to her. I sat there in my own little world. She kept on and on. I was thinking to myself. My head started going wild. I felt pressure. I started getting pissed off. She was rambling on about things, about drugs, about alcohol. She asked if I had a joint. She kept asking me. I don't know why, but I told her no.

I stared at her for a second. I got into a complete rage. To be honest, I was blind with hate of myself, the whole damn thing. Not specifically mad at her but at other things. I lunged out at her, an impulse. Actually, my mind was like someone screaming in my head, just screaming. I backhanded her across the face, getting wild more or less.

She screamed a little bit. I was like an automated machine. I knocked her down, tackled her. She was hollering, screaming. I hit her hard in the face. I don't know why. It wasn't a planned-out deal. She got dazed. I brought out my knife, from my pocket. It was like I was a machine. I started stabbing her. She put her arms up and started hollering how she loved me. Then I yelled out, "No, you don't." I felt real weird about that. It was a major surprise. I don't know what possessed me to say "No, you don't." Then I stabbed her quite a few times. I had enough. Then I cut her throat. She was dying. I assumed she was dying. I kept going through with it. I was in motion.

I asked myself a thousand times why I did it. It didn't seem real. It seemed like a bad dream. The whole thing didn't seem real. Part of me was seeing myself doing it. I could see me doing what I was doing like I was being supervised. I was watching myself. I was like watching myself like I was elevated above myself and watching. I wasn't in control, like I was watching myself. That's the best I could do to describe it.

I stood up, watched her for a second, looked off to my left and thought something was approaching me. So I took off. It didn't even hit me until I took off in my car that what happened, happened. I washed off by the boardwalk. My mind was calm and quiet after this. I washed off with cold water. It made me feel clean then. I started getting nervous, so I took off. I went home, went to sleep. I had a dream where something had happened. I took a shower and went to work in the morning. I was thinking of what happened, couldn't have happened.

While at work, I noticed a wound. That was a crash to reality. It reminded me it had happened. I worked the whole day at the carwash. Later on, I called my friend and told him what happened. I told him that I killed a man. It was a disgrace that I killed a woman.

EE was subsequently arrested, and he gave a detailed statement to the police.

The offender's background included being abandoned by his mother at age 3. He was raised by his father and had a somewhat troubled adolescence, getting into minor school difficulties but nothing very serious beyond a number of fights. He described lifelong problems relating to females. "When I'm sober, I can't talk to women. I like older women because it's easier to relate to them than girls my own age." He explained that he had been with exactly 18 women sexually but "only two when sober." He also reported a chronic belief that "my penis is too small." "I can tell that's what they [the women] are thinking. I ask them, and they say it's about average size." He also reported intrusive sexual thoughts "that make me sick." "I think of doing things with other guys, oral sex on them." EE was a rigid, political and cultural conservative, who deplored taking drugs and being sexually promiscuous even though he had engaged in this conduct "with trash."

On the urging of EE's maternal aunt, he reunited with his mother 4 months prior to the homicide. He was devastated from the moment he met her.

I hated her. I couldn't stand who she was. She looked like a full-blown alcoholic. As soon as we met, she grabbed my ass a few times, constantly looking down at my crotch. When she drank, she pointed to my ass and said to her friend, "That's mine." I think she wanted my ass. The first night I met her, she put her hands down my pants. That about made me lose my mind. But it was the first time I met her.

She would wear real skimpy clothes and cut-off shorts. I had thoughts of sex with my mother. One night she was lying in the back of her van. I walked up and laid above her, over her. She grabbed around me. She pulled me around her. I locked my elbows and didn't go down. Her boyfriend saw some of it, but he said nothing. After that day, my migraines blew off the charts. I got sexual thoughts about my mother. I have thoughts now. I had thoughts of killing my mother. I'd watch her cook, and I'd think. I thought of going over there and breaking her fucking neck.

EE described having sexual relations with one of his mother's neighbors.

She came over. She and my mother were drinking. They were both staring at me. Then I hanged around outside for a while. We went to a bar, and I started dancing with my mom's friend. We went back to the house. She was rubbing against me all night. There was no per-suasion. We got in the house, and we started kissing and took off our clothes. She gave me oral sex, and from there I was going to do the same with her, but she didn't want anything to do with that. We went at it. She seemed into it. She wanted me to pull her hair for some reason. I really thought my mom was watching the whole time from the living room. I felt her presence. I am not sure. After this, we went to sleep. My mom arranged all this. We'd sleep on the floor together. The next morning I talked to her a little bit, but I didn't like it at all.

EE had average intelligence with a history of a mild learning disability. The Rorschach and the TAT showed characterological disturbance but no evidence of any psychosis or problems with reality contact. Projective figure drawings (see Figure 5.2) reflected inner tension, self-image disturbance, and low self-esteem, evidenced particularly by drawings of people without any facial features.

The most revealing psychological test findings were several TAT stories in which EE graphically described the dynamics of the homicide.

Card 18GF:

She is a total disappointment and an alcoholic, a liar, and everything. He is trying to rip his mother's throat out. He can't believe that that's his mom. They have nothing in common.

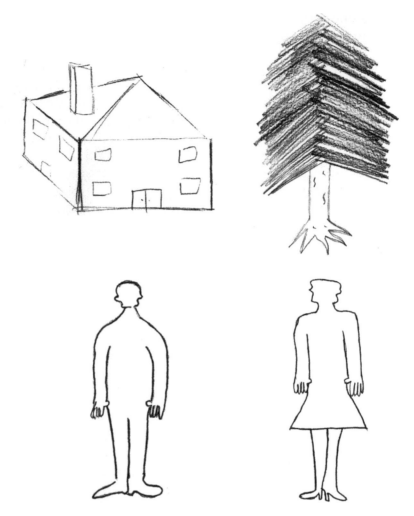

Figure 5.2 Sketches by offender who committed a displaced matricide.

They are two different people. She embarrasses him in front of everybody else—her conduct in front of other people, just the way she maintains herself in front of everybody else. She is a drunk. The picture screams out "I hate you." He is trying to kill his mom. He is choking her to death, trying to rip her throat out. The throat is a vulnerable area. All animals do it there, strangulation. He is tired of her being a disappointment. It makes him feel disgusted.

His mom is a weak person—emotionally weak and a liar. The mother's activities throughout her life is what that person is totally against—drugs. Talk, talk, like everything is a big party. Conversations are all about something funny—no intelligent conversation. When you talk about getting high or getting fucked up, that's important. If you try to discuss past events in your life, no response. Try talk about the news, no response. He can't believe that that's where he came from. How the hell can you be my mother? All your life you are told your mother was a good person, and there she is, a total opposite of what you are told. She discards you at birth.

You see her for what she is. She tries to befriend you by telling stories. She is checking you up and down all the time, looking at your ass all the time, staring at your crotch, grabbing your damn ass when she is drunk, pointing your ass out to her friends. On a level such as this, he could have had a sexual relationship with his mother. She couldn't acknowledge that's her child. You want to throw your hands up, smash her head against the wall, especially when you have sex with her friend and she watches. Her presence was there.

Card 13MF:

He is ashamed of what he's done. It looks like he killed her. They didn't have sex because he is fully dressed. A woman like this is a class of evil. The sole objective is herself—nothing more. To see who she is sickens himself. She was talking about evil spirits, ghosts, demons, all that shit. That's the type of possession that ruined your life. They took your mom from you—drugs and the whole lifestyle.

It reminds him of his mother. That's the type of person she is. He didn't mean to do it. That irritating sound colliding in your mind, hearing your own life calling you, everything hit you in the head. It looks like she'd got a neck wound, there in the picture. You can see it right there. Look what he has become. Look what he is reduced to. I imagine there is a lot more to it.

This case involves not only maternal rejection but EE's lifelong fantasy that his mother was "a good person" and his view that women who act out sexually are "trash." When he met his mother, his fantasy was shattered, as his mother epitomized the opposite of what (conservative) EE stood for. His mother not only was involved in alcohol and drug abuse but was sexually provocative in her behavior and came on to the offender sexually as well. She even arranged for the offender to have sex with her friend while she allegedly watched. It is unclear whether EE actually had sex with his mother (in the van); he denied it, although it was suspected at the time of the investigation.

The victim's behavior reminded EE of his mother, as both were "into drugs, drinking, and promiscuous sex." When the victim began discussing drugs and alcohol, maternal images flooded the offender's consciousness, and the emotions were displaced on the victim. The victim thus resurrected major maternal conflicts, and EE transferred his anger from his mother to a mother substitute whom he killed.

Case 5.6: Displaced Anger Stemming from Maternal Neglect

A 28-year-old man (FF) suddenly attacked and killed a young woman while he was working in her home. He was cleaning the homeowner's rugs and was alone in the house with the victim and her 18-month-old child. After about half an hour, FF heard the baby "screaming and crying" from the second floor. Out of concern, he told the mother. The woman acknowledged his remark but returned to her activities without seeming very concerned about her child. FF then walked upstairs, with the victim right behind him.

Suddenly, FF took a handgun from his waistband, turned, and pointed it at the woman. (He said he always carried a gun because it made him "feel stronger" emotionally.) The woman was at first incredulous, remarking, "Is this a joke?" He then grabbed her around the waist, dragged her into a room, and knelt over her, straddling her legs. The victim said, "Don't hurt me or the baby. I'll cooperate. I'll do whatever you want." The offender unbuttoned her blouse and tied her hands in front of her with a cleaning rag. She said, "You don't have to do that. I'll cooperate." He then tied another rag around her head and mouth so that "I wouldn't have to hear her keep saying, 'I'll cooperate, I'll cooperate.'" He pulled her pants and underwear off and turned her over on her stomach. Without any hesitation, he put his gun to the back of her head and shot her.

FF recalled hearing the bubbling sound of blood spilling on the floor, which "fascinated" him. When this sound stopped, he felt angry and shot her again a second time. He then turned on all the lights, looked at the crime scene, and felt horrified at what had happened. He quickly exited the house, leaving all his cleaning equipment behind. FF drove to his place of employment, cashed a check, and left some money for his wife and two children. He then drove to a friend's house and revealed what had happened. His friend contacted the police and FF was quickly arrested.

At the age of 14, the offender entered a state-sponsored youth program because of repeatedly running away from home. He had a terrible family situation; his mother, who had been married several times and lived with many men, drank to excess and spent child-support money on alcohol. While incarcerated at another juvenile institution (for various behavioral problems), he received further rejection from his parents and grandparents. Following his release, FF lived with his father and stepmother for a time, but he believed that they were unconcerned about him, and he described his stepmother as rather punitive. He believed that his stepsiblings disliked him and that they told other kids he was "no good." FF was also unhappy when he lived with his mother. He claimed that her live-in boyfriend punished him brutally. He alleged his mother hit him with a whip and the boyfriend bathed him in alcohol after the beating.

As an adolescent, FF wanted to be a police officer, a position he associated with "goodness" and morality. He believed that girls did not like him; they refused to date him, but they went out with other boys. He regarded himself as ugly and said that girls teased him about having big ears. On a couple of occasions, he was expelled from school for antagonizing teachers and for carrying a knife. The weapon "made me feel strong."

In this case, the victim's conduct—specifically, not responding to her screaming child—evoked images of maternal neglect stemming from FF's own disturbed background. In addition, because he was always bothered by his own mother's sexual promiscuity and indiscreetness, he was angered and disgusted by the victim's pleading with him in promising to cooperate (i.e., to submit to him sexually)—actions that led to her death. As is often the case in acute catathymic murders, the offender was horrified by his behavior. He left a note and money for his wife and children, behavior that illustrated his concern for them.

Case 5.7: Displaced Anger Stemming from Unspecified Dislike of Mother

An unprovoked sexual attack by a 16-year-old boy (GG) on a 22-year-old (who was 9 months pregnant) occurred in broad daylight at a train station. According to the police report, the offender grabbed the woman from behind in order to lift her skirt and pull down her underwear. He threw her to the ground, touched her genitals, and was quickly apprehended before being able to injure her further or kill her. The attack itself was triggered by the victim's obvious pregnancy which upset GG. "It made me angry. I don't know why."

The adolescent came from an intact working-class family; his father was employed as a carpenter and his mother was a housewife. He had no prior criminal involvement and no disciplinary problems in school. His intelligence fell within the low-average range, but, clinically, he appeared empty and rather dull with flat affect. His figure drawings reflected emotional detachment. For example, he drew a picture of a house with a sign on the front "do not enter" (Figure 5.3).

The offender reported conflicts with both males and females, but he was particularly disturbed by girls "who call me crazy." He had difficulty discussing sexuality. When the

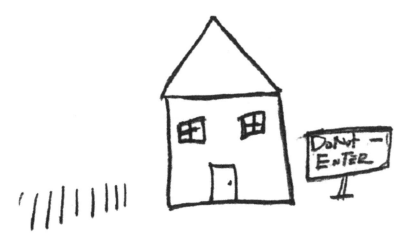

Figure 5.3 Drawing done by a 16-year-old who assaulted a pregnant woman reflects social isolation. The sign reads "do not enter."

topic was brought up, he responded, "Everyone just has sex on their mind." Some hostility was noted toward his father, but particular anger toward his mother for unclear reasons. ("I don't know if I hate her, but I dislike her.") One of his drawings was of a male running after an older female with a stick in hand, about to hit her (see Figure 2.7, Chapter 2).

Case 5.8: Displaced Anger Stemming from Multiple Conflicts Regarding Sex, Inadequacy, and Morality

This case illustrates an unprovoked sexual attack by an introverted adolescent. He was hostile toward females, preoccupied with sexual morality, had fantasies of sexual purity regarding his mother, and had strong feelings of inadequacy stemming partly from a distorted body image.

The 14-year-old offender (HH) choked and stabbed (but miraculously did not kill) a 10-year-old girl who came to his house to visit his sister. He described the attack as follows:

> When I heard her knocking at the door, my stomach was all upset; my mouth was dry, and my head was spinning all around. Then I remembered calling her in. Then I took the knife, and I attacked her, choked her, and cut her neck. When I awoke, like from a dream, I let her go. Then I went to my room and prayed.

A few hours prior to the incident, HH had had an argument with his mother because she had inadvertently broken one of his toys. He revealed fantasies of maternal sexual abstinence (even from having sex with his father) "because it's forbidden." He avoided girls at school, especially those who behaved "indecently," and expressed general dislike for girls because some of them made fun of him.

The victim of the attack did not symbolize his mother as in Case 5.5. Here, the generalized anger and conflict at HH's mother was transferred to the victim, who evoked erotic feelings in him (as his mother possibly did). In fact, HH's sister had told him that the victim "liked me." When the young girl entered the house, HH became anxious. By attacking her, he actually attacked an image of sexual impurity. He felt he took "revenge on girls" for their real or imaginary rejection of him. The violence made him feel more in control and reduced feelings of inadequacy.

5.2.3 Sexual Matricide

Most acute catathymic murders that involve conflicts with maternal conduct and maternal images result in a displacement of emotion from the mother to a victim substitute. However, in a much smaller number of cases the offender actually kills the mother rather than a substitute. Although there are no national statistics on the number of matricides, it is a relatively rare event. When it occurs, matricide is usually perpetrated by an adult male (Heide and Frei, 2009). In fact, most of the men are schizophrenic who are living alone with their mothers at the time of the act (Campion et al., 1985). The crime is fairly well known in literature and myth, but it is not seen that frequently in forensic practice (Meloy, 1996a).

Matricides are committed mostly by adults, but a few cases have involved adolescents. For example, Scherl and Mack (1966a) described the case of a 14-year-old who, disgusted by his mother's overt sexual relationship with another man and her sexually promiscuous conduct, shot her while she was sleeping. He then went to a local priest to confess the crime. There have even been a few reported cases of matricide following mother–son incest. MacDonald (1986) briefly described the case of a 14-year-old who killed his mother following sexual relations with her. Brown (1963) discussed the case of a 19-year-old who killed his mother after an 8-year incestuous relationship. Here, the homicide occurred hours after the offender was unable to consummate sexual relations with a prostitute.

The following case, of an acute catathymic matricide following years of mother–son incest, was reported in detail by Schlesinger (1999). To the offender, the murder itself, which included vaginal and anal necrophilia, was sexually arousing.

Case 5.9: Adolescent Sexual Matricide Following Repeated Mother–Son Incest

---

A 16-year-old high school student (II) was involved in a sexual relationship with his mother that began when he was about 7. The mother was sexually promiscuous, possibly even a nymphomaniac. She made sexual comments to II's friends, frequently brought boyfriends to the family home when her husband was absent, and even walked around town completely undressed (except for a fur coat), exposing herself to local merchants.

About 6 months prior to the homicide, as he approached 16 years, II began feeling uncomfortable about the frequent and ongoing sexual relations with his mother. After he told her he no longer wanted to have sex with her, she became angry and insistent. "She kept trying and she kept yelling. I told her, 'If you don't leave me alone, I am gonna tell someone.'" About 10 days before the murder, he had oral sex with his mother. "In the middle of oral sex I said 'I don't want to do this no more,' and I pushed her away. She said 'No. We're gonna have to do this some time. What's wrong with you, now?'"

On the day of the homicide, II woke up at his usual time and began to get ready for school. He observed his mother dressing in the bathroom, with the door open, as was her custom. She was wearing only underwear and a partially buttoned shirt. II described an overpowering urge, which was sexually arousing. He stated that he obtained an erection.

> I took her and pulled her out of the bathroom. I pulled her out and shoved her upstairs. I was real aroused. She said, "What are you doing? I am your mother. What are you doing?" I felt like I was out of control. My body was responding to the anger. All the anger that was bursting out from me. I shoved her in her bedroom and put my hands around her neck, and I got really excited. I choked her, and I didn't say a word. After she was dead, I tore the clothes off.

I had sex with her after she was dead. At the time, I thought maybe she was just unconscious. I was aroused by her.

II engaged in vaginal and anal necrophilia.

I felt in control of her now. She was in control of me. I was like her play toy. I felt like I was getting back at her by doing this. I did it to her. I laid her on the bed.

He was unable to explain the acts of necrophilia, particularly anal penetration, except to describe a feeling of domination and control. Following the homicide, he threw a T-shirt over his mother's face "because the eyes didn't close. They were staring at me."

His description of the homicide itself was typical of a dissociative state, so common in acute catathymic murders.

I knew what I was doing, but it was like a movie, watching myself almost in motion. It was like a movie and the camera was my eyes. I was aware of everything, but I was just not thinking. I really didn't think I was killing someone. The whole thing seemed like a dream.

Immediately following the murder, II felt relief. He denied ever having had a prior thought or fantasy of killing his mother, although such ideas are common in similarly abused children (Richards and Goodwin, 1994).

The offender had above-average intelligence with no history of any overt psychological problems. He was introverted and had some social anxiety and lack of self-confidence but nothing that seemed to warrant referral to a mental health professional. His figure drawings are displayed in Chapter 2, Figure 2.3. They are not remarkable except perhaps for some slight sexualization of the human figures.

II's central conflict clearly stemmed from the extremely rare mother–son (as opposed to the more common father–daughter) incest. At the time of the homicide, II had never had any other female contact "because somehow they'd know about me and my mom; or it might slip out when I was talking to them." Following the homicide, and after release from 2 years in prison, II briefly dated a few times, but he ended the courtships quickly as he feared loss of control once some sexual behavior was initiated (by the girl). Following several years of treatment, II improved and seemed relatively stable at a 10-year follow-up. Perhaps II resolved his conflict when he killed his mother.

5.3 Differential Diagnosis

Acute catathymic homicides are more complex acts than murders triggered by stressful situations, anger, temper, or jealousy. Much deeper feelings are tapped in the acute catathymic process, where powerful conflicts regarding inadequacy—primarily sexual inadequacy—are the causes of the violent outbursts. Individuals who experience a catathymic explosion often do not have a background of violence or impulsivity but, instead, are secretly struggling with a more ominous underlying issue. Notwithstanding these distinctions, diagnostic problems often occur in differentiating catathymic homicides and catathymic attacks from severe violence that is simply a result of anger and loss of control.

Diagnostic clarification is not helped by reference to the literature on impulse-control disorders. In fact, the many classification systems of dyscontrol syndromes have been

Table 5.2   **Monroe's View of Episodic Dyscontrol**

Primary Dyscontrol	Secondary Dyscontrol
Neurophysiological deficit	Disturbed life experiences
"Faulty equipment"	"Faulty learning"
Absence of reflective delay	Hesitation and resistance of impulse
Epileptoid dyscontrol	Hysteroid dyscontrol

inconsistent, confusing, and sometimes even incorrect. The earlier work of Monroe (1970, 1974, 1978), which expanded on Menninger and Mayman's (1956) initial description of episodic dyscontrol, is an example of confusion in terminology. Monroe described two general types of dyscontrol based on different causes. One type involves a complete absence of "reflective delay"; Monroe referred to these spontaneous acts, without much cognitive modulation, as being cases of "primary dyscontrol." In the other type, the offender hesitates and resists the impulse, so there is some premeditation; Monroe labeled these acts "secondary dyscontrol." He believed that primary dyscontrol is a result of "faulty equipment," mainly a neurophysiological deficit. "Faulty learning," found in secondary dyscontrol cases, is a result of life experiences, which can also lead to aggressive outbursts absent neurological disinhibition. He argued that primary dyscontrol can also be called epileptoid dyscontrol, while secondary dyscontrol can be referred to as hysteroid dyscontrol (see Table 5.2).

Although the *Diagnostic and Statistical Manual* is only a guideline, its coverage of impulse-control disorders since 1980 has also been quite confusing and perhaps even, at times, inaccurate. Coles (1997), among others (e.g., Cartwright, 2001), also commented on the lack of clarity in the *DSM* with regard to the explosive disorders. For instance, the *DSM-III* (1980) described "isolated explosive disorder" as involving an individual's "failure to resist an impulse that led to a single violent externally directed act which had catastrophic impact on others, such as severe assault or homicide" (p. 297). As an example, it described a person who starts shooting at others for no reason. The *DSM-III* noted that this type of explosion had previously been referred to as catathymic crisis. However, the brief description and the example of isolated explosive disorder are inconsistent with any prior description of catathymic crisis; the *DSM-III* seemed to view both catathymic violence and general unprovoked explosiveness as equivalent, which they are not.

In the *DSM-IV-TR* (2000), an impulse-control disorder is described as a

> failure to resist an impulse, drive, or temptation to perform an act that is harmful to the person or others; … the individual feels an increasing sense of tension or arousal before committing the act and then experiences pleasure, gratification, or relief at the time of committing the act. (p. 663)

But under this general diagnostic category are listed—in addition to intermittent explosive disorder—kleptomania, pyromania, pathological gambling, trichotillomania, and impulse-control disorder not otherwise specified.

The diagnostic criteria for intermittent explosive disorder are qualitatively much different from those for catathymic violence. Intermittent explosive disorder refers to a general deficit in the offender in terms of overall ability to control impulses, resulting in repetitive (intermittent) violent acts. Catathymic violence is not often found in individuals who are generally impulsive. (Impulsivity as a personality trait, however, does not preclude the possibility of a catathymic explosion.) In fact, those who experience a catathymic episode of aggression are often timid, overcontrolled people whose outburst is triggered by a strong conflict involving (sexual) inadequacy.

Kleptomania is not an impulse-control disorder. Rather than being a spontaneous, impulsive reaction to an external stimulus, kleptomania is the result of an internal drive (or urge) to steal objects not needed for personal use or for monetary gain. Pyromania, a need to set fires, often for psychosexual gratification, is also a result of an internal drive to act rather than being a behavior triggered by an external event or circumstance. Both kleptomania and pyromania are not impulses; they are the result of internal pressure to commit the act, which is usually well thought out and planned. Accordingly, their placement under impulse-control disorders in the *DSM* is unhelpful, confusing, and incorrect.

In addition, pathological gambling is generally thought of as an addiction rather than an impulse-control disorder. In fact, the treatment of choice for pathological gambling is an addiction model (Rosenthal and Lesieur, 1996). Trichotillomania—repetitive hair pulling—is considered a symptom of an obsessive–compulsive disorder rather than an impulse-control disorder (Miltenberger, 2001). Finally, the *DSM-IV-TR* diagnosis of impulse-control disorder, not otherwise specified, is also incorrectly placed. The *DSM* uses skin picking as an example. But, rather than being an impulse-control disorder, repetitive skin picking is connected to trichotillomania and obsessive–compulsive symptoms.

The *DSM-5* (2013) made a number of changes that do not help further our understanding of impulsive/explosive violent outbursts. In the latest edition, disruptive, impulse-control, and conduct disorders are in the same group, which is characterized by problems of emotional and behavioral self-control. Oppositional defiant disorder and conduct disorder (which are typically found in children and adolescents) are now grouped with intermittent explosive disorder. Intermittent explosive disorder now requires not only physical aggression but verbal aggression and nondestructive, noninjurious physical violence as well. Although there are behavioral similarities between conduct disorders in children and adolescents and violent outbursts in adults, they are similar only superficially. The new classification ignores the complexity and finer nuances of the various conditions that result in violent behavior.

The conclusion that an individual experienced an acute catathymic explosion can be reached only after careful evaluation of the offender (and the offense), so that the depth of the inner conflict and the triggering event can be fully understood. Unless the offender is questioned carefully regarding feelings of inadequacy, particularly sexual inadequacy, complete understanding of the case will likely remain illusive. For example, Ratner and Shapiro (1979) reported an interesting case of a 20-year-old who, following sexual relations with a girlfriend, choked her to death and inflicted multiple stab wounds with a knife. Both offender and victim were having sex at the victim's house while her husband was at work. She teased the offender and said that if her husband walked in, she would say she was being raped. The victim also laughed at the offender, which triggered enormous rage. He tried to control his anger by counting, but further laughter precipitated the assault. When this case was evaluated, a number of nonspecific neurological signs were detected, including an abnormal EEG and an abnormal CAT scan and MRI. The offender also apparently had had some type of head trauma years earlier.

Although Ratner and Shapiro considered this case to be an example of episodic dyscontrol, with the offender's defenses weakened by organicity, closer examination reveals that the homicide would probably not have occurred if it were not for the teasing within a highly charged sexual context. Whether this case should be considered an example of an acute catathymic homicide is uncertain and difficult to know from a distance. But, given the triggering event and the taunting regarding sexuality, a catathymic process should be strongly considered. This case is an example of an incomplete, rather than an incorrect, diagnostic formulation, with incomplete understanding of what actually occurred, not uncommon when the murder is sudden and the dynamics are unclear (Holcomb and Daniel, 1988). The authors' evaluation focused almost exclusively on the offender's weakened controls due to organicity rather than on the underlying motivational or psychodynamic process.

Case 5.10: Differentiating Acute Catathymic and Noncatathymic Homicide

A 17-year-old male became involved in a 2–4-month sexual relationship with a 24-year-old woman, initiated by her. A.J. was involved in high school athletics and was well liked by peers and teachers. He had a prior arrest for possession of a firearm and shooting at a neighbor's window, which resulted in 1-year probation. A.J. also had anger and temper problems since childhood but no history of any mental health evaluation or treatment. The sexual relationship between the victim and offender was somewhat lopsided. It seems that the young woman was involved with A.J. primarily for sexual gratification, while A.J. quickly developed strong feelings of a romantic nature toward her. The victim told A.J. repeatedly that he was too young and that their sexual involvement was wrong, yet she continued to contact him and engage with him.

One evening, while out with a group, the victim became intoxicated and was flirting with the bartender. A.J. walked her home; they engaged in a consensual sexual encounter, and he got into an argument with her. The victim did not want to become his "girlfriend" but wanted only to engage in periodic sexual relations. The victim told the offender repeatedly that he was "too young" and he should look for a girlfriend elsewhere. A.J. said, "I loved her, I didn't want no one else to have her. She said I should look for someone else; she didn't want to be with me, too young."

The defendant told the victim that he had thoughts of killing her that night and mentioned that he previously had thoughts of killing her when she kept telling him he was too young to be in a committed relationship with her. When A.J. said to her "I feel like killing you," she said, "Go ahead." "I was thinking should I kill her or not." He decided to kill her. She left the bedroom to get a glass of water and then went to the living room to lie down on the couch on her side, facing away from him.

A.J. obtained a large knife from the kitchen and stabbed her once in the head. The victim awoke and said, "Are you serious A.J.?" He then stabbed her in the head eight more times,

> as hard as I could, and the last one, I twisted the knife to make sure she was dead. I didn't know why I did it; it was just anger. I was just pissed. I got the knife and I just stabbed her.

Following the homicide, he put a plastic bag over the victim's head, dragged her nude body into the bedroom, washed off the knife and his hands, and put on the rest of his clothes. He fled the scene in a surreptitious way to avoid any contact with people. He turned his cellphone off so he would not be able to be "tracked."

After his arrest, he was taken to a juvenile detention center where he was housed prior to the legal proceedings. While there, A.J. had temper outbursts and "difficulty with female staff." One social worker noted that he was

> extremely disrespectful and demanding when angry with them [women]. When A.J. gets angry, it can last a long time. ... A.J.'s lack of impulse control and prior judgment can become dangerous to others if it is not addressed.

The defense expert incorrectly believed that this was an acute catathymic homicide. Killing someone because you do not get what you want, marked by prior thoughts of killing the individual out of anger, is not indicative of a catathymic explosion. Although there is a sexual component to this homicide, the primary underlying motivation for the homicide was that the victim would not become his girlfriend. "I guess I didn't want anyone else to have her, it would hurt to see her with somebody else." She never rejected him, never made fun of him, and he said the sexual involvement never triggered any feelings of inadequacy. It was just that he did not get what he wanted, and he decided to kill her out of anger. When questioned, A.J. said that he did not believe he did not satisfy her sexually (because she said he did); he did not feel rejected, and he said often that the reason he killed her was "due to anger."

5.4 Comment

Sudden loss of control resulting in an unplanned explosive homicide has obvious psycho-legal implications. Mental health professionals retained to assess a defendant's mental state at the time of the crime are almost always required to supply a traditional *DSM* diagnosis as a necessary—but not sufficient—condition for a legal defense. Catathymic process, particularly an acute catathymic process, can be used to supplement a traditional *DSM* diagnosis, especially where the motive is unclear. Just as a traditional diagnosis alone can never establish that a defendant met a specific legal standard, neither can a finding of catathymia, which is not a diagnosis but rather a psychodynamic or motivational process. The pure form of an acute catathymic homicide is relatively rare, but many cases of explosive violence have catathymic features. The specific facts and circumstances of each case, in addition to a diagnosis, form the basis of a forensic opinion.

Viewpoints have varied widely regarding the connection between sudden disintegration in psychological functioning and the issue of legal insanity. Meloy (1992) argues that in order to qualify for some type of mental-state defense, acute catathymic cases have to be diagnosed as a brief reactive psychosis. If the clinical diagnosis were intermittent explosive disorder, such a defense would probably not be applicable. Medlicott (1966) comments that brief psychotic episodes—defined as "brief breaks or interruptions in normal ego control, so that its integrating, reality testing and controlling functions are seriously disturbed" (p. 971)—should fall under the rubric of temporary insanity. Shenken (1966) believes that individuals who commit various acts of violence connected with psychotic episodes are often suffering from schizophrenia; he based his judgment on (clinical) signs such as flattened affect and indifference following the act. But lack of emotion in connection with such violent crimes is quite common, especially in bizarre murders. When these offenders are examined years later, they do not show the typical signs of schizophrenia in either a Schneiderian or a Bleulerian sense.

Notwithstanding the semantics used in legal proceedings where an offender's state of mind is at issue, an understanding of acute catathymic homicides can prove helpful in explaining such violence in the face of seemingly minimal overt provocation. A clear description of the syndrome to a jury can often enable the members to gain an insight into the complexity and depth of many of these cases and an understanding of how they are different from common acts of impulsive aggression triggered by resentment, fear, envy, or anger, as described in Case 5.10.

Many offenders who commit an acute catathymic homicide have been evaluated by mental health professionals prior to the explosion. Unfortunately, the depth of the disturbance is either well masked by the offender or is not understood by the examining clinician or, more likely, the offender was not properly questioned. Accordingly, mental health professionals, law enforcement officers, physicians, and other individuals who have some responsibility for assessing people in crises should be alert to the ominous significance of young men who secretly struggle with feelings of sexual inadequacy, particularly when associated with a background of maternal sexual indiscretion. A few brief questions directly put to a patient before he becomes a defendant should be part of the risk-assessment interview. Not only might such an examination prevent tragedy, but an exploration of these topics can be cathartic and can serve as a beginning step in treatment.

Chronic Catathymic Homicides 6

The chronic form of catathymic process as conceived of by Revitch and Schlesinger (1978, 1981, 1989) is an updated and simplified version of Wertham's (1937) catathymic crisis. Revitch and Schlesinger reduced the process to three stages: (1) incubation, (2) violent act, and (3) relief (see Table 6.1). During the incubation phase, the future offender becomes depressed and obsessively preoccupied with the future victim. His behavior at times may appear bizarre, while at other times his outward conduct or demeanor does not change. At this stage, he may have suicidal thoughts that later become mixed with homicidal ideas involving the future victim. The idea to kill slowly emerges, takes hold, and then becomes fixed. The future offender may notify friends, family members, his therapist, or even a member of the clergy. His pleas are frequently ignored or rationalized as the offender often reassures the confidant that he will not act out and that he is in control. But despite his inner struggle and efforts to seek help, he carries out the deed.

Following the violent act—usually a homicide—the offender experiences relief as the catathymic tension is discharged. Occasionally a chronic catathymic homicide may be followed by suicide or a suicide attempt. The event is often recalled in a detached, remote manner. In fact, the violent act—and even the offender's thoughts and activities during the incubation period—impresses him retrospectively as being dreamlike and ego-dystonic. The inexperienced examiner may take such a lack of emotion to be an indication of callousness or indifference, especially given the often close relationship between the offender and the victim.

Although there are many similarities between the acute and the chronic catathymic processes, as noted in Chapter 5 (see Table 5.1), there are a number of differences as well (see Table 6.2). For example, acute catathymic homicides are unplanned, while the chronic are planned, often in the form of an obsessive rumination. The acute process is triggered by underlying emotionally charged conflicts that flood consciousness; often these conflicts involve feelings of sexual inadequacy or a transfer of emotion from a symbolic figure— typically, a mother figure—to the victim. The chronic process is triggered by a buildup of tension, a feeling of frustration, and conflicts involving inadequacy, usually extending to the sexual area.

The acute process has a short incubation period, typically several seconds, while in the chronic process the incubation period can last for days and even up to a year or somewhat longer. Here, the offender often becomes obsessively preoccupied with the victim and sometimes stalks her. Stalking rarely occurs in the acute process.

In the acute process, the attack is usually some type of sudden, violent assault involving strangulation or stabbing. The chronic process also involves violence, but it is not sudden; it is planned in the form of obsessive rumination. The crime scene in an acute attack is disorganized, a reflection of the lack of planning. The crime scene in the chronic process is less disorganized, a reflection of planning but not planning to avoid detection. Postmortem behavior in the acute process sometimes involves (vaginal or anal) necrophilia

Table 6.1   Stages of the Chronic Catathymic Process

Stage	Description
Incubation	The subject becomes depressed and obsessively preoccupied with the future victim. Suicidal thoughts may emerge, but slowly the subject develops an idea to kill. The thought grows in strength, takes hold, and becomes fixed, rootlike, and intractable.
Violent act	The violence is usually homicide, but other forms can occur (e.g., arson, assault, and a variety of other aggressive acts, including self-mutilation).
Feeling of relief	Once the catathymic tension is discharged, the offender typically feels a sense of relief, although he is simultaneously horrified by what he has done. If all the catathymic tension is not completely released, the homicide may be followed by suicide or a suicide attempt.

and occasional dismemberment. Postmortem sexual activity and dismemberment are rare in the chronic process. Sexual activity occasionally occurs before the attack in the acute process; sometimes the offender's inability to perform (sexually) triggers the attack. Sexual activity at the time of the homicide is rare in the chronic process. Following an acute catathymic homicide, the offender typically experiences a flattening of emotions and poor memory of the event as a result of its explosive nature. In the chronic process, the offender usually feels relief while often preserving the memory.

Most victims of acute catathymic homicides are strangers, while the victims in the chronic form of the process are close relations, former intimate partners, family members, acquaintances, and only occasionally (usually in catathymic mass murder) strangers. In fact, the authorities may cite jealousy and anger over the victim's distancing herself from the offender as the motivation for the chronic catathymic homicide. Here, however, the victim's detachment is more likely the result of the offender's obsessive preoccupation

Table 6.2   Differentiating Characteristics of Acute and Chronic Catathymic Processes

Characteristic	Acute	Chronic
Activation of process	Triggered by a sudden overwhelming emotion attached to underlying sexual conflicts of symbolic significance	Triggered by a buildup of tension, a feeling of frustration, helplessness, and inadequacy, sometimes extending into the sexual area
Relationship to the victim	Usually a stranger	Usually a close relation such as an intimate or former intimate partner
Victim symbolization	Often a displaced matricide	Rarely a displaced matricide, but victim may have symbolic significance
Incubation period	Several seconds	One day to a year; may involve stalking
Level of planning	Unplanned	Planned, frequently in the form of an obsessive rumination
Method of attack	Sudden and violent; often overkill	Violent but not sudden
Crime scene	Very disorganized, reflecting complete lack of planning	Less disorganized
Sexual activity	Occasional sexual activity just before attack; impotency common	Sexual activity rare at the time of homicide
Postmortem behavior	Sometimes necrophilia and occasionally dismemberment	Rarely necrophilia or dismemberment
Feeling following the attack	Usually a flattening of emotions	Usually a feeling of relief
Memory of event	Usually poor	Usually preserved

and attempt at control, stemming from his disorganizing conflicts; the offender's behavior leads the future victim to remove herself. Thus, often the relationship itself shatters the perpetrator's psychological homeostasis; the released emotion then disrupts his logical thinking and contributes to his obsessional preoccupation.

Recently, Sinnamon (2015) and Sinnamon and Petherick (2017) noted that in some cases the entire catathymic process might repeat itself, as the resolution of the conflict (through violence) is more apparent than real. These authors also elaborated Wertham's (1978) original concept, emphasizing the delusional nature of the offender's ideation. The idea to kill the future victim, "becomes increasingly obsessional with related thought processes becoming increasingly irrational, reinforcing the delusional thoughts and validating the obsession" (Sinnamon and Petherick, 2017, p. 53).

6.1 Literary Illustrations of Catathymia

Two literary works describing the chronic catathymic process—Feodor Dostoyevsky's (1886/1955) *Crime and Punishment* and Yukio Mishima's (1956) *The Temple of the Golden Pavilion*—are illustrative. *Crime and Punishment* is based on an actual case reported in the Russian press at the time. The main character, Rodion Raskolnikov, is preoccupied with the question of why almost every crime is so easily solved, and the clues left behind by the criminal are so quickly discovered. Raskolnikov reasons:

> [The answer lies] not so much in the physical impossibility of concealing the crime as in the criminal himself; the criminal himself, at least almost every criminal, is subject at the moment of the crime to a kind of breakdown in his reasoning faculties and of his will power, which are replaced by an amazingly childish carelessness just at the moment when he is most in need of caution and reason. … If only I succeed in keeping my will and my reasoning faculties unimpaired, all the difficulties will be over. (p. 9)

Raskolnikov subsequently develops an idea to kill an elderly pawnbroker who practices usury, an act considered morally reprehensible at the time. He views the victim as socially useless; therefore, he reasons it would not be unethical to kill her and to use her wealth for higher purposes, such as helping his impoverished sister and mother. The idea to kill the pawnbroker develops into an obsessive rumination that eventually becomes fixed and intractable. Raskolnikov withdraws socially and neglects his schoolwork and his appearance. His appetite decreases, and he spends a great deal of time just lying in bed in an overt state of depression, preoccupied with the possibility of getting away with crime, in general, and with killing the pawnbroker, in particular.

He eventually picks up an axe in the house where he lives, enters the victim's apartment, and brutally kills her, along with her sister who unexpectedly enters the room. Following the killings, Raskolnikov searches the apartment and takes a few objects and a minimal amount of money; later he throws away what he has taken. He questions his motives and purpose:

> If you did this business conscientiously, not like a fool, but if you really had a firm and definite purpose, why is it you have not looked into the purse, why is it you did not even know what you have got? You don't know why you put yourself through all this trouble, don't know why you consciously started out on such a vile, base, low business. (p. 104)

Raskolnikov's belief—that by killing the pawnbroker, he will free society of a useless and harmful being and, at the same time, make a contribution to the general welfare by distributing her wealth—is an obvious rationalization. The crime's compelling character grows out of his fixed idea, an idea that eventually becomes inaccessible to logic. Once the idea enters his consciousness, it builds until he has to follow through with the act. His throwing away of the money clearly reveals that material gain was not part of the central motivation.

Several motives for the homicide are possible. The most superficial is Raskolnikov's idea of robbing for personal gain and general welfare, bolstered by his belief that "great men [dare] to cross ethical barriers" (p. 309). A sociological view of the homicide might focus on the social disintegration in Russia at the time, as evidenced by the spread of atheism and of the liberal philosophy espoused by Russian intellectuals.

Freud's (1916) theory that criminal behavior stems from a sense of guilt can also be used to explain Raskolnikov's behavior. For instance, Schneck (1966) argues that Raskolnikov exemplifies Freud's general notion that criminal acts are performed because they are forbidden.

> Paradoxical as it may sound, I must maintain that the sense of guilt was present prior to the transgression, that it did not arise from this, but contrary-wise—the transgression from the sense of guilt. These persons we might justifiably describe as criminals from a sense of guilt. (Freud, 1916, p. 42)

Freud believed that guilt stems "from the Oedipus complex, and is a reaction to the two great criminal intentions of killing the father and having sexual relations with the mother" (p. 323). In fact, in his paper "Dostoyevsky and Parricide," Freud (1928) stated, "It is a fact that large groups of criminals long for punishment. Their superego demands it and so saves itself the necessity for inflicting the punishment itself" (p. 17). Building on Freud's insights, Florance (1955) offered a somewhat different psychoanalytic interpretation of Raskolnikov. She theorized that the murder was triggered by the offender's deep-seated sexual problems, specifically incestuous feelings for his mother and sister as well as latent homosexuality. Revitch and Schlesinger (1981) noted that Dostoyevsky may have named his hero Raskolnikov from the Russian word *raskol*, which means split or schism, as the main character's behavior was contrary to basic notions of morality and was even detached from his conscious will.

But notwithstanding the theory of the crime, the development of Raskolnikov's obsessive rumination to kill, followed by a feeling of relief after the act, is typical of the chronic catathymic process. Because the catathymic process is a motivational one that describes and explains the offender's actions, it can coexist with any theory of crime, as well as any psychiatric diagnosis.

In Yukio Mishima's (1956) *The Temple of the Golden Pavilion*, the author—a brilliant but psychologically disturbed person who eventually committed suicide by disemboweling himself—provides a vivid step-by-step description of the chronic catathymic process. Like Dostoyevsky, Mishima created his novel on the basis of actual events. The central character is a young man, Mizoguchi, who is plagued by a strong sense of his own ugliness, plus feelings of social and sexual inadequacy. He becomes obsessed with the beauty of a historic Buddhist temple that has been considered a national treasure for over 500 years. After destroying the structure by setting it on fire, he feels relief, and his long-standing psychological conflicts are resolved.

Mizoguchi's severe stuttering makes it almost impossible for him to relate to others, especially women, since his anxiety increases with interpersonal contact. He is taunted by his peers and feels unlovable. At the same time, he envies a handsome classmate who is athletic and well liked. On several occasions, Mizoguchi attempts intercourse with prostitutes but finds that he is impotent. One of his masturbatory fantasies involves visualizing a pretty female classmate naked; however, the image quickly dissipates as he immediately envisions himself as an ugly insect. In one incident, Mizoguchi meets up with the attractive young woman, the object of his sexual fantasies. Instead of being friendly, she mocks Mizoguchi; he is crushed when she calls him a stutterer.

Mizoguchi is also plagued by recurrent recollections of maternal sexual infidelity that greatly disturb him. On several occasions, he observed his mother having sex with a visiting uncle. Mizoguchi's father, who was quite ill, unsuccessfully tried to shield his son from his mother's sexual conduct. At another point, Mizoguchi mentions to his mother that he might like to enlist in the army, but she teases him and says that if the army takes "stutterers like you" then Japan's military is finished. He hates his mother for her behavior and wants nothing to do with her.

In contrast to his feelings of self-disgust, Mizoguchi forms a strong obsessional attachment to, and envy of, the well-known temple and its beauty. The obsession with the temple grows. Just like Dostoyevsky's Raskolnikov, Mishima's Mizoguchi becomes depressed and withdrawn, neglects his schoolwork, and for a period of time, feels aimless.

> During all these hours I did not read any book, nor did I have money to spend on amusements. Sometimes I would talk to Kachewagi, but most of the time I stayed by myself doing nothing. This sort of inactivity was perhaps my own special form of Zen practice. (p. 195)

During these states of depression, Mishima's central character thinks that he, with all his inadequacies, and the temple, with all its beauty, cannot exist in the same world.

> If there was no chance that the Golden Temple would be attacked [by the Americans during World War II], then for the time being I had lost my purpose in living, and the world in which I dwell must fall to pieces. (p. 81)

Mizoguchi then suddenly develops the idea that he has to destroy the temple by setting it on fire.

> This notion would suddenly come to life within me, revealed the meaning that had flashed through my mind earlier, and it made me shine brightly inside. I still did not try to think it out deeply, but was barely seized by the notion, as though I had been struck by light. Yet that idea, which until then had never once occurred to me, began to grow in strength inside as soon as it was born. Far from containing the idea, I myself was wrapped in it. And this was the notion that entrapped me. I must set fire to the Golden Temple. (p. 285)

Mizoguchi's resolve to burn down the temple becomes stronger. He attempts intercourse with several women, but on each occasion, a vision of the Golden Temple appears and makes it impossible for him to sustain an erection. However, once he begins to make definite plans to set fire to the temple, Mizoguchi feels a sense of liberation. He goes to a prostitute and finds that the vision of the temple is no longer present; he is finally able to consummate sexual relations.

Mizoguchi finally sets fire to the temple and watches it burn. "I noticed the pack of cigarettes in my other pocket; I took one out and started smoking. I felt like a man who settles down for a smoke after finishing a job of work. I wanted to live" (p. 285). As he runs away from the fire, burning timbers sound to him like the crackling of people's joints, an image with strong sexual connotations.

The sexual dynamics in this case are much more pronounced than in the case of Raskolnikov. Freud (1900, 1905, 1914, 1925) commented many times on the traumatic effect of a child witnessing adult intercourse, which he referred to as the primal scene. Freud felt that observing this event is traumatic since it not only elicits overwhelming sexual excitement, but the youngster also may misinterpret the act of sex as an assault on the mother. Arlow (1978) discussed the impact of Mizoguchi witnessing the primal scene as a central motivation for his fire setting, a sort of retaliatory act against his mother. Whether observing the primal scene is the main motivation for Mizoguchi's behavior is debatable. In fact, just as in the case of Raskolnikov, many levels of motivation may be operative. But, notwithstanding theory, the case graphically illustrates the development of the chronic catathymic process with the three stages of incubation, violent act, and subsequent feeling of relief.

6.2 Meloy's Psychodynamic Contributions

J. Reid Meloy, a contemporary forensic psychologist, has made significant contributions to further our understanding of the catathymic process. He clarifies the personality structure of such offenders, the complexities of the incubation phase, the posthomicidal feelings of relief, and the connection of catathymia to disorders of attachment (see Table 6.3).

Meloy (1988, 1992) believes that anyone who commits a chronic catathymic homicide has, at least, a borderline personality organization. Traits such as the lack of an integrated identity, difficulties in reality testing, and the use of primitive defenses are characteristic of individuals who commit catathymic homicides and suggests that these individuals have underlying borderline personalities. In fact, Meloy found the lack of an integrated identity, which hinders interpersonal relationships, to be rather common among the group of offenders he evaluated. As an example, the author cites one individual who stated, "Either he or I must die, something has to give"; this remark illustrates the homicidal–suicidal wish that emerged during the incubation phase in this subject. Meloy views this dichotomy—a wish to destroy the "bad self" or the "bad object"—as a resolution to an internal problem or conflict. Such shifting of the violent wish is one type of primitive defense mechanism

Table 6.3   **Meloy's Psychodynamic Contributions to Catathymia**

- Offenders who commit a catathymic homicide have a borderline or psychotic personality organization.
- A central defense mechanism of such offenders is projective identification.
- The future offender attributes malevolent and controlling characteristics to the future victim.
- The feeling of relief following the violence has a physiological and a psychodynamic basis.
- The mode of violence is affective, but there may be an extended period of planning and preparation.
- Some of the planning in the incubation phase has ego-syntonic and ego-dystonic characteristics.
- Catathymia stems from a disorder of attachment.

that offenders often employ. The idea to kill either is projected onto the victim in the form of homicide or is introjected and results in suicidal ideas.

> The aggressive wish follows: if he dies, I destroy the pain; if I die, I destroy the pain. The suicidal or homicidal nature of the aggressive wish depends upon the perceived origin of the emotional distress, which may rapidly oscillate. (Meloy, 1992, p. 59)

Meloy refers to other defense mechanisms indicative of borderline personality such as splitting ("either he or I must die"). Splitting may occur during alternating emotional states toward himself and the victim. In addition, defenses of primitive idealization and devaluation are also used by these offenders. Such opposite notions are similar to splitting and are typical in individuals who fall within the borderline spectrum but who have pronounced narcissistic traits characterized by a sense of entitlement along with severe dependency. Frequently, such offenders have a wish to be admired and, at the same time, to be taken care of. They are vulnerable to slight criticisms or narcissistic injuries.

Problems in reality testing are yet another indication of borderline personality organization: "Impairments in the patient's ability to distinguish between internal and external reality are expectable when defenses are utilized that distort, negate, deny, split off, and grossly alter whole sectors of experience" (Meloy, 1992, p. 63). The author also finds that the catathymic individual's defenses can fall apart completely with the emergence of a psychosis. For instance, one offender remarked with significant loss of logic, "I am legion and must die." In this offender's thinking, "the remedy is found in the action, not through a more internal modulated process of change" (p. 59).

Most central to understanding catathymic violence, in Meloy's view, is the concept of projective identification, which, he notes, has two necessary components: attribution and control. In catathymic violence, projective identification serves a defensive function. During the incubation phase, the offender feels confused, depressed, and controlled by the future victim. The concomitant feeling is that he must control the future victim, thereby eliminating feelings of helplessness.

> Projective identification, in this sense, is functioning within a borderline level of personality wherein demarcation between self and objects is retained, but confusion is apparent around the origin of psychological content and motivation: Who is doing what to whom? Am I feeling a certain way or is he? This state of mind is often apparent to others in the incubation period, when the patient becomes more intrusive, overt, and confused in her behavior towards the object, but perceives this behavior only in the object who will eventually be victimized. (p. 61)

Thus, the explosion of violence in a catathymic homicide is a result of projective identification stemming from a need to control.

> The tension build up, usually lasting months to a year, is finally cathected, and the intolerable feeling of being controlled by the malevolent object [the victim] is reversed. Absolute control of the object, as the source of persecutory distress is acted out through violence. (p. 62)

In discussing the feeling of relief experienced after the catathymic homicide, Meloy points out that both physiological and psychodynamic components are operative. The strong emotion that has been released results in "a parasympathetic return to baseline autonomic functioning, and a subjective feeling of relief because the perceived threat has been removed" (p. 62). From a psychodynamic perspective, the victim has been destroyed, and the defense of projective identification is no longer necessary. The author observes that some individuals, following the homicide, wish for an idealized relationship with the victim. This wish should be considered an indication of a psychosis because the offender refers to the victim in the present tense, as if she were still alive.

Meloy views catathymic violence as primarily affective (inasmuch as there is an explosive outburst that results in death or serious injury to the victim), but it can also be predatory (in that planning does occur). During the incubation phase, the thought to kill can be either ego-syntonic or ego-dystonic. Ego-syntonic ideas to kill the victim are "conveyed with pleasurable or comfortable affect, without fear or trepidation, in a threatening or grandiose manner, in the absence of conscience or superego constraint, and without reference to the unwanted or obsessional quality of the thoughts" (p. 56). Thus, ego-syntonic behaviors include conscious planning, experimenting with weapons, constructing alibies, and planning legal defenses. Ego-dystonic ideas are conveyed differently:

> [They are recognized by] displeasurable or anxious affect, perhaps with fear and trepidation; maybe a genuine cry for help to a professional or close friend; [are] absent any sense of grandiosity or omnipotence; may emphatically be felt as impending loss of control; [are] accompanied by fears of punishment and anticipated remorse; and ... refer to the unwanted nature of the thoughts. (p. 57)

Ego-dystonic actions might include obtaining a weapon for unexplained reasons, not practicing with the weapon, and not thinking about mitigating future events from a legal perspective. Meloy (2010) provides an interesting case of a 37-year-old male who developed a fixed idea to kill his 13-month-old son by drowning him in the bathtub. After he called the police to report the homicide, he felt relief and calm.

Perhaps Meloy's most significant contribution to understanding catathymic homicides is his relating catathymic violence to attachment pathology. He concludes that catathymic violence is, in general, a disorder of attachment that has its roots in the offender's early life. In catathymic violence, threats of abandonment are important in understanding the development of projective identification, as the victim "is perceived as abandoning, and therefore controlling the perpetrator" (p. 64). The victim's behavior triggers memories of early experiences of abandonment and neglect. "In other words, the victim of catathymia, during the incubation phase, is perceived as a threat, and in extreme cases, a predator, who in a magnified and mad sense is doing irreparable harm to the individual" (p. 64). The explosive outburst in catathymia is the end of the symbiotic attachment to the victim.

6.3 The Predominance of Depression

Over the years, some clinicians have linked depression and homicide, but relatively little research on this connection has been conducted in comparison to the voluminous amount of study of each of these conditions individually. Although mental health practitioners automatically consider suicide to be related to depression and therefore always assess it in a fairly detailed fashion in a depressed person, they often do not make the same connection to homicide. In their review of 17 randomly selected psychiatric textbooks, Rosenbaum and Bennett (1986) found that 11 (64%) did not even mention homicide at all, and only 2 noted that homicide might have a relationship to depression. Contemporary clinicians' disregard for the association between depression and homicide (Malmquist, 1996) continues a situation first noticed by Batt (1948) years earlier. In fact, Muncie (1939), who was well aware of the concept of catathymia, described "catathymic depression" with "catathymic ideation" leading to suicide rather than to violence.

Depression alone, however, cannot explain an offender's criminal acts; it is the change in thinking that results in action. Although catathymia is often manifested in symptoms of depression (sleep disturbance, diminished appetite, and somatic complaints), it is a dynamic-motivational process that can explain violent behavior. During the incubation phase of the chronic catathymic process, the future offender experiences low mood, and his thinking becomes obsessive, ruminative, and egocentric. Early in the incubation phase, suicidal thoughts predominate, but later they may recede or intermingle with homicidal ideas, which gain strength and become fixed.

Therefore, to understand the offender's criminal behavior, a motivational or dynamic process (the catathymic process) is much more useful than a diagnosis of depression alone. In fact, many authors have reported cases of depressed individuals who committed homicides that had many of the classic signs of the catathymic process but were not labeled as such. For example, Malmquist (1996) found that depression is directly related to some homicides, especially those depressions where there is a disturbance in thinking. "In the transition to the homicidal state is the emergence of the idea that somebody must pay for one's suffering" (p. 247). Such an idea often becomes a "fixed belief" which Malmquist believes reaches delusional proportions. Whether such thinking is delusional or quasi-delusional is a matter of clinical judgment. But Malmquist's description of the future offender's thinking is exactly the kind of thought process Wertham (1937, 1978) described in the catathymic crisis.

In West's (1967) classic study of murderers who commit suicide (common in catathymic homicides), he differentiated a subgroup of depressed offenders, who were unable to live with their financial or sexual inadequacies. In fact, West cited Wertham (1937) and agreed with his contention that many such offenders experience violence as a solution to a feeling of inner tension and frustration; once the victim is killed, the aggression is turned inward if the inner emotion is not dissipated by the act of violence.

Dorpat (1966) also studied murder–suicide in depressed men, who had been enmeshed in prolonged, tumultuous relationships with their victims. He concluded that many murderers who had committed suicide under such circumstances entertained a fantasy that they would die and reunite with their deceased loved ones. Such a fantasy helps them achieve a sense of control over a situation that they feel no control over—a theory similar to that was espoused by Meloy (1992) years later in explaining some catathymic homicides.

In yet another study of murder–suicide, Berman (1979) examined a group of offenders whom he labeled "erotic-aggressive." These individuals had disturbed love relationships with long-standing "love–hate" patterns including repetitive separations and accusations of infidelity. He described a man who, after shooting his girlfriend three times in the head with a rifle, bent over and kissed her before committing suicide. This action illustrates the obvious ambivalence he felt toward her, a feeling typical in many chronic catathymic offenders.

Rosenbaum (1990) found that individuals who murder and then attempt to commit suicide are mostly (95%) men who have a clinical diagnosis of depression (about 75% of the time). This group was different from a group of offenders who committed homicide but did not attempt or commit suicide in that the nonsuicidal offenders were not found to be clinically depressed. And, in the murder–suicide group, the most important distinguishing feature other than depression and gender was the presence of pathological jealousy, likely stemming from deep underlying feelings of sexual inadequacy. In fact, ideas of sexual infidelity also differentiated depressed men who killed their partners from those who did not in a prior study by Rosenbaum and Bennett (1986).

Harrer and Kofler-Westergren (1986) consider many cases of homicide or extreme violence by depressed individuals as displaced suicides. Many of their subjects wanted to commit suicide, but, because of various circumstances, acted out in a violent—as opposed to a self-destructive—fashion. For instance, the authors report an interesting case of a 50-year-old depressed woman who had thoughts of committing suicide by setting her house on fire, but instead only scratched her eyes out with her fingernails because of intense guilt over incest with her son. The woman felt relief after the self-blinding, believing her incestuous acts would be forgiven. Harrer and Kofler-Westergren also find that "anxiety, inner tension, resentfulness and latent aggression may lead to an undefinable need for discharge and eventually to a sudden acting-out of suppressed emotion" (p. 218). Such a process, together with a strong sexual dynamic, is exactly descriptive of chronic catathymia. In fact, years earlier, Woodis (1957) found that in many cases of murder associated with depression, "sometimes, especially after acts of violence, all the clinical signs of depression may disappear, as if the very explosive nature of the act had worked as a cathartic and the patient had cured himself" (p. 85).

A number of other researchers also studied the relationship between depression and homicide (Bourget, Gagne, and Moamai, 2000; Hirose, 1979; Reinhardt, 1973; Stone, 1993; Tang, Sun, Li, Fang, and Fan, 1999) but focused primarily on the clinical diagnosis of depression. The descriptions of their cases, however, suggest the strong likelihood of catathymic dynamics in some of the offenders.

The following cases are typical descriptions of depressed men who committed homicide. In most such instances, the depression was recognized, but the motivational dynamics—the catathymic dynamics—that led to the killings were, unfortunately, ignored.

Case 6.1: Killing of Wife by a Depressed Individual

A 29-year-old man (AA) killed his wife of 3 years following repetitive separations, during which the victim returned home to her parents. AA was previously married to his childhood sweetheart, but the marriage ended after a year. He stated that he felt uncomfortable with his second wife (the victim) because "she was overly protected as a child. She was weak-minded. Her parents were very dominant. She always went back to her parents when we had an argument or problem." AA had been steadily employed as a salesman for many years and was well liked by friends, neighbors, and co-workers. He had a good work record and no prior involvement with the law.

About 9 months before the homicide, marital difficulties increased, and the couple sought counseling at a local mental health center. His wife found the therapy ineffective and decided to divorce. Although the marital counseling ended, AA continued in individual therapy with a psychiatrist who also prescribed medication for depression.

Over the course of 9 months, AA's depression deepened, with the emergence of suicidal thoughts. He also developed a vague idea to kill his wife—an idea which, at first, seemed distant and unreal. After toying with the thought for a week or two, he decided to tell his psychiatrist, who dismissed it as insignificant "because he expressed it. If he didn't express it, he would be dangerous." AA explained that slowly the idea to kill his wife increased in intensity and "no longer seemed crazy." "I purchased a gun. I thought of suicide." He went to his wife's place of employment to show it to her.

> I talked to her for a final time with the gun in my car, and then I put the gun to my head and told her I am going to kill myself. She promised that she would come back to me then.

His wife quickly brought threat charges against AA, and he served 30 days in jail "with animals." He was released on bail without any forensic evaluation; the court simply recommended he return to the mental health center where he had been treated.

AA maintained hope that he and his wife would reunite despite her insistence on the divorce and her filing a criminal complaint. After several more months, AA bought another gun which he intended to use to commit suicide. "I felt weak, and the gun made me feel stronger." The approach of the Christmas season made him feel worse. "I tried to contact my wife. I felt bad. People were happy, but I wasn't happy. I cried, and I could feel that something was happening."

"On Christmas Eve I decided to go to midnight mass and see my wife." AA knew that she and her family would attend church services as it had been their custom over the years. "I saw encouragement in her eyes. I tried to talk to her, but her mother intervened. I followed them home. I had the gun in my car." He indicated that while he was riding in his car, "things didn't look real to me. The trees didn't look real. I actually saw myself driving. It was weird."

> I followed them to their house into the garage. They pulled in the garage, and I went in behind them. I asked to talk to my wife. Her father hit me with a broom handle, and her mother went in the house. I pulled out the gun. I put numerous shots into my wife. I wanted them to know I meant business. The parents were all scattered. I stepped into the driver's seat, shot her in the head again and again. She fell out the passenger side. I saw no blood on her. I said to her that I loved her, and I kissed her on the lips. Then I shot her again from close range directly in the head. I think I fired two more shots. I walked away and felt I would throw up. I pulled the hammer back again and pointed it to my head. My hand shook so bad I couldn't pull the trigger. I looked in her eyes. I felt ill. I saw the police coming so I dropped the gun. I was afraid that my father-in-law would go for it and start shooting me. I yelled at the cops to pick up the gun that I had dropped.

When evaluated in the county jail, AA showed no clinical signs of psychosis, although he was clearly very depressed. AA admitted to suicidal preoccupation both before and following the homicide. He expressed great remorse over the murder and said he felt the need "to kill myself and join her." Concomitantly, however, he said that the "horrible feeling" he had had for several months prior to the homicide lifted following the shooting.

AA had average intelligence with no evidence of any organicity. Borderline personality characteristics were noted on the Rorschach by lack of inner integration and cohesiveness. He used rigid, compulsive-like defenses, appearing neat, orderly, and quite controlled.

The following TAT excerpts provide insight into some of AA's inner thoughts and emotions:

- *Card 3BM*:

We have a person here. A woman leaning against a bench, in a deep depression of some kind. Crying or mourning something, obviously hurt. The shoulder shows this person to be tense. She suffered a rejection of some sort. Her and her fiancé had an argument, and he called off the marriage. She is reliving the pain by letting out an emotion. I don't know if she will get back together.

- *Card 4*:

Man and a woman. Woman is looking into a man for moral support. He's turning away from her. The man is disinterested. Something casual, she is asking him. They are married. Having a communication problem. He is ignoring what she wants. I don't know how it turns out. The dominant person is the man. He will win due to his dominance.

- *Card 14*:

Not a pretty picture. A man peering out a window. Could be on the brink of suicide. Looking for someone to talk to. Maybe talking to God. He is all by himself. It is a shadow of a man. He could have suffered a major setback. He had lost his job, and he loved it. He was a success-oriented person. He can't take the thought of rejection, of being unsuccessful.

- *Card 5*:

A mother holding her lifeless child. No wound or injury. The child has taken a drug overdose. The mother was caring. She is hurt and concerned. It is a tragedy. A very sad ending. It doesn't turn out good. The person is obviously dead, and she will mourn for a long time.

- *Card 13M*:

A man. No weapon. His wife is dead. He just murdered her. He hates himself. He cannot face the sight of seeing her dead. I can't tell why he killed her. Maybe she was unfaithful to him. She is unclothed. He came home from work in a state of tension. He strangled her about the neck. He has a lot of regret. He hates himself. He is very guilt-laden. This is the man who jumps out the window. He is confused and doesn't know why he did it.

In this case, the incubation phase of the catathymic process was accompanied by depression with suicidal preoccupation that later mixed with and was finally dominated by homicidal thoughts. At first, the idea to kill his wife seemed vague, far off, and "crazy." But it slowly built to a point where he became obsessed with the thought and believed it was the only way to solve the problem. Unfortunately, AA's psychiatrist dismissed the revelation to kill the victim. The revelation was actually a plea for help, as AA felt ambivalence due to the ego-alien nature of the thought.

This offender's marital difficulties stemmed partly from his own conflicts over the relationship with his wife. These conflicts were graphically illustrated by his ambivalent feelings of love and hate: he kissed her on the lips after having shot her several times in the head. The closeness of the marital relationship created a state of confusion and helplessness, feelings of abandonment and sexual inadequacy, and a sense of failure that he could not tolerate. He explained that he felt his wife had left him because he was "unable to satisfy her sexually. She did not say this exactly, but you could tell it was true." The breakup of his first marriage was also due, in part, to his perceived sexual shortcomings.

As the catathymic tension built, he believed he could reduce the internal pressure only by elimination of the source of the tension through homicide or by removing himself through suicide. In studying homicides in marital relationships, Cormier (1982) found that men often develop the idea that

> murder is the only way to dissolve a union that other people terminate by more normal means. The murder occurs at a point of intense emotions and a feeling that to continue is inconceivable and to give up is impossible. (p. 190)

Although the clinical diagnosis of AA was major depression, depression alone cannot explain his actions. In such cases, the authorities typically look for a logical motive, often citing anger because of an impending divorce. But such a simple explanation does not begin to penetrate the depth of these offenders' conflicts, nor does it explain all levels of motivation. As in this case, it is not the offender's lowered mood but the emergence of the idea to kill—with the accompanying pressure to act—that resulted in murder.

Case 6.2: Killing of Fiancée by a Depressed Individual

A 26-year-old male (BB) shot and killed his girlfriend of 8 months while he was a passenger in a car she was driving. Following the homicide, he ran to a phone and called his clergyman. The tragedy began about a year before the homicide, when he met his first girlfriend (not the victim). After 6 weeks of intensive dating, the couple was engaged. But BB soon became jealous, imagining that his fiancée was sexually interested in a neighbor. He became confused, and the feeling of closeness to his girlfriend left. He began to act strangely, discontinued school, and finally the fiancée broke the engagement, an act she viewed as a solution to the "dilemma."

Several months later, while on a new job, BB met the future victim (C) and was immediately attracted to her. They dated, and within a short time became engaged, a pattern identical to that with his first girlfriend. The relationship grew in intensity, but by the 4th month, BB developed feelings similar to those he had had previously. He felt C was distancing herself from him: "I thought things were deteriorating." At this time, he became preoccupied with discussing sex to the point that his new fiancée asked him to change the subject. He believed that she was disappointed in him, and he told a friend he was thinking of joining the military. At the same time, BB pressed his fiancée regarding marriage to such an extent that she, like the first fiancée, had second thoughts. C said that she still loved him but decided to postpone the wedding.

BB developed a depression that increased in intensity and fluctuated with occasional feelings of euphoria. He told the future victim that either he would not like to see her at all or he wanted to be with her constantly. He repeatedly asked her whether she still wanted to marry him, and she replied that she did. Yet, at the same time, he felt his desire for her diminishing. "One day it entered my mind to end it all. I had continued sadness." In spite of BB's conflicted feelings, he continued to date the future victim.

His depression increased, and BB developed ideas of killing himself. On one occasion, he told C about his suicidal thoughts, and she became very upset. Around the 5th month of the relationship, he had a feeling of "total chaos." Although BB functioned at work, he had strange, intrusive thoughts that his girlfriend smiled more at others than at him. By the 6th month, he had lost weight, and his family doctor referred him to a psychiatrist for treatment of depression. He thought more and more about committing suicide, but "I had enough life left in me to want to live." He obtained a gun for suicidal purposes, and while thinking about suicide, he fired several shots into C's front lawn. On another occasion, he punctured the tires on her car.

During the 7th month of the relationship, BB went to the beach, called his fiancée, and told her he was going to commit suicide. He shot into the water and then returned home. Following this episode, he gave the gun to his psychiatrist as he felt a loss of control. He then told a few friends that he was going to shoot his girlfriend, but they apparently took it as a joke.

A week later, BB returned to his psychiatrist and asked to have his gun back since he felt better and in control. The gun was returned, and he immediately drove to C's home with the intention of shooting her. He stated that the idea of killing her took "such hold" of him that he was unable to cope with it. He had a feeling that "it had to be done." This idea, at times, came in spurts and then receded. By the 8th month, he thought of contacting a professional hit man to kill her.

BB explained that he was in a good mood the night before the homicide. He went to work with the loaded gun in his briefcase. Throughout the day he felt depressed, but periodically he felt mild elation. He had strong thoughts of killing his fiancée, but at other times, he thought about dropping the entire matter. By the end of the workday, he decided that he would kill her and himself. He called C and asked whether she would drive him to a gas station where his car was being repaired. During the car ride, he took the gun out of his briefcase and discharged all the bullets into her.

Shortly after the homicide, when evaluated in the county jail, BB felt a sense of relief, and his depression dissipated. He explained that at the time of the shooting, he had "an incredible inferiority complex." He said that he was too dependent on the victim, and that in killing her, he solved two problems: he achieved freedom, and she would not have to live in a hostile world. Sex with her seemed to him to be immoral and against his religion, "like having sex with my mother."

In fact, BB's entire life was filled with sexual conflict and disturbance. He had overall average intelligence, but with superior verbal skills. The Rorschach was typical of borderline structure, filled with repetitive sexual references illustrating the intensity of this offender's sexual preoccupation. The following Rorschach perceptions are illustrative:

> I see two animals of the Paleolithic age, almost like in mythology, fighting, or it could be an act of fornication with the blood there, with the girl being a virgin. That could be blood from the battle. Stomachs. These could also be some type of sex organs. Maybe they are homosexuals, but that's ridiculous. They look like butterflies. I suspect there are sex organs inside. I keep thinking about sex organs today for some reason. This is a male. A young boy age twelve. He is a wreck, so make him 14 years old. For some reason, I think of a female sex organ and these are some kind of legs. These look like some kind of legs of a heavy girl about 20, and she is large. Has very large legs, and this is the lower outside leg and some kind of erection; or, this could be two lesbians having some kind of relationship. Is it called oral-anal? Maybe sixty-nine is going on. These two girls, one 20 and one 14; and this one has her mouth on her sex organ. This is a woman's womb up here. A clitoris and these are eggs. That's a flame. A hot flame. Down here are the testes. A penis in the womb. Those are supposed to be some kind of an erection. A vagina down here. Looks like two rats here. A woman's womb. Supposed to be an unsatisfied penis that's not achieving climax. Looks a little limp. This is some kind of sex. The act of intercourse. Some kind of climax or satisfactory climax. The woman is in

her period, so they can't be too old. Not over forty-two. A penis again. Female sex organs. The pink, I guess the woman is in her period again. Is this symbolic of all the anxieties and thoughts that go through her mind when she is having her period?

TAT stories were also filled with themes of sexuality, many of them rather disturbed: "Lesbians. No. Maybe they are just jealous of each other." "Two men kissing. Age 18 and 40." "He is thinking about sex and the enjoyment of it." "This woman has been killed by him. It's his mother. No. She wouldn't let him have sex." "This is a house of prostitution. He has a great desire to have sex, but, at the same time, he has an element of discipline." "Surgeries being performed on a young man. He is having some evil cut out of him."

The following TAT story (Card 13MF), given after BB's release from prison (8 years after the murder), provides additional insight into the dynamics of the homicide:

A young man who is lamenting the fact that he killed his girlfriend or had sex with his girlfriend. He went to prison for seven years. The killing was a mistake. He should not have had guilt about having closeness with her. He was emotionally dependent upon her. When she tried to break up, it resulted in her death. His emotional dependency drove her away. There was a reluctance to have a closeness to someone else. Now he wants an emotional closeness, but he remains autonomous.

Projective figure drawings displayed in Figure 6.1 reflect not only inadequacy (the tiny house, tree, and human sketches) but also sexual preoccupation, as the offender was sure to incorporate genitalia.

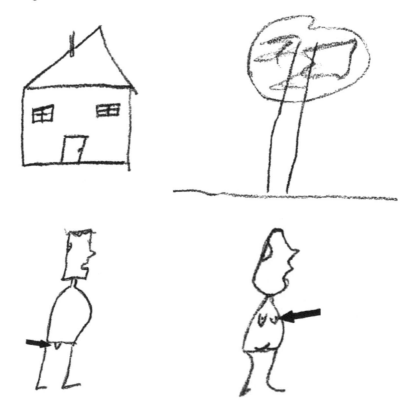

Figure 6.1 Drawings by an offender who committed a chronic catathymic homicide. Inadequacy and sexual preoccupation are obvious.

This is a typical case of a chronic catathymic homicide occurring within the framework of an ego-threatening relationship. BB was experiencing a clinical depression, but it was the catathymic motivational process—not the depression—that resulted in the murder. The incubation phase was marked by suicidal ideas which finally culminated in a strong homicidal idea that became fixed. BB struggled with the urge to act violently but eventually did. Following the homicide, he felt a sense of relief, and the depression quickly dissipated. The ambivalence, sexual preoccupation, and repetitive pattern with his first and second girlfriend illustrate, as noted earlier by Wertham, that if the underlying complex is not resolved, it is likely to recur, and another catathymic event can result. BB received several years of psychotherapy following his release from prison, and he seemed to achieve some degree of insight into his ambivalent and conflicted feelings regarding the opposite sex. He had less difficulty in yet another relationship following release from prison. This case is supportive of Wertham's contention that psychotherapy has value in these cases.

6.4 Catathymia with a Predominant Obsession

An obsession is "an idea, emotion, or impulse that repetitively and insistently forces itself into consciousness even though it is unwelcome" (Hinsie and Campbell, 1970, p. 518). Although obsessive features often accompany depressive states, some depressed individuals also have a distinct and pronounced obsession beyond that associated with the affective disorder. Frequently, obsessions appear as ideas "which are strongly charged with emotions" (p. 518), and sometimes there is a strong urge to act, such as in "impulsive obsessions which are repetitively intrusive ideas that lead to action" (p. 519).

The case of Ricardo Lopez (Schlesinger, 2006) is illustrative. Lopez was a young man who became obsessed with a rock star and attempted to kill the celebrity by sending her an acid bomb. He then committed suicide, videotaping his death. Prior to the suicide, he wrote a detailed 807 page diary of his thoughts with respect to his fantasy relationship with the celebrity and his plan and motive for killing her. The 21-year-old offender became obsessed about 2 years before the attempted homicide and suicide. His idolization of the celebrity turned to anger when she left her long-term boyfriend and quickly developed a relationship with another man and moved in with him. Lopez was depressed, withdrawn, fairly intelligent, and quite insightful with respect to many of his own psychodynamics. He felt extremely inadequate, based on having gynecomastia (enlargement of breasts in men), and on his belief that a woman would never want to be with him, as he considered himself "a freak." He initially saw the celebrity as "so angelic, elegant, and sweet," a view that was shattered when he learned of her new boyfriend, whom he considered to be "unacceptable." The incubation phase of the catathymic process lasted about 3 months. Because he did not actually kill her, the emotional (catathymic) tension was not fully released and he shot himself in the head.

Cases of filicide (the murder of one's child) frequently involve obsessional states. In many instances, the homicide is essentially a catathymic murder. Neonaticides (the killing of newborns), as well as early filicides (the killing of young children) and late filicide (the killing of older children or adult children), are committed in states of depression, dissociation, or sometimes psychosis, or as a result of fear or panic (Sadoff, 1995). Many such homicides occur during postpartum depression (Gold, 2001; Haapasalo and Petaejae,

1999) in which an obsessional altruistic idea becomes fixed. Here, the parent kills in order to relieve the child from suffering or to spare the child from some ominous fate (Bourget and Labelle, 1992).

In a study of 120 women admitted to their forensic hospital, McDermaid and Winkler (1955) found that 12 were charged with some form of infanticide. Three of these cases were triggered by social pressure; three cases involved a clear-cut psychosis, but six women were considered to be suffering from a condition the authors termed "child-centered obsessional depression." Symptoms included long-standing tension, depression, and obsessional pre-occupation with the child's health; the obsessions were "produced in a ruminating man-ner" (p. 36). In essence, the parent became preoccupied with the child's appearance, health, safety, or future. The murder was followed by suicide or a suicide attempt, as is found in many catathymic acts of violence. In such cases, the parent–child relationship becomes so intense that the parent overidentifies with the child. "It is the combination of the catathy-mic thinking, the obsessional fears, and the depression with suicidal tendencies which was considered as causative in the formation of short-circuit reactions leading to infanticide" (p. 38). The mother is usually the offender, but in a minority of cases, the father develops an obsessive rumination that leads to a fixed idea to kill the child and results in a catathymic homicide.

The following case of a father who shot his son after a prolonged period of preoccupa-tion with the boy's allegedly deformed mouth is illustrative.

Case 6.3: Filicide after Prolonged Obsession

Following oral surgery (to extract a superimposed tooth) on his 7-year-old son, a 54-year-old man (CC) developed an obsessive preoccupation with the child's "mutilated" mouth. He believed that the youngster would "suffer" when he grew up as a result of the perceived deformity. Initially, his obsessive preoccupation was of a recurrent nature and diminished after discussion with either his wife or the dentist.

The obsession continued for several years in a mild form, but after his wife died of breast cancer, CC's symptoms grew in intensity. CC was exceptionally close to his son, particularly following his wife's death. All his emotion and affection were concentrated on the child. He blamed himself for making the wrong decision in allowing the oral surgeon to extract his son's tooth and believed that, through this decision, he had "mutilated" the child. He suddenly developed an idea which appeared ego-alien at the time—that it was necessary to kill his son in order to free him from future suffering. CC thought of discuss-ing this idea with a clergyman, but he realized it sounded so absurd that he feared he would not be believed.

The idea subsided in intensity for several months but then increased again and grew stronger. CC became depressed and preoccupied with the bleak future his son would have, and he concluded again that the only solution was to kill the child to prevent his suffering.

The offender bought a rifle and hid it in his room. For the next several days, he waited for the "proper time" to commit the act. He finally shot his son while the child was asleep. Immediately afterward, he felt that he "did the right thing." He did not believe his act was wrong or criminal. In fact, he felt no remorse and was interested only in the salvation of his son's soul. The tortured feelings he experienced prior to committing the homicide dissipated after the shooting. However, several months after the murder, CC realized that he had made "a stupid mistake" and came to believe that he had "exaggerated" the idea that the mild deformity of his son's mouth would somehow interfere with his life. CC was found legally insane and spent 2 years in a psychiatric hospital, followed by outpatient psychotherapy.

As a child, CC had been unpopular and teased in school. He described himself as rather rigid and orderly, always fearful of making mistakes or hurting another's feelings. He worked as an accountant, a profession in which his personality traits were useful. CC's intelligence fell within the superior range; projective testing reflected a rather bland, unoriginal, and practical approach to life with no signs of structural disorganization.

This case is typical of a child-centered obsessional depression, culminating in a catathymic homicide. The treating psychiatrist concluded—after 6 years of therapy—that the extremely close relationship with the son and the quasi-delusional preoccupation with the child's mouth pointed to a deeper source of disturbance and conflict. Although unable to document or substantiate his conclusions in a direct way, the psychiatrist believed that incestuous homosexual conflicts were at the root of CC's disturbance.

6.5 Stalking and Catathymic Homicide

Stalking has been described as the quintessential crime of the 1990s (Goldstein, 2000). During this decade, a great deal of interest was generated in stalking, and numerous clinical and empirical studies were carried out. In Meloy's (1998) compendium on the topic, he summarized 26 fairly definitive research findings on every aspect of stalking perpetrators and victims. Most research has found that, although stalkers are a heterogeneous group of offenders, common to all stalking behavior is an obsessive (pathological) attachment to the victim. Some stalkers are unable to give up a prior intimate relationship (Zona, Sharma, and Lane, 1993). Some develop delusional beliefs about the target (Goldstein, 1987), while others develop strong obsessional thoughts about virtual strangers (Spitzberg and Cupach, 1994). Meloy (1992) and Kienlen (1998) believe that a disturbance of attachment begins in the offender's early childhood and stalking starts when some type of loss in adulthood resurrects these early conflicts.

Intimate relationships often involve a great deal of violence, including homicide. The percentage of females involved in violent relationships, who were eventually killed by their mates (about 30%), has remained fairly constant since 1976 (U.S. Department of Justice, 2000). It is not clear how many of these aggressive and homicidal acts involve prior stalking, however. In fact, the prevalence of homicide among stalkers is unknown, and estimates are unclear. Meloy (1996b) reviewed the scientific literature between 1978 and 1995 and found that out of 180 cases of stalking, only 4 of the subjects committed a homicide—an incidence of 2%. However, this finding may underestimate the prevalence of homicide among stalkers because (1) the vast majority of cases were not reported in the scientific literature and (2) as Meloy (1998) has subsequently pointed out, when there is a homicide, individuals are frequently not charged with stalking.

Moracco, Runyan, and Butts (1998) provide a methodology that may obviate these problems. These researchers determined the percentage of femicides in a jurisdiction in which stalking was involved by reviewing police and medical examiners' reports and by interviewing law enforcement officers. Using this method as opposed to simply looking at whether the perpetrator was legally charged with stalking, Moracco and colleagues found that 23% of the women were stalked prior to their deaths. In a subsequent study

(McFarlane, Campbell, Wilt, Sachs, Ulrich, and Xu, 1999), the researchers not only used medical records and law enforcement information but also conducted interviews with proxy informants (victims' family members and friends). This procedure revealed that 76% of female victims were stalked prior to their death, and 42% of these women had not reported the stalking to the police. It therefore seems clear that the prevalence of homicide among stalkers may be greater than previous estimates indicated.

The following case of a stalking homicide involved a young man who quickly became obsessively attached to his girlfriend. He followed her, broke into her home, and ultimately developed a fixed idea to kill her in a manner typical of the catathymic process.

Case 6.4: Stalking Homicide of a Girlfriend

A 22-year-old male (DD) killed his girlfriend (A) by multiple stabs to the neck during a car ride. Immediately following the homicide, the offender had fleeting thoughts of committing suicide but lacked the impetus to carry it out.

DD grew up in a working-class family with five siblings. The father was a lay preacher who was preoccupied with religion, as was DD. His mother was described as heavy set, aggressive, and the one "who ruled the roost." DD dropped out of high school in the ninth grade, served 6 months in the military, but was administratively discharged because of emotional instability and various psychosomatic manifestations. Diagnostically, he fell within the spectrum of severe personality disorders with schizotypal and paranoid traits.

Throughout DD's life, he was a loner with few friends. He felt shy and inferior and had serious difficulties relating to females. As a young boy, he was involved in a forced homosexual relationship that he equated to "a big sin." Following this experience, he felt that sex was dirty, and he claimed it made him feel even more inferior. "I couldn't make out with girls like the other guys; I liked to be alone by myself." He had three prior sexual contacts before meeting A, but he was unsure whether he had intercourse since he was uncertain as to whether he had penetrated the woman. Several times DD attempted to sexually touch his younger sister. During his preteen years, he recalled hitting a girl cousin in the stomach but could not explain why he did it. When he was 15 or 16, a girl insulted him, and he grabbed and twisted her breast until she started crying.

DD and A dated for about 9 months before the homicide. When DD met A, she seemed to accept him immediately; he was surprised because of his previous experiences with members of the opposite sex. The courtship was marked by DD's obsession with A and his attempt to control her. He not only stalked her but continuously tested her love and her interest in him. The relationship became intense shortly after they met, and he immediately became insecure, possessive, and threatening. He would check on A's whereabouts, also requesting that she provide him with details of her past activities and friendships. He got angry if A went home from work a different way than usual or disobeyed one of his "orders." On one occasion, the offender went to the home of A's former boyfriend and told him that he had had sexual relations with A and that "she was no good." On another occasion, he told A's father "she is no good. She is a whore. She had sex with me and with E." DD felt that he had to "own" A completely. He also broke into the cellar of A's home to see whether he could find an alleged letter from a prior boyfriend in the garbage can. He even tried to check on A's faithfulness by asking his friend to call her and attempt to make a date. Although she did not accept the date, A made some remarks damaging to DD, which also angered him. He always felt that she lied to him, told "fishy stories," and may have been seeing another man.

There was frequent hitting, cursing, and yelling. Once DD hit A when the car in which they were driving came to a red light; she tried to jump out of the car, and he kept hitting her. He then asked her forgiveness. On another occasion, "I hit her out of the clear blue sky." There were several other incidents of unprovoked minor assaults on A, followed by feelings of remorse. In general, DD found his relationship with A confusing. Her actions often enraged him and made him feel insecure and distressed.

The homicide was preceded on DD's part by several weeks of strange fantasies, obsessional ideas regarding suicide, murder, and stalking. One afternoon, while driving with A over a bridge, DD told her jokingly that he would throw her off. On another occasion, he was in the car with her and her mother. He drove both to a local tavern, and after some talk, he felt like crashing the car. Several weeks prior to the homicide, he borrowed a knife, sharpened it, and told his friend to stay with him while he visited A. He did not want to go alone because "I was afraid I was going to hurt her." DD increasingly experienced intrusive violent thoughts in which he felt like smashing A in the head with a bottle. He also had a bizarre fantasy of catching a snake, throwing it at A, and having the snake bite and kill her. He had daydreams of shooting A and of taking A to a reservoir and shooting and killing her, as well as other fantasies of hitting A's younger sister with a belt. On another occasion, while he was kissing A, he bit her lip so hard that she bled. "I wondered why I was thinking about all this. Maybe I should have shot her and made an excuse when the cops came. I can't understand it."

The homicidal thoughts were becoming overpowering, and DD said he was "trying to fight them." He threw his gun and bullets into the woods in an attempt to remove any weapons from his possession that could lead to A's death. He later returned to pick up the gun. While he was there, he was rather surprised at his actions: "Holy cow! What am I doing in the woods with my shotgun? It was like a dream. Then I put the shotgun in my car and went back home."

Three weeks prior to the homicide, DD cried in church.

> When I am in church, I think of God, then I cry. I thought of leaving God out of my life. I still have sin in me. I asked my pastor if I could see him. He told me to call him the next afternoon. So I told my father I wanted to use his car. I started crying. My father said, "What's the matter?" I told him the devil was in me. Then I told the pastor what I had in mind. I also thought of shooting myself. The pastor prayed for me. All this came into my mind just like that.

The day before the homicide he put the shotgun in his father's car and thought, "I am going to kill A." All evening, while driving the car, it seemed to him that the scenery was moving but he did not move. He also felt that he had no sense of balance. While all these thoughts and actions were gaining momentum, he went to see his friend in order to reveal his plan. He still did not believe it was possible to act on his thoughts. His friend thought DD was joking.

On the day of the murder, DD brought a sharpened knife with him to a planned date with A. He had homicidal thoughts intermingled with some vague suicidal ideas, but the homicidal intention was now dominant and fixed. He picked up A; they changed cars, and he got into her car.

I don't even know what was said. I grabbed her by the hand and told her to drive. Then I started unbuttoning her coat. I had her by the hair at the same time. Then I said I meant business. I felt different. I felt as if someone else was doing my movements. Then I said that we are going to drive on. I had my knife. I felt as if I was in a predicament. I didn't know what to do or what to say. I was looking at her. Looking at her throat. Then something happened. Like a bad dream, when you fall off a fence.

I was trying to stab her in the head. I felt like the weakest person in the world. Then a car blew the horn. I was in the driver's seat then. I put the car in neutral. She yelled for help. I pulled her. My hands felt real cold. She grabbed the wheel. I was driving fast. It felt like there was no time at all. When she asked me to take her to the hospital, I asked, "A, what happened?" She said, "You stabbed me." Then I put the knife between my legs. She said, "Please hurry." I started going towards the hospital. She said, "Honey." I said, "God will tell me what to do." Then I asked her to show me the wound. There was a cut on her neck and on her arm. I asked myself what I was gonna do. I was afraid. I put my arms around her. I asked her to kiss me and she kissed me. Then I saw a police car.

I started driving again. But instead of going to the hospital, I went around the park. Then I saw a sign and went into the park. I was afraid. She said, "Honey, let's go." I picked up the knife. My heart was pounding. I had the knife in my hand. She said, "Stop. I am dead already."

Then the knife fell out of my hand. I started reaching for the knife, but immediately I was afraid. Then she fell and sighed. Everything looked so different. I stopped the car and picked her up. She felt very light. All of a sudden she fell on the floor. I looked at her, and I thought it was a joke. What the heck did she try to prove. I said, "A," but she didn't answer, so I started cleaning up the blood. It was thick. It stunk. My mouth felt dry and hot. It never was like that before.

A was still lying there. Then I realized that she was dead. I was afraid. I did not remember stabbing her. I took my shotgun out of my car and put it in her car. Then I thought about getting a soda or about going to my pastor. Suddenly the thought came to my mind. "Now you have to kill yourself." I loaded my gun and went on, but everything looked funny. I went to a cliff. I shot off the gun. I looked at A, touched her pulse, but there wasn't any. I saw cigarettes on the floor. I finished my last cigarette, put the gun in the back, and went to the police. I told them I had killed my girlfriend. I left a note. "A and I have sinned together. I hope God will forgive us." DD explained that the sin he referred to was "having sex."

Following the murder itself, DD expressed a feeling of relief. "Now I don't have A to worry about any longer." He was emotionally flat during the evaluation and was most upset about having sinned by having sexual relations. He even claimed that he would fast on A's birthday since he loved her so much. He was quite upset by the prosecution theory that he had planned the homicide. "They all think that I planned it. It was just in my mind. I never thought it would happen. I never really meant it."

After serving 17 years in state prison for the homicide, DD was paroled. Within a year of his parole (at age 39), he succeeded in establishing a romantic relationship with another woman. A press report noted that he went to his new girlfriend's home when she was out. There, he attacked a 27-year-old woman who lived in the same house, bound and gagged her, and put her in an upstairs bedroom. DD then waited for his new girlfriend's return. When she entered the home, he shot and killed her and then committed suicide.

Unfortunately, the details of this new relationship remain unclear. Perhaps this was another catathymic homicide or, perhaps, it was the breakthrough of an underlying compulsion to kill, unleashed by the first homicide. The prior sadistic fantasies and unprovoked attacks against A, as well as other women, are typical of compulsive offenders.

The stalker who kills has been rarely studied and remains poorly understood, but the stalker who kills a relative stranger is even more enigmatic. Unlike cases in which there had been an intimate relationship between the stalker and the victim, relatively few instances of stalking homicide in which no such prior relationship existed have been reported. Schesinger and Mesa (2008) studied 17 cases of celebrities who were killed by their stalkers and found catathymic process to be an aid in differentiating those who are at the risk of actually acting out violently from those who had similar obsessive ideas but managed to control their behavior.

In the following case, described in detail by Schlesinger (2002a), a stalker kills a casual acquaintance, following months of obsessional preoccupation that developed into a fixed idea to kill the woman.

Case 6.5: Stalking Homicide of a Casual Acquaintance

A 28-year-old male (EE) stabbed and killed a 23-year-old female (B) whom he had stalked for less than a year. EE met the victim at church about a year prior to the homicide. He was immediately attracted to her. After several weeks, he drove by her home and began to "watch" her and her boyfriend. "I thought of her all the time. I could not get her out of my mind. It was her charm and smile. She was perfect. I was supposed to be her boyfriend."

During the next 6 months, EE followed B to her job, began to telephone her with increased frequency, and repetitively asked her on dates which she politely declined, explaining that she had a boyfriend. One month prior to the homicide, EE called the victim three to five times a day asking her to go out with him. About 2 weeks before the homicide, an idea to kill B emerged spontaneously

> when I was driving by her boyfriend's house. I saw her car parked. It was right there I got the idea to kill her and kill myself. It was just an idea. I didn't think it was possible for me to kill somebody. The idea was just a little bit; but the idea kept building. My life was pretty much empty without her.

About a week prior to the homicide, following an increase of stalking and telephone calls, B sent EE a letter. She explained that she had a boyfriend, planned to get married, and although she would like to have EE "as a friend," she was not in love with him and did not want any type of romantic relationship. This letter triggered anger and a deep feeling of rejection in EE.

> It belittled me. It made it look like there was nothing. I loved her. … I kept thinking of killing the both of us as the only thing to do. Now I felt I had to do it. There was no choice. The urge was so strong.

On the day of the homicide, EE went to B's boyfriend's house and spotted her carrying an infant.

> I went to my car and picked up a knife I had in the trunk. Then she came out and said, "What's going on?" She put the baby down that she was carrying and ran away. That's when I stabbed her in the back. I don't even know why. Then I started stabbing myself because I felt I wanted to die I wanted to put an end to it. I loved her so much. I was angry that she wasn't mine. I

thought about killing the both of us all the time. It's better for both of us to die because I loved her and I didn't want nobody to have her. I couldn't imagine my life without her.

Not only did EE stab himself, but he resisted aid and tried to injure himself further by inserting his fingers into his abdominal wounds in an apparent attempt to pull out his internal organs. He was eventually placed in custody and transported to a local hospital, where he underwent surgery and recovered completely. Initially, EE told hospital and legal authorities that he killed his "girlfriend because she broke up with me for another man." Finally, he told the truth, described a feeling of relief after the murder, but revealed embarrassment over what now seemed to him to be illogical thinking at the time.

Psychological testing was consistent with clinical impressions indicating that EE fell diagnostically within the schizotypal spectrum, characterized by introversion, excessive social isolation, and feelings of interpersonal alienation. Figure drawings were meager and revealed depression, inadequacy, and immaturity (see Figure 6.2).

TAT stories were quite illuminating, with repetitive themes of sexual inadequacy leading to unfaithfulness and subsequent violence. The following TAT stories are illustrative:

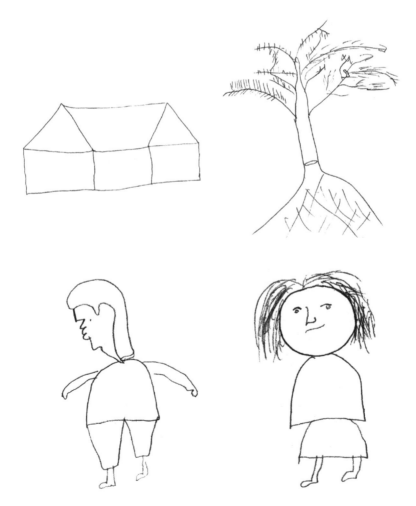

Figure 6.2 Sketches by a man who stalked and killed a relative stranger. Depression, inadequacy, and immaturity are noted.

"Infidelity. She cheated on him. She cheated on him for sexual satisfaction. He probably beats her up when he finds out because he is insecure. He is not sure of himself." "It looks like her husband is abusing her due to infidelity. She was unfaithful because he didn't satisfy her." "She is sexually bored. She will find somebody else. She will find another man to keep her happy. The new man will give her more sexual satisfaction."

> She has been raped and sexually abused. She left him because of his sexual performance. She underrated his performance. She didn't get sexual satisfaction from him. He ends up killing her because she laughed at him. She said, "You are half a man." He raped and killed her because she was about to leave him. He is insecure about finding another girlfriend for himself as beautiful as she is.

Interestingly, EE previously had thought to kill a former girlfriend but was able to control himself because "I didn't love her as much [as B]." The obsessional ideas in the prior relationship were not as strong as with the current victim, and the stalking behavior associated with the first relationship was not as extensive. The homicide itself is a classic example of a chronic catathymic process within the context of depression. Applicable here is Meloy's (1992) belief that the murder in such cases reverses an intolerable feeling of being controlled by the victim. Here, EE viewed the victim's rejection of him as the ultimate form of control, and he attempted to regain some degree of control through violence.

6.6 Catathymic Mass Murder

Mass murder is the killing of many individuals at a single time in a single location. Although there are no U.S. crime statistics on mass murders, such incidents seem to have been rather rare in the first half of the 20th century but not that uncommon since the 1950s. Dietz (1986) refers to three types of mass murderers: set-and-run killers (who set bombs and leave the scene before the explosion); pseudo-commandos (who dress in paramilitary garb and typically kill relative strangers); and family annihilators (who kill their entire families). Disgruntled employees and disgruntled students can be added to the list, along with the most frequent type of mass murderer, the one who shoots multiple strangers. Douglas, Burgess, Burgess, and Ressler (2013) describe the prototypical mass murderer as "a mentally disordered individual whose problems have increased to the point that he acts out against groups of people who are unrelated to him or his problems, unleashing his hostility through shootings and stabbings" (p. 114).

The six types of mass murder delineated above do not encompass every type of multiple murder, as human behavior is exceptionally complex and defies rigid classification with specific boundaries. The case of Levi King, a Missouri man who murdered five people and severely wounded another, is an example. A series of murders such as his were previously referred to as spree killing—killing multiple people in two or more incidents without a cooling-off period. However, spree killing has been eliminated as a separate, stand-alone category (Morton and Hilts, 2005), as the concept offers little help to investigators and "cooling off" is difficult to measure. This case can best be understood as a catathymic homicide.

An examination of King's thinking indicates a long incubation period in which he fantasized about killing people and felt tremendous relief afterward. "I was extremely angry

… [after killing] I felt relief, peace. I was enjoying it." After he killed a couple in Missouri, he wanted to experience a sense of relief again, as the pleasurable feeling dissipated after about four to five hours. "I wanted to feel that peace again. … I wanted to kill again." When evaluated following his apprehension, he did not appear particularly angry or upset; in fact, he seemed relaxed and happy. Although he was diagnosed as having many conditions such as bipolar disorder, paranoid schizophrenia, psychopathic personality, and antisocial personality disorder, none of these diagnoses explain his behavior. The offender said that earlier in his life, he killed animals, which made him feel good but not good enough; he set fires ("I enjoy doing it"), but that also was not enough. Killing people satisfied him, but the feeling of relief and peace—which was very pleasurable for him—lasted only for several hours. Following his trial, he displayed no remorse whatsoever. He blamed his father for many of his problems.

Hempel, Levine, Meloy, and Westermeyer (2000) detected social isolation, recent loss, depression, anger, pathological narcissism, and paranoia (often with psychosis) to be typical traits of the mass murderer. Cantor, Mullen, and Alpers (2000) found their group of seven mass murderers to be "socially inadequate and self-absorbed individuals who have lived for years resenting their subordinate status" (p. 63). Hershman and Lieb (1994) note that manic depression is related to some forms of politically motivated mass killing. But despite such traits and symptoms, Milton (1992) was struck by the mass killer's relatively normal facade, which seems to mask his chronic sense of failure.

Some mass murders, particularly family mass murders, are best understood as catathymic explosions. Kretschmer (1934) described explosive reactions that occur during states of depression and lead to extreme acts of violence—especially the murder of the offender's own family—which he referred to as "raptus melancholicus." Here, an accumulation of catathymic tension, caused by a sense of helplessness and confusion, fuels the outburst. Dietz (1986) describes the typical family annihilator as a man who is depressed, drinks excessively, kills his family by shooting, stabbing, or strangling them, sometimes kills himself, and occasionally sets the house on fire. Wilson, Daly, and Daniele (1995) describe the despondent—in contrast to the paranoid—familicidal offender as depressed, brooding, and someone who "anticipates impending disaster for himself and his family and who sees familicide followed by suicide as 'the only way out'" (p. 288). Despondent familicidal offenders are not at all angry with the family members they kill but instead view them with sympathy.

Although depression is the most obvious clinical symptom in this group of family mass murderers, an individual's fixed idea that killing his whole family is the only possible solution to his problem cannot be explained by the depression alone. Here, the concept of catathymic process is particularly relevant. Brinded and Taylor (1995), for example, described a familicide committed by a 24-year-old male, who bludgeoned and stabbed to death several people and wounded two others. The victims were his three sons, his sister-in-law and brother-in-law, their 3-year-old son, and another individual home at the time. The offender later attacked his wife and his father-in-law but was restrained and arrested before these victims were killed. This man experienced a "build-up of intense frustration, anger, and despair" and then "arrived at his decision to kill his family" (p. 319). Following the act, the depression and tension dissipated.

Nesca and Kincel (2000) also report a case of a familicidal offender which they explained in terms of the catathymic process. Here, a middle-aged man brutally murdered his partner and his two oldest daughters with an axe. These authors found in the offender evidence of conflictual traits of dependence and entitlement which they considered "central to the catathymic process" (p. 43), in addition to finding a link between catathymic violence and depleted narcissism.

Vinas-Racionero, Schlesinger, Scalora, and Jarvis (2017) conducted a study of youthful familicidal offenders. The study involved 16 family mass murders (19 offenders, ages 14–21). The findings indicate that half the offenders reported to others their intent to kill their families; all the victims were specifically targeted, and most of the murders (75%) were planned shooting attacks rather than spontaneous eruptions. In about half the cases, the offenders called their friends to report the murders and then planned leisure activities; almost all of them quickly confessed to the homicides. In many of these cases, the offenders felt compelled to carry out the act—their behavior progressed to the development of a fixed idea, typical in chronic catathymic murders, that the homicide was the solution to their problems.

The following case of familicide, depression, and catathymic process, reported previously by Schlesinger (2000c), is illustrative. In this case, there is some suggestion of a sexual component, but in many catathymic mass murders, sexual dynamics cannot be elicited.

Case 6.6: Catathymic Familicide

A 46-year-old male (FF) killed his wife and three children with multiple stab wounds in order to protect them from enduring the humiliation he thought they would experience following his inability to properly install a home heating system. The offender was employed by a public utility and was described as "well liked, industrious, quiet, and even tempered" by his supervisors. He and his wife of 8 years, along with their three children (ages 5, 4, and 4 months), lived in their own home. FF was active in his church, an elected member of the local zoning board, and had served in the National Guard, as well as the Air Force Reserves following his discharge from the Air Force several years earlier. He also worked part-time in a construction company to earn additional money.

Six months prior to the homicides, FF added to his home a family room with its own heating system. Unfortunately, he was unable to get the heating system to work properly, and he refused to seek help from a plumber or heating specialist. FF had always prided himself on being able to solve these types of home-improvement problems and considered it humiliating to ask for assistance. He was quite defensive about having never attended college and compensated by emphasizing to others that he earned as much money as individuals in his company who were college graduates. Unlike them, FF was always able to solve such mechanical problems on his own.

About a month prior to the homicides, FF sank into a deep depression with an obsessive idea of "failure on my part" because of his inability to solve the problem with the heating system.

> I couldn't face the failure. I got so worked up; I couldn't figure any way to keep my family from being hurt by my failure. The failure was the heating system. I couldn't get it to work. There was no way to handle this. I couldn't face the failure.

His sleep became disturbed, and he awoke early in the morning. He developed agitation characterized by pacing the floor, along with preoccupation about both the malfunctioning heating system and his failure to solve the problem. FF expressed overwhelming feelings of failure and humiliation and an inability to explain the situation to his family.

> In a split second I thought to get a knife and do it. Myself was telling me, if we all go, I wouldn't have to face this problem and they wouldn't be left behind to handle the problem for me.

Once this idea emerged, he "could not let it go. I kept thinking of killing us all. It became stronger and stronger, clearer and clearer."

On the morning of the killings, FF awoke at 5 o'clock. He was "so upset" by his inability to figure out the heating system that he "became overwhelmed" with the idea that he had to kill his entire family and himself to spare them the humiliation of his failure. He took his hunting knife and stabbed his wife 37 times. He also killed his 5-year-old daughter by stabbing her 34 times in the back and chest and his 4-year-old son by stabbing him 18 times in the back, chest, and abdomen. He then went to the nursery and stabbed his 4-month-old daughter 21 times in the back. After these killings, FF stabbed himself 26 times in the chest and abdomen and cut his wrists. He miraculously survived; a neighbor who had come to take one of the children to school spotted him on the floor in the kitchen.

When evaluated several weeks later, FF was exceptionally depressed and overwhelmed by the act he had just committed. Psychological test findings were interesting. Projective figure drawings reflected depression, a poor self-image, and feelings of inferiority, evidenced by tiny figures without any elaboration (see Figure 6.3). There were suicidal themes on the TAT, with one story about a man who committed suicide because "he couldn't handle the problem in his life, an everyday problem. It was easier to face death. It could be done so quickly. He is gone now and no more problems." The MMPI indicated major depression, including feelings of weakness and low self-esteem. Two interesting Rorschach perceptions suggest underlying inadequacy extending to the sexual area: "a man's tiny penis" and "two penises that are very small."

FF's inability to solve the heating problem resurrected long-suppressed conflicts regarding his intellectual competence and lack of a college education. Inability to solve the problem overwhelmed his defenses because he had always prided himself on being able to handle such tasks. Although he was clearly depressed, depression alone is unable to account for such a conduct. Even psychotic depression is merely a description of the intensity of symptoms and does not explain the dynamics or motivational process leading to the homicides. FF was found not guilty by reason of insanity, sentenced to a psychiatric hospital, and released after about 10 years. While in the community, 2 years following his release from a halfway house, he committed suicide, according to press reports.

6.7 Comment

The chronic catathymic process has been recognized as a clinical entity for almost a century; however, its usefulness in both forensic and clinical practice has been greatly undervalued. Not only can the catathymic process inform forensic practitioners in cases of extreme violence such as homicide, but it can also inform nonforensic clinicians (Schlesinger, 2002b) in cases of stalking, suicide, and even self-mutilation (Greilsheimer and Groves, 1979; Simpson, 1973). Perhaps because catathymia is not listed in the latest edition of the

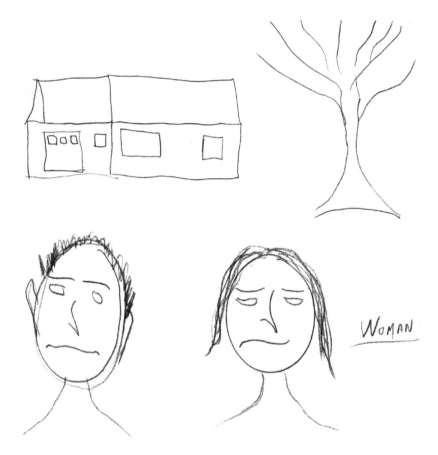

Figure 6.3 Deep depression is obvious in drawings by a man who killed his entire family.

diagnostic manual or perhaps because it is a psychodynamic construct (which may not be easily understood), its applicability has been relatively limited.

In some instances, the catathymic process is incorrectly applied to cases of interpersonal violence involving symptoms of brooding, depression, and a conflicted relationship with the victim. Schlesinger (1996b) discussed the differential diagnosis of the catathymic process and argued "not all explosions of violence directed against the partner, in a long term conflictual relationship, are necessarily catathymic reactions. Many primary psychiatric conditions may also result in explosive/homicidal behavior" (p. 131), as well as simply anger and jealousy. The catathymic process has also been incorrectly used as an explanation for serial murder (Garrison, 1996) and to explain other forms of behavior such as male battering (Dutton, 1998).

Both acute and chronic catathymic processes can also be useful in courtroom proceedings as a supplement to a traditional *DSM* diagnosis, especially in cases where the offender's motive is unclear. Catathymia is not meant to replace a diagnosis but rather to accompany it. A clinical diagnosis is a description of symptoms. The catathymic process helps explain the individual's behavior. Neither a diagnosis nor a psychodynamic explanation can directly satisfy the requirements of a legal standard; however, various disorders, conditions, and syndromes that relate to the loss of control are always of interest to the court. And as noted in Chapter 5, a catathymic homicide in its pure form may be relatively rare, but features or elements of the process can be found in many cases.

An insanity plea is usually rejected by the jury in chronic catathymic homicides, essentially for three reasons: (1) there is often no clear-cut psychosis, a necessary condition to establish mental disease; (2) the jury does not fully appreciate the frequently accompanying dissociative state; and (3) the jury often considers obsessive rumination to be the equivalent of premeditation. Nevertheless, a clear explanation of the catathymic process can enable jury members to gain additional insight into the complexity and depth of many such cases. Sentencing options, capacity for rehabilitation, and the potential for repetition if the underlying complex is not adequately addressed are additional issues of importance to the court.

The devastating consequences of a catathymic homicide underscore the need to develop effective risk-assessment strategies. Recognition of the clinical manifestations of the process helps to identify individuals at risk, particularly when a person reveals a belief that a violent act is a solution to an internal conflict. Practitioners, therefore, should routinely question their patients regarding homicidal thoughts with the same level of conscientious detail they use in assessing thoughts of suicide. Those found to be at risk need immediate intervention and treatment, including the option of hospitalization (possibly involuntary). Meloy (2010) notes that in cases of catathymic homicide, "the act is inexplicable by those who investigate it, and the prior absence of any violence completely obliterates the usual phenomenological explanations for intentional killing" (p. 1395). Nesca and Kincel (2000) believe that individuals in the incubation phase of the catathymic process can be effectively treated by "an aggressive focus on mood stabilization and relationship issues" (p. 52). They found pharmaceuticals as well as individual and conjoint psychotherapy to be of help. In addition, these authors stress the need for consultation with a forensic specialist who has expertise in this type of clinical syndrome.

Many suicidal threats often mask homicidal risk, while those who make homicidal threats often wind up committing suicide (MacDonald, 1968; Pokorny, 1966; Rhine and Mayerson, 1973). Thus, both types of threats, no matter how indirect, require careful assessment. The uncovering of catathymic ideation is always a foreboding sign that needs to be recognized and properly treated in an attempt to prevent tragedy. The effectiveness of restraining orders and antistalking laws is, at this point, unclear. Such measures hold promise, however, if a potential offender can be identified and referred for mandatory assessment and treatment rather than just handled legally without any mental health intervention. But the first step in prevention is the recognition of risk.

Compulsive Homicides in Historical Context

7

The word *compulsion* is derived from the Latin *compellere*, which means to compel, force, urge, or drive on. Unfortunately, the term *compulsion*—or *compulsive*—has been used to label very different forms of behavior and symptoms: the compulsive offender, the compulsive personality, and the obsessive–compulsive neurotic (see Table 7.1). The compulsive offender lies on the extreme endogenous end of the motivational spectrum (see Chapter 3) and is least influenced by external or sociogenic factors. From a clinical perspective, the compulsive offender has a powerful urge to act out his violent thoughts and fantasies, with a strong potential for repetition. He knows that the urge is dangerous and often plans his actions first in his mind and then perhaps through some behavioral tryouts; finally, often years later, he commits a criminal act. Other times, the compulsive offender acts out his fantasies in an unplanned, spontaneous manner when a victim of opportunity crosses his path.

The individual with a compulsive (or obsessive–compulsive) personality is totally different from the compulsive offender. The compulsive personality is characterized by inflexibility and a preoccupation with orderliness, perfectionism, and mental and interpersonal control. Individuals with this personality disorder are rigid and difficult to get close to since they often have detectable anger right at the surface that emerges easily in interpersonal situations. They may be excessively devoted to work and productivity, overly conscientious, stubborn, scrupulous, and unbending regarding matters of morality and ethics.

Both the compulsive person and the compulsive offender are different from individuals who have an obsessive–compulsive disorder, or what has sometimes been referred to as an obsessive–compulsive neurosis. Freud (1895) described this neurosis under the name *Zwangneurose*, which comprises both obsessions and compulsions. Clinically, this condition is characterized by rituals such as repetitive hand-washing, checking and rechecking, counting, or repeating words silently—intrusive, inappropriate obsessional thoughts, which are ego-dystonic, concern contamination, doubts, or what Rado (1959) has referred to as "horrific temptations." "In his fit of horrific temptations the patient, suddenly beset by the urge or idea to kill someone (characteristically a close and loved relative), shrinks back in horror from a temptation so alien to his entire being" (p. 325). The obsessive–compulsive neurotic does not want to act out and knows that he will not act out his "horrific temptations"; however, he fears that he might and so seeks reassurance from strong and supportive figures. Revitch and Schlesinger (1981) reported the case of a man so obsessed with the idea that he might kill his entire family that he left a ceremonial sword at another location in order not to be tempted to act on his horrific temptation.

The compulsive offender, however, does not have ego-alien temptations but rather has a compelling urge to act out dangerous fantasies. Here, the criminal act, such as murder, is itself eroticized (or sexually gratifying). These homicides do not necessarily involve rape or genital contact, as the murder itself is sexually arousing and sufficient. Thus obsessive–compulsive neurotics and compulsive offenders both have an urge for some type of

Table 7.1   Differing Uses of the Terms *Compulsion* and *Compulsive*

Terms	Symptoms and Behavior
Obsessive–compulsive neurosis Obsessive–compulsive disorder	The individual experiences obsessional thoughts as intrusive and inappropriate. He also exhibits repetitive behaviors, the goal of which is to prevent or reduce anxiety. Self-doubts and rituals (e.g., hand-washing) are common. Occasionally the individual has "horrific temptations" to hurt a loved one, which he realizes he will not act on.
Compulsive personality Obsessive–compulsive personality	The individual exhibits traits such as rigidity, orderliness, perfectionism, neatness, control, inflexibility, and interpersonal anger.
Compulsive offender	The individual has a powerful urge to act out dangerous fantasies, with a high potential for repetition. The offender knows this urge is dangerous and plans his actions methodically, or the compulsion may break through spontaneously when a victim of opportunity is present. The criminal act itself is sexually gratifying.

behavior, but the clinical features of the acting out and the underlying psychodynamics have nothing in common. In the obsessive–compulsive neurotic, defense mechanisms of isolation and undoing separate emotion from ideas. The same may occur with compulsive offenders, but their compulsions stem from a fusion of sex and aggression, quite different from those of the neurotic. Both, however, should generally be considered a repetition compulsion as described by Freud (1920), inasmuch as they involve an obligation to symbolically repeat a traumatic situation through action in order to avoid anxiety by gaining mastery of the repressed memory of the trauma.

7.1 Compulsive, Sexual, or Serial Murder?

Compulsive murders, where there is an internal drive or force to kill, are sexually motivated. The vast majority of psychiatric, psychological, and criminal investigative researchers agree that murders such as these, which sometimes involve multiple victims, are sexual murders (e.g., Geberth and Turco, 1997; Grubin, 1994; Lunde, 1976; Myers, Reccoppa, Burton, and McElroy, 1993; Ressler, Burgess, and Douglas, 1988; Revitch and Schlesinger, 1981, 1989; Warren, Hazelwood, and Dietz, 1996). Compulsive offenders have a disturbance in the sexual instinct that results in aberrant sexual fantasies in which gratification is achieved through various forms of aggression. After a period of fantasy, usually lasting several years, the subject begins to act out through various sadistic acts toward animals, perhaps fire setting, or even unprovoked attacks on females. In some cases, the subject engages in repetitive ritualistic behavior that provides him with a perverse sense of psychosexual gratification that is not achieved by the homicide alone. Such offenders have an inner drive to act out their thoughts and fantasies; once they kill, the killing is frequently repetitive if the offender is not apprehended.

Many cases of compulsive, repetitive murder do not involve overt manifestations of genitality, a phenomenon that has led a few researchers to question whether the motivation in these offenders is sexual (Egger, 1990b; Levin and Fox, 1985; Storr, 1972; West, 1987). And lack of clarity of what exactly makes a murder "sexual" is a continuing problem (Chan and Heide, 2009). For example, Egger (2002) has argued that sex is only an instrument used by the killer to obtain power and domination over his victim. … [The sexual component is] frequently present in a serial murder, [but] it is not the central motivating factor for the killer, but merely an instrument used to dominate, control, and destroy the victim. (p. 30)

We believe that the domination and control of the victim is what is eroticized and gratifying sexually. Genital contact or ejaculation is not necessary for sexual satisfaction, a conclusion widely held by authorities on sexual behavior for quite some time (e.g., Freud, 1905; Socarides, 1988).

Since the early 1980s, the term *serial* has become the popular and accepted adjective for describing the offender who kills repetitively in this manner (Morton and Hilts, 2005). It is an appropriate adjective because it aptly describes what the individual is doing (i.e., killing a series of people) and because it is much easier to understand than the term *compulsive*, which has several different meanings, as we have seen. The use of the term "serial" also obviates the problem of calling these offenders sexual murderers.

However, the term "serial" does not clarify the many cases of individuals who kill a series of people solely for profit rather than for sexual gratification—such as contract murderers. Almost every state prison has inmates who have killed multiple people in the course of their criminal career, for a variety reasons such as anger and during another felony. And the number of victims necessary to apply the term "serial" (2, 10, or 40) is arbitrary. Moreover, the killing of multiple victims is often the result of a number of factors that have little to do with the drive or urge to kill. For example, the offender's degree of planning, his level of intelligence, his geographic mobility, his posthomicidal conduct, the type of victim (prostitute or child), various investigative problems, plus the major component of luck, all contribute to the total number of victims. Thus, the serial nature of the crime often has more to do with various circumstances outside the offender rather than the main mechanism resulting in murder, which is a compulsion to kill. If Ted Bundy, who is alleged to have killed over 40 women (Rule, 1988), had been apprehended after the first victim (for whatever reason), he would not be considered a serial killer. Bundy still would have had the same inner drive or compulsion to kill, but he would have been prevented from acting on the compulsion because of his incarceration.

Accordingly, we believe the term *compulsive murderer* reflects more accurately than *serial murderer* the main dynamic mechanism or motivation within the offender—the mechanism that pushes him to murder. Also, although we strongly believe that compulsive murders are sexually motivated, the underlying sexual component is not explicit in the term, a convention that will perhaps satisfy those who have a more concrete view of sexuality in this regard. The term "compulsive murderer" also excludes those who commit multiple homicides in which the motive is profit or revenge rather than an inner drive to act.

7.2 Premodern Examples of Compulsive Homicide

Compulsive, repetitive, sexually motivated homicide is by no means a modern or even an American phenomenon (Proulx, Beauregard, Carter, Mokros, Darjee, and James, 2018). Ancient Roman emperors, with their absolute power and control over subordinates, expressed their sexually sadistic proclivities without much hindrance. For example, Caligula, whose real name was Gaius Caesar, found sexual gratification through exercising his power and domination (Barrett, 1990). Some of his sadistic behaviors resulted in murder. It was not uncommon for Caligula during a banquet to order the wife of a guest to his room, where he would rape her. The ruler would then discuss her sexual performance and techniques in front of others, achieving a great deal of sadistic pleasure from watching the couple being humiliated. Caligula had underlings act as virtual slaves; he cut out people's tongues for minor infractions or sometimes for no reason at all. He is also reported to have had incestuous relations with three of his sisters. Caligula's grandiosity was displayed by his having a temple built in his name; there, sacrifices and prayers were directed to him as if he were one of the ancient gods. As a child, Caligula displayed sadistic tendencies exemplified by his enjoyment in watching executions. His physical smallness and frailty probably contributed to underlying feelings of inadequacy that he compensated for in a dramatic manner. In fact, Caligula, which means "Little Boot," was a nickname he earned as a youth.

The 15th-century French nobleman Gilles de Rais was one of the wealthiest men in France during the Hundred Years' War, in which he fought the English alongside Joan of Arc (Benedetti, 1972). With the help of subordinates, he managed to kidnap, torture, sexually molest, and kill at least 150 (according to some estimates, as many as 800) children. He was executed in 1414 after an 8-year period of murder. Rais killed the children after torturing them, using such methods as decapitation, dismembering, and breaking their necks. Often he would dress the victims in fine clothes, get them drunk, and then sodomize them, hang them, and have intercourse with them while they were dying. He preferred to ejaculate on their corpses. It was disclosed at his trial that he kissed the severed heads of the victims' bodies and sexually violated them. The bodies of most of the children were burned, but Rais kept the heads of those he considered "particularly beautiful" as souvenirs. One of his accomplices stated in court that Rais had taken more pleasure in seeing the body parts pulled from the victims and in watching them die than in having sex with them.

Interestingly, this offender is reported to have displayed a combination of both sadism and some kindness and tenderness. He was eventually apprehended and admitted his guilt in court. In an allocution prior to his execution, Rais admonished parents to raise their children with discipline and morality so that they could avoid idleness, laziness, and excesses that would result in "evils."

In 16th-century Europe, when a badly mutilated or disemboweled body of a woman was discovered, the populace could not imagine that another human being was capable of having killed someone in such a manner. These premodern individuals concluded that only some type of supernatural force, such as a vampire or werewolf, could have killed the woman with such savageness. Many times a humanlike figure was observed fleeing the crime scene, which led observers to conclude that a man must have turned into a wolf, killed and dismembered the victim, and then turned back into a man. The belief in lycanthropy—the notion that humans have the capacity to turn into wolves—was fairly widespread at the time (Hill and Williams, 1967). (*Lycanthropy* comes from the Greek words *lykos*, meaning wolf, and *anthropos*, meaning man.) There are many stories of man–wolf transformations in medieval folklore. Given that the mutilated bodies of women were often found when the moon was full, many reasoned that the lunar cycle had something to do with this transformation.

Although the church in the Middle Ages condemned lycanthropy as a form of sorcery and witchcraft, it was considered a valid medical phenomenon. Gilles Garnier, arrested in France in 1573 for a series of sexual attacks on and murders of children, is a case in point. Garnier killed a 10-year-old girl whom he cannibalized; he later strangled a 10-year-old boy and ate part of him. The accused claimed that he was a werewolf, and this defense was seriously considered at his trial (Hill and Williams, 1967).

In 16th-century Germany, Peter Stubbe raped, tortured, and committed 15 sexual murders that involved cannibalization. He was supposed to have attacked and torn apart several children using his bare hands and teeth. Stubbe also killed his own son after ripping out his throat; he then cracked open his son's skull and ate his brains. This offender also used the defense of lycanthropy, claiming he was not responsible because he was a werewolf (Hill and Williams, 1967).

One of the most notorious premodern cases of compulsive homicide was that of the Whitechapel murderer, who terrorized Victorian England in the late 1880s (Begg, Fido, and Skinner, 1991). This offender, whose identity has never been officially determined, killed between five and nine prostitutes in 1888, most in the Whitechapel section of London. He is more commonly called "Jack the Ripper." He earned this sobriquet because of letters he was supposed to have sent to the press proclaiming, "I am down on whores and shan't quit ripping them until I do get buckled." In one letter, he lamented his inability to cut off a victim's ears and send them to the police. Examination of this victim's body revealed that the Ripper did, in fact, attempt this act. The Ripper's method of assault was to knife his victims, cut open their abdomens, and frequently remove the intestines and genitals. The press followed this case closely, carefully chronicling his actions, as well as the steps taken by the police to make an arrest.

The last recorded victim was killed in her room and mutilated in a rather shocking manner. A newspaper description of this victim is vividly descriptive of the Ripper's conduct.

> The throat had been cut right across with a knife, nearly severing the head from the body. The abdomen had been partially ripped open, and both of the breasts had been cut from the body. … The nose had been cut off, the forehead skinned, and the thighs, down to the feet, stripped of the flesh. … The entrails and other portions of the frame were missing, but the liver, etc., were found placed between the feet of this poor victim. The flesh from the thighs and legs, together with the breast and nose, had been placed by the murderer on the table, and one of the hands of the dead woman had been pushed into her stomach. (quoted in Schechter and Everitt, 1996, p. 132)

Jack the Ripper was never apprehended. As a result, numerous Ripper theories have arisen in regard to his identity. There are even Ripper clubs and periodicals devoted to discussing the case. A long list of suspects includes a member of the British royalty, a local physician, a midwife, several attorneys, and judges. There is even a theory that Jack the Ripper traveled to the United States and killed several women as well (Gordon, 2003). Douglas and Olshaker (1995) and Ressler and Shachtman (1997) independently analyzed the crime scene information available and concluded that the Ripper was probably a mentally ill individual who was becoming more disorganized and psychotic as time went on; possibly he committed suicide or wound up in a mental asylum. A recent, and perhaps a most compelling, analysis is provided by Cornwell (2002) who concluded that the renowned artist Walter Sickert was the killer.

7.3 Krafft-Ebing's *Psychopathia Sexualis*

At the same time Jack the Ripper was active, Richard von Krafft-Ebing (1840–1902) was beginning the scientific study of sexual deviation. Krafft-Ebing had become interested

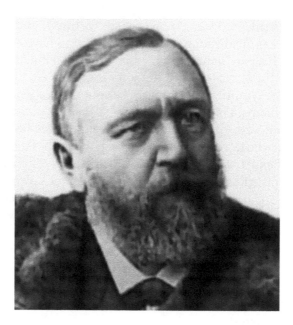

Figure 7.1 Richard von Krafft-Ebing, MD (1840–1902).

in psychiatry as a young man (see Figure 7.1). After working at a number of hospitals in Vienna, Strasbourg, Prague, and Berlin, he became a professor of psychiatry at Graz University in 1873. He was also one of the directors of a newly built state psychiatric facility at Feldhof. After a number of years at this hospital, Krafft-Ebing left to dedicate himself completely to his research. In 1876, he authored the *Textbook of Forensic Psychiatry*, in which he espoused the view that psychiatry should be a descriptive—as opposed to an explanatory—science. He also argued that the offender, rather than the criminal act, should be the focus of psychiatric investigation, a rather novel idea at the time.

Perhaps Krafft-Ebing's most important work, and certainly the one for which he is most acclaimed, is *Psychopathia Sexualis* (*Sexual Psychopathology*); originally published in 1886, it went through 12 editions before the author's death and is still being published. This book had a major influence at the time, and it was referenced by all turn-of-the-century scholars, including Freud (1905). Many consider Krafft-Ebing to be one of the true founders of the scientific study of sexual deviation. He coined the term *sadism* after the Marquis de Sade (1740–1814), who wrote extensively on the relationship of cruelty, pain, and sexual arousal. In fact, *Psychopathia Sexualis* was actually the first organized scientific account of sexual murder and sexual murderers. Recently, the original papers of Krafft-Ebing (which had been in the family home in Graz since his death), including his notes and commentary, have been made available for modern researchers. Present-day literary critics such as Stephen Heath (1986) have used the original insights of Krafft-Ebing to explain various themes in novels such as Robert Louis Stevenson's *The Strange Case of Dr. Jekyll and Mr. Hyde*, published in the same year as *Psychopathia Sexualis*.

In addition to reporting his own cases, Krafft-Ebing (1886) referred to a number of "older" 19th-century alienists, physicians who described and tried to understand the sexual murderer. For example,

Blumroder [in 1836] saw a man who had several wounds bitten into the pectoral muscle, which a woman, in great sexual excitement, had given him at the acme of lustful feeling during coitus. Blumroder calls especial attention to the psychological connection between lust and murder. (p. 57)

Krafft-Ebing also cited several cases previously reported by the well-known Italian physician and criminologist Cesare Lombroso; these cases illustrated "a desire to murder with greatly increased lust" (p. 57).

A careful reading of Krafft-Ebing's text reveals that a great deal of what we know today about the compulsive, repetitive murderer was first described by him at the end of the 19th century. Table 7.2 lists a number of characteristics of contemporary sexual murderers that Krafft-Ebing originally described. For example, Krafft-Ebing noted that sexual murder typically involves a male offender, and he even provided a theory of why this is the case. He found that such offenders lied and manipulated, took trophies and souvenirs from the crime scene, used ligatures to strangle victims, engaged in torture (often for prolonged periods of time), and reported greater sexual satisfaction in their torture and killings than in actual intercourse with their wives and girlfriends. The author also observed that such individuals had a history of animal cruelty, targeted prostitutes, revisited the crime scene, escalated the severity of their sadistic acts and criminal conduct, used pornography, and engaged in repetitive ritualistic behavior. Krafft-Ebing's subjects also often showed no overt signs of abnormality, frequently planned their murders in detail, and had disturbed relationships with their mothers.

The case of Louis Menesclou, as well as the case of a clerk named Alton, illustrates Krafft-Ebing's contention that there is a connection between murder and sexual arousal:

> The forearm of the child was found in [Menesclou's] pocket. … The genitals could not be found. … The circumstances, as well as an obscene poem found on his person, left no doubt that he had violated the child and then murdered her. Menesclou expressed no remorse, asserting that his deed was an accident. (p. 63)

Alton killed and dismembered a child whom he lured into the bushes. Following the homicide, he wrote an entry in his notebook: "Killed today a young girl; it was fine and hot" (p. 63).

The compulsive murderer Vincenz Verzeni, described by Krafft-Ebing, was not too different from many contemporary serial killers. Verzeni was initially accused of strangling three women. He then killed a 14-year-old girl and a 28-year-old woman. The 14-year-old's genitals were torn from her body, and, following her death, the offender filled her mouth with dirt. He slit open her stomach with a knife so her intestines were hanging out when the body was discovered. Interestingly, Verzeni did not kill his third victim, a cousin, perhaps because he had an emotional connection with her. Nevertheless, he engaged in a rather odd ritualistic behavior with this victim and the others: he pressed the women's hands together and then pulled out their hairpins.

When apprehended, Verzeni first lied about his involvement and tried to blame others. He then provided a detailed and insightful statement to the authorities explaining the sexual arousal he felt while killing, particularly during prolonged torture. In particular, he emphasized the sexual gratification achieved by ligature strangulation as being "greater than [that achieved through] masturbation" (p. 66). Verzeni also took some of the victims' clothing and intestines because he enjoyed touching and smelling them; he used the souvenirs to stimulate his fantasies. The offender had a background of animal cruelty as well

Table 7.2   Characteristics of Contemporary Serial Murderers as Noted by Krafft-Ebing

Characteristics	Quotes from Krafft-Ebing (1886)
Serial murder is a male phenomenon.	"Such monstrous acts … are much more frequent [in men] than [in] women" (p. 59).
Lying and manipulation are common.	"M expressed no remorse, asserting that his deed was an accident" (p. 63). "Arrested, at first he lied" (p. 64).
Murderer often takes trophies and souvenirs.	"A number of heads of particularly beautiful children were preserved as memorials" (p. 58). "I took the clothing … because of the pleasure it gave me to smell and touch them" (p. 67).
Ligatures are used.	"Her corpse [had] the mark of a thong around her neck" (p. 65). "His satisfaction in this garroting was greater than in masturbation" (p. 66).
Victims are tortured, often for prolonged periods.	"He then allowed his victims to live. … [The] sexual satisfaction was delayed, and then he continued to choke them until they died" (p. 60).
Offenders frequently do not harm wives or girlfriends.	"Two sweethearts that he had … it was very strange to him that he had no inclination to strangle them" (p. 66).
Sexual satisfaction is greater with murder than in nonaggressive sexual relations.	"But he had not had the same pleasure with [his girlfriends] as with his victims" (p. 66).
Offenders have a history of animal cruelty.	"When he was 12 years old, he expressed a peculiar feeling of pleasure while wringing the necks of chickens" (p. 67). "He killed animals himself" (p. 85).
Prostitutes are common victims.	"They were almost all public prostitutes" (p. 67).
Offenders sometimes revisit the crime scene.	"[He] fished her out again [for] renewed violation" (p. 68).
Disturbed relationship with mother is common.	"But on the way, he hid [the body] under a straw sack, for fear his mother would suspect him" (p. 66).
Crimes and sadistic acts tend to escalate.	"He obtained animals. … [But] these bodies no longer satisfied him. … He felt the desire to make use of human bodies" (p. 70).
Offenders make frequent use of pornography.	"Among his effects were found objects of art and obscene pictures painted by himself" (p. 73).
Offenders have a need to humiliate and degrade victims.	"because its effect on her is humiliating, mortifying" (p. 66). "[He took] pleasure … in humiliating her" (p. 77). "Defile[d] … women … and put contempt and humiliation upon them … with disgusting, at least foul, things" (p. 79).
Crimes may have signature aspects, revealing behavior idiosyncratic to a particular offender.	"It also gave me great pleasure to pull the hairpins out of the hair of my victims" (p. 67). "The mouth was filled with earth" (p. 65). "He pressed her hands together for some time" (p. 65).
Offenders often show no overt signs of disturbance.	"His external appearance was rather pleasing. He lived in very good circumstances" (p. 74). "23 years old, powerfully built, neat in dress, and decent in manner" (p. 79).
Some murders are highly planned and organized.	"He set about his horrible deeds with such care that he remained undetected for 10 years" (p. 67).

Source: From Schlesinger, L.B., *Serial Offenders: Current Thought, Recent Findings*, CRC Press, Boca Raton, FL, 2000, p. 6. With permission.

as lying and manipulation. Although Verzeni had several girlfriends, he found sexual violence with his victims much more pleasurable than conventional sexual relations. He also found it curious that he had no desire to hurt either of the girlfriends.

Krafft-Ebing also reported the case of Gruyo, a 41-year-old without a past criminal record, who strangled six prostitutes. He planned his crimes with such care that he went undetected for 10 years. After strangling the victims, he tore out their intestines and kidneys through their vaginas. Krafft-Ebing also described the strange case of a necrophiliac named Sergeant Bertrand. This individual initially fantasized about having sex with dead animals, later engaged in such activity, and then progressed to disinterred human bodies.

> I covered it [the body] with kisses and pressed it wildly to my heart. All that one could enjoy with a living woman is nothing in comparison with the pleasure I experienced. After I had enjoyed it for about a quarter of an hour, I cut the body up, as usual, and tore out the entrails. Then I buried the cadaver again. ... Enjoyment in doing so was greater than in using the body sexually. (p. 70)

Krafft-Ebing wrote at length about the relationship between fantasy and the compulsion to kill. He described the case of the "Girl Stabber of Bozen," who knifed girls in the genital region. This offender drew his own pornography, likely used as a fantasy aid, which was found in his home following his arrest. Another individual (Krafft-Ebing's Case 27) ejaculated the instant he stabbed a woman. Krafft-Ebing noted that the stabbing was "an equivalent for coitus" (p. 73). The connection between fantasy and the compulsion to kill is also highlighted in the case of the "Girl Cutter of Augsburg." This offender had a collection of knives in his home that gave him "an intense feeling of sexual pleasure with violent excitement. According to his confession, he had injured, in all, fifty girls" (p. 74).

The root of sadism, according to Krafft-Ebing, is the offender's feeling of power and control over others. "The idea that she might feel the power I had over her" is sexually arousing (p. 76). The author reported the case of an individual who felt sexual pleasure only by "humiliating [and] mortifying" women; [she should] "feel that she is completely in his power. One of the hidden roots of sadism—the impulse to complete subjugation of the woman, which here became consciously entertained" (p. 78). Krafft-Ebing also described several individuals who engaged in sadistic acts with animals, rather than humans, for fear of being arrested. One man had ejaculations when he killed chickens or pigeons by wringing their necks. Another person enjoyed "committing sodomy with geese, and cutting their necks off *tempore ejaculationis*" (p. 85).

Although some women also have sadistic proclivities, Krafft-Ebing noted that most sadistic acts are committed by men. Drawing on his medical background, the author reasoned that the "active or aggressive role" in sexual relations belongs to the man—"women remain passive, defensive" (p. 59). He concluded that men have an inborn aggressive character that is also seen in the animal kingdom, where the male always pursues the female. Thus, in cases of abnormal sexual aggression, men's natural aggressive character becomes "excessively developed, and expresses itself in an impulse to subdue absolutely the object of desire, even to destroy or kill it" (p. 60). The author further noted that in the early history of civilization, premodern men often used violence and aggression to obtain female partners for propagation. Thus, contemporary males' similar acts represent "outbreaks of sadism [that] are atavistic" (p. 60). Accordingly, sexual murder is a throwback to, and an exaggeration of, behavior that was common much earlier in the evolutionary development of the species.

7.4 Compulsive Homicides in the First Half of the 20th Century

In the early years of the 20th century, a number of compulsive murder cases were reported with fairly accurate detail. A case in point is that of Peter Kürten, who terrified Düsseldorf, Germany, in the late 1920s (Wilson and Pitman, 1962). Born in 1883, Kürten was the third of 13 children who were raised in poverty (all family members lived in a single room) and in an environment where alcoholism, brutality, and pathological sexuality were common. He frequently watched his father rape his mother; his father also engaged in sex with one of his daughters.

Kürten had sex with his sisters; however, his preferred form of sexual activity in his developing years was bestiality. He became friendly with a dog catcher who taught him how to torture and masturbate animals. From ages 13 through 15 he engaged in numerous sexual acts with pigs, sheep, and goats, sometimes stabbing the animals to death while having intercourse with them.

At age 9, Kürten committed his first murder by throwing a boy off a raft and preventing another youngster from rescuing the child. Kürten was also a thief and a burglar, and he spent a number of years in prison for assorted offenses. While there, he poisoned several inmates in the prison hospital. After his release, the offender attacked 29 people and killed several others including a 5-year-old girl. He also broke into the home of a 13-year-old girl, strangled her, and killed her by cutting her throat with a knife.

In 1921, Kürten married a woman who had previously killed her husband. She agreed to marry him after he threatened to kill her if she did not do so. Despite Kürten's background and behavior, the marriage appeared reasonably stable to most who knew the couple. However, during this period, Kürten became preoccupied with fire, burned down a number of buildings, and experienced sexual excitement while watching the flames. He had hoped that homeless people living in the buildings would die in the fires.

In 1925, and for the next 5 years, until he was apprehended, the compulsion to kill became overwhelming. Kürten attacked men, women, and children, killing them by knifing, choking, and cutting their throats. On one day alone he killed two girls aged 5 and 14. The offender engaged in necrophilia and stuffed the genitals and rectums of these victims with some material. He set one little girl on fire after her death. The varied pattern and the high number of victims led the police to believe, at first, that the murders must have been committed by more than one offender. In addition, Kürten was a vampire, gaining sexual gratification through drinking the blood of his victims. Kürten's vampiristic behavior is typical of clinical vampirism—as distinguished from vampire myth—with sexual (Bourguignon, 1997) and various psychodynamic etiologies (Jaffe and DiCataldo, 1994).

When finally arrested and evaluated psychiatrically, Kürten displayed little resistance and was exceptionally cooperative, even having a fairly good rapport with the examining doctor. He spoke of his obsession with blood and said he hoped to hear the sound of his own blood running into the basket while the executioner cut off his head with an axe. Kürten also reported that one time he became excited by watching the sunset because the red sky reminded him of blood. His preoccupation with blood was so intense that he once killed a swan and drank its blood.

> I used to stroll at night through the Hofgarten very often, and in the spring of 1930, I noticed a swan sleeping at the edge of the lake. I cut its throat. The blood spurted up and I drank from the stump and ejaculated. (Schechter and Everitt, 1996, p. 155)

In addition, he revealed having fantasies of becoming a chief of police and saving the town from monsters. Kürten accepted his execution (in 1931) calmly and ate well before his death.

Around this same time, Germany endured the deprivations of another compulsive killer, Fritz Haarmann, who murdered between 27 and 50 young males, mostly refugees who had flocked to his city during World War I (Nash, 1973). His methodology included luring a young boy to his room, providing him a meal, and then, with an assistant, overpowering the child and chewing through his throat until the head nearly separated from the body. He described the experience as providing great sexual arousal. Following a homicide, Haarmann cut up the body parts and peddled some of them on the black market as beef. He disposed of inedible body parts in a nearby canal and gave the boy's clothing away.

As a child, Haarmann was made to dress as a girl. He served time in prison for child molestation and engaged in petty crime, pickpocketing, burglary, and smuggling; at one point, he was even a police informant. Although he was briefly engaged to a young woman, Haarmann seems to have been homosexual, and he committed some of the murders with a homosexual prostitute with whom he was involved.

Perhaps one of the most bizarre cases in the annals of crime is that of Albert Fish, who operated in New York during the 1920s (Nash, 1973; Schechter, 1990). Although this offender looked like a genteel grandfather, he was a compulsive murderer, sadist, masochist, pedophile, and cannibal. Fish was raised in an orphanage with fairly brutal caretakers, who beat the children while they were naked. From an early age, he gained sexual gratification by inflicting pain on himself. For example, Fish shoved rose stems up his penis; he had his wife beat him with leather straps and nail-riddled paddles; he ate his own excrement; and he even shoved sewing needles into his groin. In fact, after his arrest, an X-ray was taken of him which distinctly showed about 24 needles around his bladder.

In 1910, Fish killed a man, and in 1919, he tortured and killed a mentally retarded boy. He was apparently responsible for the murder of another young male at the same time. In 1927, he sexually violated and killed a 4-year-old boy as well. He was also alleged to have killed several adolescent boys by castration, gaining sexual gratification from watching the youngsters die a slow and painful death.

Fish was married several times, once to a woman who had six children. He was employed as a handyman and painter and responded to "lonely hearts" advertisements from women who wanted to meet a man for companionship or marriage. When he met the women, he told them that he did not want to be married but instead wanted to be spanked.

Fish became interested in cannibalism and developed a taste for raw meat. This preoccupation led to one of Fish's most disturbing offenses—the murder of Grace Budd, a 12-year-old girl he abducted through a clever manipulation. After befriending the child's parents, Fish asked them whether he could take Grace to a birthday party he was having for his niece. The parents consented. He took the child from New York City to Westchester County, where he had already picked out a vacant house. Once there, Fish killed the little girl, cut up the body, and ate her over a 10-day period as part of a stew that included potatoes and vegetables.

The case remained unsolved for 6 years, as Grace's family did not know Fish's true identity. Twice during the time of Grace's abduction (1928) and his arrest for murder (1935), Fish was a patient at Bellevue Hospital, committed for sending obscene letters. In both instances, he was found to be "harmless" and was released (Oshinsky, 2017). During that period, Fish probably fantasized about the crime many times and, after several years, he needed increased sadistic satisfaction. Accordingly, he wrote a graphic letter to the victim's mother, with enough detail so that Mrs. Budd was certain that Grace's killer was the author. Fish explained how he first developed an interest in cannibalism and then described Grace's murder:

> I took her to an empty house in Westchester I had already picked out. When we got there, I told her to remain outside. She picked wild flowers. I went upstairs and stripped all my clothes off. I knew if I did not, I would get her blood on them. When all was ready I went to the window and called her. Then I hid in a closet until she was in the room. When she saw me all naked she began to cry and tried to run downstairs. I grabbed her and she said she would tell her mama. First I stripped her naked. How did she kick—bite and scratch. I choked her to death, then cut her in small pieces so I could take my meat to my rooms cook and eat it. How sweet and tender her little ass was, roasted in the oven. It took me nine days to eat her entire body. I did not fuck her tho I could of had I wished. She died a virgin. (quoted in Schechter and Everitt, 1996, pp. 165–166)

A New York City detective who never stopped trying to solve the case managed to trace the letter to Fish. Once arrested, he was examined psychiatrically by Fredric Wertham, who considered him psychotic and legally insane. Wertham was very critical of his colleagues prior evaluations of Fish which he considered superficial and incorrect (Oshinsky, 2017). Although the jury acknowledged that the offender was mentally ill, they believed he deserved to be executed. Fish was reported to have said, "What a thrill it would be to die in the electric chair! It would be the supreme thrill—the only one I haven't tried" (Schechter and Everitt, 1996, p. 92). At 65 years of age, Fish was electrocuted in 1936.

Another interesting case is that of Earl Nelson, executed in 1928 for strangling 20 women in a period of about a year (Nash, 1973; Wilson and Pitman, 1962). All the victims (ranging in age from 14 to 60) were killed in their homes. Reportedly, Nelson would choke the women to death, engage in necrophilia, and place the corpses in various hiding places. One body was stuffed in an attic trunk, one under the victim's bed, while others were placed in basement furnaces.

At about age 10, Nelson had been hit by a trolley car, and he remained unconscious for several days; perhaps this trauma caused some type of organic pathology. He was raised by an aunt who stressed religion and Bible reading; in fact, Nelson carried a Bible with him at several of his murders. As a young man, he was involved in voyeurism, once attacked his female cousin and was also arrested for rape. In his early 20s, he married a 60-year-old woman and was pathologically jealous. He once raped his wife while she was hospitalized and then accused the doctor of having sex with her. Once Nelson began to kill, he could not contain the compulsion and murdered almost twice a week. He traveled throughout several parts of the United States and was finally arrested in Winnipeg, Canada.

During World War II, there were many sexual murder cases; however, they were not extensively publicized, perhaps because of preoccupation with the war. Jenkins (1988, 1989) researched newspaper clippings from this time and found many cases that seem, at least from a distance, to have been sexually motivated, compulsive homicides. For example, an English mailman named Gordon Cummins committed multiple sexual murders, particularly in the blackouts during the war (Schechter and Everitt, 1996). His first victim was a female pharmacist whom he strangled in an air-raid shelter. The next day he killed a prostitute by slitting her throat; he then mutilated her genitals with a can opener. Additional victims followed on succeeding nights. After several more killings, he was finally arrested.

Around the same time, William Heirens terrorized Chicago (Freeman, 1956). Heirens was apprehended while attending college, but he had begun his criminal career years earlier. As a youth, Heirens developed a fetish for female underwear, and he committed numerous home burglaries in order to obtain the fetishistic objects. On some occasions, he urinated or defecated on the premises. At the time of his arrest, Heirens was suspected of committing hundreds of burglaries. He had also killed two adult women in their homes and had then abducted a sleeping 6-year-old girl from her bedroom. After killing the child, he cut her body into pieces and deposited them in sewers and garbage cans around the Chicago area.

This case is particularly instructive as an illustration of the underlying compulsion to kill, as evidenced not only in the offender's actions but also in some of his statements. For example, when Heirens tried to resist the compulsion to kill, he reported developing headaches and profuse sweating. "I resisted for about two hours. I tore sheets out of place and went into a sweat. I would take out plans and draw how to get into certain places. I would burn up the plans. Sometimes this helped" (quoted in Kennedy, Hoffman, and Haines, 1947, p. 120). Heirens became well known for writing in lipstick on the mirrors in the victims' homes: "For Heaven sakes catch me before I kill more, I cannot control myself." An interesting aspect of this case is that Heirens placed bandages on wounds of his victims, possibly an attempt to undo or symbolically reverse the homicide (Russell, et al, 2018).

When arrested and evaluated, Heirens was initially uncooperative. He told the psychiatrist that his name was Joe Blow and asked for someone named William. When he was told that his name was William, and Joe was his roommate's name, Heirens then said his name was Joe Blow William. The evaluators believed that he was trying to portray symptoms he thought a mentally ill person would exhibit. He also spoke of an acquaintance named George Murman, a fictitious individual who Heirens claimed committed the crimes. After further examination, the evaluators concluded either that he was trying to get them to believe someone else committed the crimes or that he had another personality. Heirens eventually confessed ("I'm sorry for the acts I committed," Cauldwell, 1948) and was sentenced to multiple life terms in prison. While in prison, he earned a college degree, recanted his confession, and proclaimed his innocence, arguing that the police framed him.

7.5 Examples from the Latter Half of the 20th Century

Two compulsive murderers with different abduction techniques were active during the 1950s. Edward Gein (Schechter, 1989) served as a model for Alfred Hitchcock's main character in *Psycho*. Gein had a disturbed relationship with a domineering mother, who constantly told her son stories about the sinful nature of women. Following his mother's death, he preserved a room in his house as a shrine for her. He began digging up corpses from local cemeteries and later killed and disemboweled two women at his home. After killing an older woman who owned a hardware store, Gein became a suspect and was arrested. The police discovered the victim's headless corpse hanging upside down in Gein's home. They also found chairs upholstered with human skin, soup bowls made from victims' skulls, and a collection of female genitalia in a box. Gein told investigators that he enjoyed dressing up in a vest made of human skin.

Gein's crude method of abducting victims is in direct contrast to the techniques used by Harvey Glatman (Nash, 1973). This offender was quite intelligent, yet he was lonely and socially introverted, especially with members of the opposite sex. Glatman came from a middle-class background and was a good student, but a morbidly perverse side of him emerged in childhood. For example, he engaged in the dangerous autoerotic practice of tying a rope around his neck to achieve sexual gratification (Resnick, 1997). At age 17, he ordered a girl to undress by threatening her with a toy gun. Sometime later, he was arrested for robbery and spent 5 years in prison. After his release in 1951, Glatman started a small TV-repair business.

The compulsion to kill had been building in Glatman for years, but, because of his discomfort with women, he needed a method to obtain victims that involved minimal interaction with them. In 1957, Glatman set up a photography studio in his home and placed ads in newspapers for models. He told the women that they would be on the cover of detective magazines, which were quite popular at the time. The models allowed Glatman to tie them up, as was typical in most of the pictures on the magazine covers. When they were bound, he raped them at gunpoint, photographed them, killed them by strangling them, and disposed of the bodies in the nearby California desert. He murdered three women with this technique; however, the fourth victim managed to overpower him, and he was arrested.

Albert DeSalvo, commonly known as the "Boston Strangler," terrorized Boston in the early 1960s (Rae, 1967). DeSalvo grew up in a home with significant abuse and brutality. It is alleged that his father had sex with prostitutes at the home, scenes that were witnessed by some of his children. At an early age, DeSalvo liked to place starving cats in an orange crate with a puppy and watch the cats scratch the dog's eyes out. He also had voyeuristic tendencies in his youth: "I had a lot of fun climbing up on the roof of the restaurant and watching couples go at it in the rooms, which made me come in my pants, sometimes without even touching myself" (p. 64). DeSalvo joined the army and was stationed in Germany. Here, he began a series of burglaries that were sexually motivated. He married a German woman who found his incessant sexual demands irritating. "I wanted Imgard to make the first move. She never could see her way clear. I felt less than a man in bed with her. She would say I was dirty and sickening, and called me an animal" (p. 75). Notwithstanding marital conflict, DeSalvo maintained a fairly normal family life—at least as seen from a distance— and functioned as a husband and father all through the period when he committed some exceptionally shocking crimes and homicides.

Prior to his spree of strangulation murders, this offender committed a series of sexual molestations that earned him the name "Measuring Man." DeSalvo would knock on the doors of homes posing as a representative from a modeling agency, an idea he claimed he got from watching a movie. When a woman answered the door, he praised her for her figure and asked whether he could take her measurements and photograph her. He told the victims that they had a good chance of becoming models. While taking their measurements, DeSalvo fondled and molested them. The offender was shocked by the number of women who let him engage in this activity. "I am not educated and these girls was all college graduates, understand me? I made fools of them. I made them … accept me and listen to me. That was why I was around measuring them" (p. 82).

I know that they look down on people who come from my background. They think they are better than me. They was all college kids and I never had anything in my life, but I outsmarted them. I was supposed to feel that they was better than me because they was college people. (p. 85)

At the age of 29, DeSalvo was apprehended for a burglary attempt and sentenced to prison for 2 years.

When he was released (in May 1962), he began knocking on the doors of homes dressed in green work clothes, claiming to be a repairman. This methodology earned him his next title, "Green Man." The offender told the women who came to the door that he was sent to repair a leaky faucet or a broken appliance. When they let him in, he overpowered them and raped them. DeSalvo's first rape victim was a 55-year-old woman.

> We talked about the work, and she'd let me in. As she walked and I was behind her, I hit her on the head with a lead weight. She fell. I reached over the back of her and I put my arms around her neck, and we fell to the floor together. Her blood was all over me. I got up, took her robe. I had the robe belt, a blue one, and I put it around her neck and it gave me two turns—tightened it good and knotted it and I think it caught into kind of [a] bow, you understand? I left it on her. I think she was alive when I had intercourse with her. (p. 7)

DeSalvo was alleged to have killed 13 women during the 18-month period following the Green Man rapes. He said that the compulsion to kill was irresistible: "When this certain thing comes on me, it's a very immediate thing. I get up in the morning and I get this feeling, and I tell my wife I am going out on my job, but I am not" (p. 7).

> If you ask me why I did that, I would have to say I don't know. It does not seem that it was me, and yet I know that I did that. But I can't understand why and no one has ever been able to help me understand it. (p. 54)

The offender described an episode with one victim who was reluctant to open the door since she did not know him. "The door opened a little more. So help me, this thing going to my head, this pressure. I want to say, don't open the door, but still I want it open, it's funny" (p. 19). Another time a victim hesitated to let DeSalvo in because she was ready to go out. He told her that the "repairs" would not take much time, and she eventually consented. "I closed the door behind me and even though I fight it all the way, it's funny, I didn't want to go in there in the first place. I just didn't want it to happen" (p. 19).

Another victim, whom he considered rather attractive, opened the door without hesitation when he said he was a repairman. She invited DeSalvo to have coffee and was nice to him.

> I really wanted to get out of there and don't want to do anything to her. She has been very nice to me and I don't want to hurt her, but I can feel the urge on me like a real push. It is me and I don't want to hurt this nice person who has been good to me and treated me like a man. (p. 7)

Nevertheless, the compulsion overpowered DeSalvo.

> She turned her back on me. I rose. I didn't really want to do it, but the next thing before she knew it, I had my arms around her neck from in back. She didn't say anything, she couldn't. She fall back on top of me. She passed out. I think that she was so surprised and shocked when she see what I do, that she just can't stand it. She passed out on me. I put

her on the bed and looked at her. Naturally, when I saw her the sex thing came on strong. I opened the robe. I don't think I took it off. I just think I just opened it. I wanted to see her breast, as I am … I don't know exactly but I did reveal her busts. I remember seeing her strip naked on the bed. She was stripped naked. Her leopard pajamas was ripped off or pulled away from her busts and her privates, up over her busts and down around her ankles. Now I say I had intercourse with her while she was unconscious but still alive. I was thinking about how nice she had been to me and it was making me feel sad. I am sorry about that one, really sorry but she shouldn't have asked me to stay and then there was the thing I felt. (pp. 109–110)

DeSalvo described his interaction with a 68-year-old victim who triggered hostility in him. He choked her in his usual way when she turned her back and then violated her sexually. But instead of feeling a sense of relief, he became angry.

It was later, right then, when I strangled her with a stocking. I was very, very angry at her, this woman, I don't know her and she never done nothing to me, but I am very angry and pulled them stockings awful tight. Then I got up and went through the place. Whew! I was mad and went through the place yanking out drawers and throwing clothes around. (pp. 33–34)

His last victim was a young married woman. Instead of ringing the doorbell, DeSalvo broke into her home and abused her sexually. He then apologized and left. This incident eventually led to his arrest, which ended the string of homicides in the Boston area. Following this arrest, he was connected to the prior rapes and molestations. While in jail, DeSalvo told another inmate that he was the Boston Strangler. DeSalvo's attorney had him plead guilty to the stranglings in order to avoid the death penalty. As part of the plea agreement, the offender gave a detailed statement to the authorities. He was killed in prison by another inmate in 1973.

DeSalvo's family now questions the validity of his confession. While they concede that he committed the rapes, they do not believe he was capable of multiple murders and contend that he made a false confession for various legal and perhaps psychological reasons. Although most rapists do not progress to sexual homicide (Podolsky, 1966; MacDonald, 1986) and those rapists who do kill mostly murder their victims in order to escape detection, a small subgroup of rapists do escalate their activity to sexual murder (Ressler, Burgess, and Douglas, 1983). DeSalvo certainly could fall within this category. Moreover, he had the background characteristics of a potential sex murderer (Schlesinger, 2001b). It is not completely certain that DeSalvo was the Boston Strangler; but if the detailed statements he gave to the authorities were lies, his is probably one of the most dramatic cases of false confession of all time.

During the 1970s, the public, largely as a result of media coverage, became increasingly aware of the repetitive sexual murderer. A well-publicized case was that of the highly intelligent Edmund Kemper, who killed multiple individuals including his grandparents and his mother (Chaney, 1976; Strentz and Hassel, 1970). As a child, Kemper was treated in a cruel manner by his mother, who was a respected college administrator. She made the young Kemper live in the basement and ridiculed him for his enormous (6 ft, 9 in) size. During his youth, Kemper killed cats with a hatchet and kept the dismembered parts in his closet. He once buried a cat alive, then cut off its head and kept it in his bedroom. At age 15, he stabbed his grandparents to death for no apparent reason and was subsequently hospitalized for 6 years and then released as rehabilitated.

Following this disturbed childhood and adolescence, Kemper committed eight sexual murders. Typically, he would pick up hitchhiking women (usually coeds), drive them to a remote location, and stab them to death. He also photographed the corpses, dissected, and had sex with the bodies, and, on several occasions, he decapitated the victims. Although Kemper enjoyed the killings, he described the postmortem paraphiliac activity as even more arousing.

Kemper eventually killed his mother by smashing her skull with a hammer while she slept and then cutting off her head. He raped the decapitated body, cut out the larynx, and threw it down the garbage disposal. He then killed his mother's friend by smashing her skull with a brick and followed the murder with necrophilia. Afterward, he called the police and confessed.

Notorious multiple murderer Ted Bundy (Rule, 1988) became so well known that his name has almost become synonymous with serial killer. The case became highly publicized for many reasons including the high number of alleged victims (over 40), his geographic mobility, and his pleasing, clean-cut, conservative appearance, superior intellect, and law school background. As a youth, Bundy was obsessed with pornography and progressed to voyeurism, sexual burglary, and sexual homicide. He used a variety of techniques to abduct victims. For example, he would put a fake cast on his arm in order to appear weak and defenseless. After gaining the future victim's confidence and asking her assistance, he would attack her. Bundy eluded law enforcement for years. He eventually changed his modus operandi (MO) and began randomly breaking into homes and attacking women. Finally, he broke into a sorority house and attacked a number of coeds; this act demonstrated his complete loss of control over his compulsion to kill, as sometimes occurs in compulsive offenders at the end of a killing cycle. Bundy represented himself at his trial and was executed 10 years after his conviction.

Gary Heidnick was a financially successful and self-appointed church bishop who tortured a total of six women in the basement of his home (Englade, 1988). The victims were killed slowly in various sadistic ways. For example, one woman was forced into a pit filled with water and then electrocuted with a live wire. He put dog food and human remains in a food processor and made his victims eat it. Another woman was hung by her wrists and died a slow death over a period of about a week. He drove screwdrivers into the ears of other women and raped and tortured some while forcing others to watch. One woman managed to escape, and Heidnick was apprehended. At his trial, he told the judge that "the women were already there when he first moved into the house. For some reason, the judge failed to believe him" (Schechter and Everitt, 1996, p. 113).

During the 1980s, Andrei Chikatilo committed over 50 murders in the Soviet Union (Lourie, 1993). The Communist authorities wanted to believe that murderers of this type were a product only of the decadent West. However, they were disabused of this notion after arresting the 42-year-old teacher who was married with children. Chikatilo targeted boys, girls, and young women. He lured them away from bus stops or train stations with the promise of a meal. After leading them into the woods, he killed them, often cutting out their tongues, slicing off their noses, gouging out their eyes, and eating their genitals. In one month alone, this offender was alleged to have killed six victims. Chikatilo was arrested in the early 1990 and was charged with 53 murders. When questioned, he said the motive for the killings was not exactly sexual, but they gave him "peace of mind." He was executed 4 years after his trial.

Another dramatic case of compulsive murder is that of Jeffrey Dahmer (Dvorchak and Howlewa, 1991; Schwartz, 1992), who killed 17 men, most of whom he picked up in gay bars. He drugged them, dismembered them with a saw, and engaged in cannibalism as well as necrophiliac rape. In an attempt to make some victims zombies, he drove holes in their skulls (while they were living) and injected muriatic acid into their brains with a turkey baster. Dahmer was eventually arrested when a young victim managed to escape from his residence. When the police officers went to Dahmer's home, they found a human head in the refrigerator, several skulls in a closet, various body parts in a barrel, and decomposed hands, bones, and various organs in the freezer. Dahmer had also taken pictures of his victims and their corpses.

As a child, Dahmer dissected roadkill, butchered small animals, nailed cats and frogs to trees behind his house, and once put a dog's head on a stick. At 18 years of age, he picked up a hitchhiker, killed him, and dismembered the body. The compulsion to kill emerged 8 years later, when he committed his second murder. Two years later, he committed his third and fourth murders; the fifth murder, the next year; 5 years later (in 1991), he killed four people, and he killed eight more the following year.

Dahmer reported wanting "complete control" over his victims and was fascinated by the idea of "the captivity." He was sexually aroused by eating parts of the bodies; he described this activity as a further step toward achieving gratification—"just as an escalation, trying something new to satisfy" (quoted in Ressler and Schactman, 1997, p. 139). He also engaged in vampirism but did not find it as stimulating as anthropophagy. After serving only several years in prison, Dahmer was killed by another inmate.

7.6 The Study of Compulsive Homicide in the Modern Era

Psychoanalysts have never had any significant interest in sexual murder, notwithstanding their immense contribution to understanding sex and aggression, Freud's (1930) two basic instincts. Only a few psychoanalysts have described and commented on cases of compulsive homicide. Karpman (1954) studied several offenders and found them to be psychotic and often impotent. He theorized that the state of excitement that results from the killing energizes the offender neurologically, which helps him achieve an erection. Williams (1964) treated a number of sexual murderers from a psychoanalytic perspective. He described several cases and concluded that the offender has an "encapsulated, split off, murderous part [which] constitutes the blue-print of murder" (p. 356). The offender projects intolerable internal conflicts onto the victim and then kills the victim to get rid of these conflicts. Michaux and Michaux (1963) and Lindner (1982) also treated sex murderers from a psychoanalytic perspective and utilized traditional analytic concepts to understand their patients' behavior.

In the 1950s and 1960s, several psychiatrists became interested in the study of homicide and briefly described and discussed some cases of sexual murder. De River (1958) offered a theory of sadomasochism and sexual murder.

> Many sadistic acts finally culminate in lust murder, or they are accompanied by acts of perversion such as vampirism, cannibalism, necrophilia, etc. Not every lust murderer, however, is a sadist and lust murderers may be found among homosexuals as well as among heterosexuals. (p. 40)

He concluded that the sadistic lust murderer often tortures his female victims or cuts their genitalia, rectum, or breasts because these body parts contain

> strong sexual significance to him and serve as a sexual stimulus. They may be symbolic of his particular sexual fixation. Very often he has a fetish for a particular part of the body, and it demands expression through his mutilation and destruction of the part that most fascinates him. (p. 41)

DeRiver reported sexual offenders who jabbed or stuck women with sharp, pointed instruments, and he insightfully realized that the feeling of total possession and domination of the victim is a significant element of sexual arousal for this type of individual. DeRiver also described offenders who planned their crimes in detail to avoid apprehension. Interestingly, he commented on the sex murderer's legal responsibility: "he may know right from wrong, but he is unable to appreciate it" (p. 42).

Guttmacher (1960) found that those whom he, like deRiver, called lust murderers were quite rare. He noted that offenders in these cases typically have a background of abuse and of involvement in animal cruelty. For example, he reported the case of a man who buried a dog alive and cut off the legs and head of a horse prior to burial. Guttmacher confirmed Krafft-Ebing's findings: such offenders

> give vent to their hostile impulses through cruelty to animals. Their real hatred is not against animals, but, of course against their fellow man. Animals are mere substitutes, they serve as scapegoats. Furthermore, dumb brutes cannot file complaints with the police and in some quarters a certain degree of cruelty to animals is accepted as a sublimation of sadistic impulses. Certainly, this is true of hunting. (p. 100)

Bromberg (1961) listed various types of homicidal offenders including those who commit sadistic and thrill murders, which are basically sexual homicides. "Lust murder is one in which the act of killing or maiming (through strangulation, stabbing, crushing, eviscerating, suffocating), ... and witnessing suffering in the victim, stimulate or potentiate sexual impulses in the offender" (p. 148). Bromberg accurately differentiated the sexual murderer from the rape-murderer. The sexual murderer achieves sexual gratification from the killing itself, while the rape-murderer is "usually motivated by a rush of guilty feelings and panic which follows a realization of the enormity of the offense [rape] just concluded" (p. 149).

The few compulsive murderers whom Bromberg evaluated seemed to him to be psychotic "or so severely perverted (psychopathic) as to be compulsively driven to crime" (p. 149). He also noted that sex murderers do not typically have a background of sexual crimes and that the sexual gratification achieved in such a homicide is not the traditional sort of gratification achieved in intercourse. The author cited a number of sexual murder cases where males, as opposed to females, were victimized. For example, he reported the case of an individual who (over a 10-month period) killed five young men ranging in age from 13 to 39, including three under age 19. The victims were struck from behind and were found nude, face down in the mud, with their skulls bashed in. One victim's head was nearly decapitated. The offender, who was arrested a year later, had a history of voyeurism. Bromberg reasoned that this man achieved sexual gratification from undressing his victims, as opposed to engaging in ordinary sexual acts with them.

MacDonald (1961, 1986) described his experience with sex murderers in both editions of his well-known text. He concluded that the sexual element is present in all sadistic murders and motivates these acts. Interestingly, MacDonald also noted that "the great majority of rapists do not murder their victims" (1986, p. 168). Like Bromberg, he astutely differentiated the sex murderer, who gets gratification from killing, from the rape-murderer who kills his victims in order to escape detection. MacDonald also discussed the psychodynamics of necrophilia and commented that several of the sex murderers he studied had a background of minor sexual offenses, specifically voyeurism and exhibitionism.

As a result of his association with the New Jersey Diagnostic Center, the state's forensic facility, Revitch gained considerable experience with cases of sexual homicide and sexual aggression. In 1957, he categorized these offenses into four groups: (1) murder as a prerequisite for sexual satisfaction, (2) murder not as a prerequisite for sexual satisfaction but as a result of frustration, anger, or fear during an attempted or completed rape, (3) nonsexual acts such as knifing, choking, or battering as an expression of aggressive sexual needs, and (4) fantasies as an expression of aggressive sexual needs. Compulsive homicides fall into the first category, while the second category essentially covers situational murders associated with a sexual offense, such as a rape-murder. Revitch's third group contains sexually motivated aggressive acts, where the sexual element is often covert. The last group includes individuals with sexually aggressive fantasies who have not acted out.

Revitch (1957) concluded that prediction of the potential sex murderer should be based on a combination of factors, including a history of assaults on women or girls, dislike and resentment of females, sadistic fantasies, sexual preoccupation (particularly fetishism for female underwear), and schizoid traits or a well-defined schizophrenic processes. He also theorized that the psychodynamic factor leading to these forms of sexual aggression is "resentment of a maternal figure transferred to womenhood in general" (p. 522). He called for more clinical research, the necessity for courts to refer for evaluation of individuals who commit unprovoked assaults on females, and the need for family physicians to be alert to—and not casually to dismiss—children who commit violent acts against girls, especially when these acts are connected with sexual preoccupations.

Several years later, Revitch (1965) completed a descriptive study of 43 adult and adolescent males who attacked women; this group included 9 murderers. He found that 18 offenders (42%) knew their victims, while 25 did not. Of the 43 offenders, 30 (69%) had previously committed offenses, but only 3 of these were overt sexual offenses, while 12 (40%) involved breaking and entering. The backgrounds of these offenders included noticeable hostility to women, preoccupation with maternal sexual conduct, overt or covert incestuous preoccupation, guilt over sex and rejection of sex as impure, sexual inferiority, and occasionally a need to completely possess the victim. Hostility toward women was more predominant in the adult offenders, while sexual preoccupation, particularly preoccupation with maternal sexual behavior, was more striking in the adolescent group. Tendencies toward introversion, along with feelings of isolation and detachment and blurring of reality boundaries, were also common findings. Nineteen offenders (44%) were considered schizoid, nine (20%) overtly schizophrenic, five (12%) mentally defective, and ten (23%) were classified as having a personality disorder. Revitch's finding that only 3 of the 43 attackers had a record of previous sex offenses suggests that such a history is of little use to law enforcement personnel looking for an unknown offender who has perpetrated a sexual murder or an unprovoked sexual attack on a woman.

Table 7.3   Brittain's (1970) Profile of the Sexual Murderer

- Younger than age 35
- Introverted
- Rich fantasy life
- Disturbed relationship with a disturbed mother
- Concerned about sexual adequacy
- History of voyeurism, fetishism, and fire setting
- Interest in hard-core, sadistic pornography; draws his own pornography
- Interest in and collection of weapons such as guns and knives
- Interest in Nazi atrocities
- Absence of psychosis
- Jobs involving power and control over others, such as being a butcher or working in a slaughterhouse
- Manual or ligature strangulation used to cause death
- Absence of intercourse or orgasm during the homicide, but sometimes masturbates beside his victim; often inserts objects into the vagina or rectum of victim
- Returns to crime scene
- Exhibits normal behavior following the murder
- Enjoys talking or writing about his crimes
- Knows it is wrong to kill but feels the prohibition does not apply to his case
- Potential for repetition is great

In 1970, Brittain drew a profile of the sadistic murderer from the perspectives of forensic psychiatry, forensic pathology, and crime scene observation. This profile was based on his more than 20 years of experience with such offenders and their victims. He did not rely on any psychiatric theory, neither did he refer to the psychiatric literature in constructing his profile, as he wanted to avoid any preconceptions of what such individuals would be like. His ten page article, now considered a classic, reveals the traits, characteristics, behaviors, background, and dynamics of the compulsive, sexually motivated, sadistic murderer (see Table 7.3).

Brittain noted, for example, that such an offender has a profuse inner life.

> He is typically a daydreamer with a very rich active fantasy life. He imagines sadistic scenes and these he acts out in his killings. ... The extremes of cruelty and the ingenuity he can show ... are almost inconceivable until one sees, for example, his drawings of his fantasies. ... His fantasy life is in many ways more important to him than is his ordinary life, and in a sense more real. ... Most sadists restrict themselves to fantasy and only a minority act out their imaginings in criminal acts. ... He is usually of high intelligence, which is probably necessary for a rich, complicated fantasy life. (pp. 199, 200)

Following years of fantasy, the murder itself is often triggered by an occurrence that reduces the offender's self-esteem, such as rejection by a woman or loss of a job. "The sadist who has been laughed at by a woman or mocked by his acquaintances, particularly in his sexual contacts, or who has been demoted or discharged from his employment is likely to be at his most dangerous" (p. 199).

Brittain found that such an individual frequently has an ambivalent relationship with his mother. He may be close to her or hate her, and sometimes he kills her. "He often tells of having, as a child, seen his mother undressed" (p. 202). The author observed that when mothers of incarcerated sexual murderers come to visit their sons, "they bring books or magazines [that] deal with matters of a sadistic, criminal or pornographic nature" (p. 202).

The method of killing is almost always asphyxiation, either manually or by the use of a ligature.

> By increasing or decreasing the pressure, they have it in their power to give their victims their lives or to take their lives from them. They can feel this as a godlike power, and they can play with their victims like a cat with a mouse. ... If the victim resists they become the more determined and brutal. (p. 204)

These men have explained that shooting is too sudden and too quick a method.

Following the crime, the offenders often behave normally, going home to eat and sleep without feeling remorse. They return to the crime scene, and some

> seem to enjoy talking of what they have done and to get satisfaction of an exhibitionistic kind from this and would often say they feel better after talking thus freely. A few will take plea- sure in writing a detailed account of what they have done. (p. 205)

Brittain found such individuals to have deep sexual disturbance, including multiple sexual perversions—transvestism, performance of sadistic acts toward animals, fetishism, voy- eurism, and fire setting, along with concerns about their own sexual potency. The murders are sexually motivated, but

> sexual intercourse or even orgasm does not always occur. Sometimes the murderer mastur- bates beside his victim. Sometimes also a phallus-substitute is used and a piece of wood, a cylindrical electrical torch or other similar object may be inserted—and this can be with great force—into the vagina or rectum of the victim. (p. 204)

Finally, Brittain concluded that the potential for repetition in such cases is quite high. "Given the opportunity the sadistic murderer is likely to murder again and he knows this" (p. 205).

The first systematic, empirically based investigation of the sexual murderer was car- ried out by Ressler, Burgess, and Douglas (1988), under the auspices of the FBI. These authors studied a nonrandom sample of 36 incarcerated sexual murderers from various geographical areas throughout the United States in an attempt to understand their per- sonality traits and characteristics, the manner in which they committed their crimes, and their crime scene behavior. Seven of their subjects (19%) had been convicted of killing one person, while 29 offenders (81%) were convicted of killing multiple victims. Information from official psychiatric, court, and prison records was supplemented by interviews with the subjects. The investigators uncovered a wealth of information on the backgrounds of such individuals. Table 7.4 lists the childhood sexual experiences of the subjects; Table 7.5 reports their various childhood, adolescent, and adult behaviors.

The investigators found examples of childhood sadistic behavior toward animals, par- ticularly cats. One individual stated,

> I killed a cat once. I can't tell you why. I was just mad and the cat came at the wrong time and I strangled this cat. It's the only animal I ever killed. ... I had a dog when I was young and

Table 7.4   Childhood Sexual Experiences of 36 Sexual Murderers

Experience	Number/Total	Percent
Witnessing sexual violence	9/26	35
Witnessing disturbing sex, parents	9/26	35
Witnessing disturbing sex, other adults, friends	11/26	42
Having sexual injuries or diseases	9/25	36
Experiencing sexually stressful events	19/26	73
Experiencing childhood sexual abuse	12/26	46
Engaging in voyeurism	20/28	71
Looking at pornography	25/31	81
Engaging in fetishism	21/29	72
Having rape fantasies	22/36	61
Having first rape fantasies between ages 12 and 14	11/22	50
Having consensual sex	20/36	56
Having no peer consensual sex	16/36	44
Experiencing sexual incompetence	14/32	44
Experiencing sexual aversion	13/30	43
Engaging in autoerotic practices	22/28	79

Source: Adapted from Ressler, R.K., Burgess, A.W., and Douglas, J.E., *Sexual Homicide: Patterns and Motives*, Free Press, New York, 1988, p. 24.

somebody fed it ground glass and we had to put it to sleep. I was very shook up over that. It was the only dog I ever had. (p. 38)

Another subject also talked of killing cats.

One time I found a kitten and it was raining. The kitten was shivering and I brought it home. About 2 weeks later the house was full of fleas. From there I just started hating cats. I don't know what happened. My father thought I did something to it, and I thought my father did something to it, because I came home from school one day and the cat just wasn't there. ... That's when I got to tying a cherry bomb to the cat's leg, light it, and watch the cat run down the street. ... I made a lot of one-legged cats. (p. 38)

The offenders were well aware of their long-standing preoccupation with, and preference for, their violent sexualized thoughts. Many offenders reported that even in childhood they had developed sexual fantasies in their play. The fantasies had a marked aggressive component, as illustrated by the case of a 12-year-old who played "gas chamber" with his sister. She tied the offender in a chair, threw an imaginary switch, and when the gas was "introduced," the youngster would drop to the floor and pretend to enter into a convulsion and eventually die.

The subjects utilized their fantasies and early sadistic activities as behavioral tryouts for their later acts of murder. For example, one murderer said, "I knew long before I started killing, that I was going to be killing. That it was going to end up like that. The fantasies were too strong. They were going on for too long and were too elaborate" (p. 42). Ressler and colleagues found that most of their subjects recognized the importance of their fantasies to their crimes. Thus, they concluded:

Table 7.5 Frequency (in Percent) of Reported Behavior of 36 Sexual Murderers in Childhood, Adolescence, and Adulthood

Behavior	Childhood	Adolescence	Adulthood
Daydreaming	82	81	81
Compulsive masturbation	82	82	81
Isolation	71	77	73
Chronic lying	71	75	68
Enuresis	68	60	15
Rebelliousness	67	84	72
Nightmares	67	68	52
Destruction of property	58	68	35
Fire setting	56	52	28
Stealing	56	81	56
Cruelty to children	54	64	44
Poor body image	52	63	62
Temper tantrums	48	50	44
Sleep problems	48	50	50
Assaults on adults	38	84	86
Phobias	38	43	50
Running away	36	46	11
Cruelty to animals	36	46	36
Accident proneness	29	32	27
Headaches	29	33	45
Destruction of possessions	28	35	35
Eating problems	27	36	35
Convulsions	19	21	13
Self mutilation	19	21	32

Source: Adapted from Ressler, R.K., Burgess, A.W., and Douglas, J.E., *Sexual Homicide: Patterns and Motives*, Free Press, New York, 1988, p. 29.

The fantasies reflect their actions based on their beliefs and patterns of reasoning. Extensive early childhood aggressive and sexualized vengeful preoccupations and sadistic acts, either indulged in by reenactment of trauma or repetitive play, not only develop their reasoning for murder but also rehearse the methods. These cognitive acts gradually lead to the conscious planning and justification for murderous acts. … These men murder because of the way they think. (p. 43)

The men often selected victims based on their long-standing fantasies. Although such victims were symbolic, others were chosen because of their conduct, such as hitchhiking or prostitution. On other occasions, a victim may have been selected because her actions elicited a certain response in the offender. For example, a woman may have reminded the offender of his belief in an unjust world. "He may feel unfairly treated, and this sets into motion the justification to kill" (p. 50).

In some cases, the murder was a direct replication of the fantasy, while in other cases the murder went beyond the fantasy. Sometimes the offender was shocked by what he had done, but many times he was not. About half the offenders raped the victim prior to the homicide; some raped their victims after the homicide, while others engaged in the mutilation of the corpse. The behavioral pattern of many murderers was rather typical, but some engaged in extremely unusual conduct, such as the man who ejaculated onto a knife wound that he made in the victim. Many offenders inserted foreign objects into the vaginal or anal cavities of their victims; others slashed the bodies, cut the genitals, bit various body parts, and engaged in torture.

Offenders disposed of the bodies in different ways including leaving the body visible, varying the victim's state of dress, or positioning the victim in unnatural ways. The final location of the victim's body was also often an outgrowth of the offender's fantasy. For instance, one subject described a heightened state of arousal while disposing of his victim's body.

> I am really rushed. My heart is beating 90 miles a minute. My blood pressure is so heavy it sounded like somebody crunching behind me. I jumped around and grabbed my gun and freaked out, but it was my blood pressure pounding in my ears. It was driving me. I thought I was going to croak while I was getting rid of the bodies or evidence. (p. 61)

Following the murder and body disposal, offenders had a wide range of reactions, including a sense of relief, a release of tension, and deliberateness in avoiding apprehension. The murderers' postcrime behavior was also found to often be an outgrowth of their fantasies. Some offenders returned to the crime scene; others observed the discovery of the victim's body; still others kept souvenirs; and some even participated in the investigation.

Finally, the murderers were apprehended in a number of different ways. Half (50%) were identified through police investigation. About 17% were identified by a surviving victim; 17% were apprehended for a crime other than the homicide; less than 1% were identified by a partner or spouse; 1% turned themselves in, and the remainder were apprehended in other ways. Interestingly, the authors found that 20% of their subjects committed a murder while out on bail for another crime.

Since the turn of the 21st century, some interesting research on sexual murder has been conducted, including studies of sexual sadism, methods of investigation, and even some attempts at treatment with both psychotherapy and pharmacological agents. A good compendium of this research is presented by Proulx et al, (2018). The various studies described are international in scope and add to our knowledge of sexual homicide. However, each study must be evaluated on its own merits, as different operational definitions of what constitutes sexual murder were used as well as different data sources (e.g., police investigative files and individual evaluations). Different methodologies can easily affect how the results are presented and interpreted. As in all research, the results of a study are what the researchers found; the problem usually arises in the interpretation of these results and, more important, their application to clinical practice.

7.7 Influence of Investigative Profiling

Although compulsive murderers have not received a great deal of attention from psychiatric or psychological researchers (relative to other disorders such as depression, anxiety, schizophrenia, and posttraumatic stress disorder), members of law enforcement agencies—especially the FBI—have become interested in this group of criminal offenders mainly from an investigative perspective. Their interest began in the 1950s, when New York City was rattled by a person the press called the "Mad Bomber." This individual set bombs at various landmarks throughout the city such as Grand Central Station, Penn Station, Radio City Music Hall, theaters, and the public library. He planned his bombing with such a high degree of detail that he went undetected for about 16 years.

Out of frustration, the New York authorities consulted James Brussel, a local psychiatrist who was interested in forensic psychiatry and criminal behavior. Brussel (1968) reviewed all the information available, including the letters that the Mad Bomber had sent to the police, photographs of the crime scenes, and descriptions of the homemade bombs. After analyzing this information, Brussel concluded that the offender was a paranoic of Eastern European descent, who lived in Connecticut with an aunt or sister. He believed he was over 40 years old, had a serious illness, attended church regularly, and was soft-spoken, polite, and exceptionally neat in appearance. A brief profile was published in the *New York Times* on Christmas Day 1956:

> Single man, between 40 and 50 years old, introvert. Unsocial but not antisocial. Skilled mechanic. Cunning. Neat with tools. Egotistical of mechanical skill. Contemptuous of other people. Resentful of criticism of his work but probably conceals resentment. Moral. Honest. Not interested in women. High school graduate. Expert in civil or military ordnance. Religious. Might flare up violently at work when criticized. Possible motive: discharge or reprimand. Feels superior to critics. Resentment keeps growing. Present or former Consolidated Edison worker. Probably case of progressive paranoia. (Brussel, 1968, p. 47)

After Brussel gave his profile to the detectives, he closed his eyes, conjured up a mental image, and said, "One more thing … when you catch him—and I have no doubt you will—he'll be wearing a double breasted suit. Buttoned" (p. 46).

As a result of Brussel's profile, the police narrowed their investigation to an individual they had suspected: George Metesky, a former employee of Consolidated Edison, who was unhappy with the company for a variety of reasons. When they went to arrest Metesky, they found that he fit Brussel's profile in shocking detail. Not only did he have all the characteristics that Brussel said he would, but he wore a double-breasted suit that was buttoned!

Authorities were amazed at the uncanny accuracy of Brussel's conclusions. Therefore it is not surprising that members of the FBI—whose job it is to investigate unknown offenders—were quite curious as to how Brussel arrived at his findings. The psychiatrist explained his thought processes as a series of "deductions." For example, psychiatrists, psychologists, and other mental health professionals regularly evaluate people and offer predictions regarding how such individuals might behave in the future. After an evaluation, a psychiatrist might conclude that the patient is likely to experience periods of depression; make unsuccessful suicide attempts; have difficulty with authority; or endure unsuccessful relationships with members of the opposite sex. These types of psychiatric predictions are not uncommon; in fact, they are rather ordinary in day-to-day mental health practice.

In drawing a profile of an unidentified offender, Brussel simply reversed the process. Instead of offering predictions about a person he examined, he offered deductions about the type of person who committed the crime. Thus, the profiler examines (in detail) the behavior an individual engages in and then constructs a profile of the type of person who would behave in this manner. Rather than studying the person and predicting his behavior, the profiler studies an individual's criminal behavior and predicts the type of person who would have acted in that manner.

Mental health professionals know, for example, that individuals with compulsive personalities are typically neat, orderly, and somewhat rigid, and these characteristics are usually consistent throughout various aspects of their lives. It is uncommon for a compulsive person to live in an unkempt apartment or to drive a battered old car. Such an individual dresses neatly, lives in an immaculate apartment, and keeps his car well maintained. And if he were to commit a crime, he would probably do so in a logical, detailed, and planned fashion. He most likely would not change his pattern of thought and behavior and commit an impulsive, unplanned, and spontaneous criminal act. When Brussel reviewed the crime scene information on the Mad Bomber and noted the extensive amount of planning that went into the bomb-making, he correctly concluded that the offender must be highly organized and rigid. And a neat appearance would likely be consistent with other aspects of his personality, behavior, and lifestyle.

This reasoning process formed the basis of what later became known as psychological, criminal, or investigative profiling—or more recently referred to as behavioral analysis—which is used mostly by members of law enforcement agencies, especially the FBI. Thus, the need for a psychological investigative tool reawakened scientific interest in the compulsive–repetitive murderer, who was previously mentioned in the scientific literature only sparingly. This type of behavioral analysis has been used not only in identifying unknown offenders in serial crimes, such as serial homicide, but in other settings also, such as hostage negotiations (Reiser, 1982), and to identify anonymous letter writers (Casey-Owens, 1984), those who make violent threats (Miron and Douglas, 1979), as well as rapists, arsonists, stalkers, and other offenders. And even if a psychologist, psychiatrist, or mental health professional is not going to engage in this type of work per se, the findings this technique has generated provide a much deeper insight into the psychopathology and psychodynamics of the compulsive offender than has otherwise been achieved, by focusing on the crime scene behavior rather than solely on psychopathology or other mental health issues.

7.7.1 Profiling Basics

Douglas, Ressler, Burgess, and Hartman (1986) described five stages of the profiling process: (1) input: the profiler collects the crime scene information; (2) decision process: the profiler arranges the input into meaningful patterns and analyzes victim and offender risk levels; (3) crime assessment: the profiler reconstructs the crime and its motivation; (4) criminal profile: the profiler develops a specific description of the offender; (5) investigation: the profiler turns over the written description to law enforcement as an aid in investigation; and (6) apprehension: the profiler checks the accuracy of the description against the actual offender.

The profiler is interested in both the offender's criminal technique, or MO, and his "signature." The MO can change over time (Douglas, Burgess, Burgess, and Ressler, 1992); as an individual commits more and more crimes, he often makes changes in his technique in order to increase efficiency. Thus, a burglar, through experience, learns different burglary methods, thereby increasing his skill and reducing the chance of apprehension (Schlesinger, 2000b). In addition to an offender's MO, the profiler looks at a crime scene for evidence of repetitive ritualistic behavior that gives the offender psychosexual gratification and has little to do with the perpetration of the crime itself. In many serial cases, this "signature" is unique and acts like a "calling card" for linking various crimes which may have occurred over a period of time to the same offender, notwithstanding differences in

MO. Examples of signatures are postmortem body positioning, mutilation of the body, and symbolic gestures and written statements left behind (Keppel, 2000).

7.7.2 Crime Scene and Personality Patterns

Hazelwood and Douglas (1980) observed crime scenes of violent sex offenders and sexual murderers and divided them into two general groups: those that are "organized," reflecting a great deal of planning and in which little evidence is left behind, and those that are "disorganized," noted by a great deal of evidence left, reflecting an impulsive, unplanned crime. Over the years, these and other investigators have found a number of distinct differences between what they referred to as organized and disorganized crime scenes. For example, the organized crime scene reflects a high level of control by the offender: strangers are targeted, restraints are used, and the body is often hidden or sometimes transported from the murder site to another location. Disorganized crime scenes reflect spontaneity and a lack of planning: the victim is often known to the offender, bodies are left in plain view (usually at the death scene), and a weapon of opportunity is used.

In addition to crime scene behavior, different personality characteristics in those individuals who leave organized and disorganized crime scenes have also been found. For example, organized offenders are typically socially competent, intelligent, live with a partner, follow the crime in the media, and often leave town after the murder. They are thought to have psychopathic (Bursten, 1972; Cleckley, 1976; Hare, 1993; Schlesinger, 1980), manipulative, or narcissistic (Schlesinger, 1998) personalities. They can be charming and are neat in appearance, physically attractive, and able to speak easily with women. Disorganized offenders, in contrast, often have poor work histories, live alone and near the crime scene, have little interest in the media coverage of the case, and do not change their lifestyle following the crime (see Table 7.6). They are much more unstable mentally; they may be schizoid, schizotypal, borderline, or sometimes schizophrenic. Such individuals are likely to be physically unattractive, have little experience with members of the opposite sex, and live alone because others cannot tolerate their eccentricities.

The organized and disorganized offenders display different approaches to murder as a result of their different personality makeups. Consequently, if you categorize a crime scene as either organized or disorganized, you can draw some immediate inferences regarding the personality of the offender. The profiler cannot say who did it, but he or she can indicate the type of person likely to have done it. A profile can at least allow those conducting the investigation to narrow the field of potential suspects.

7.7.3 Need for More Research

Because theory and reality often diverge, the profiling process is much more complicated than simply matching a list of crime scene behaviors with corresponding personality characteristics. Most sexual murder crime scenes are neither highly organized nor highly disorganized; instead, they present a mixed picture. Crime scenes, like most other phenomena, fall on a normal distribution, with highly organized and highly disorganized on the extremes (see Figure 7.2). Profilers whose experience is limited to FBI cases believe that approximately 75% of serial murderers are organized (Douglas and Olshaker, 1995). However, this impression may be a reflection of the cases the FBI handles. Crimes that are highly planned are extremely difficult to detect, resulting in many victims, and therefore

Table 7.6   **Characteristics of Organized and Disorganized Offenders**

Organized Offenders	Disorganized Offenders
Crime Scene Behavior	
Plan in great detail	Do not plan
Choose low-risk abduction	Choose high-risk abduction
Display control during crime	Behave haphazardly during crime
Cleverly manipulate victim	Rarely manipulate victim
Transport body	Leave body where killed
Bring restraint devices	Do not bring restraint devices
Torture before death	Mutilate after death
Stage the crime scene	Do not stage the crime scene
Often inject themselves into investigation	Rarely inject themselves into the investigation
Geographically mobile	Geographically stable
Personality Characteristics	
Psychopathic, antisocial, and narcissistic	Borderline, schizoid, and schizophrenic
Pleasant looking and physically attractive	Strange looking, often odd, unkempt, and disheveled
Have wives, girlfriends, and experience with females	Have little experience with females
Live with a woman	Live by themselves or with family members
Good verbal skills	Poor verbal skills
History of behavior problems and conflicts with authority	History of psychiatric treatment and suicide attempts

Source: From Schlesinger, L.B., *Serial Offenders: Current Thought, Recent Findings*, CRC Press, Boca Raton, FL, 2000, p. 16. With permission.

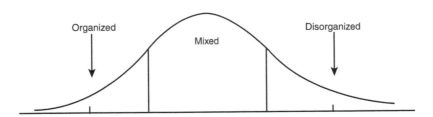

Figure 7.2 Crime scene patterns fall on a normal curve.

are frequently referred to the FBI. But sexual murderers with a compulsion to kill, who commit their crimes in less than organized fashion and leave some evidence at the scene are often apprehended after the first, second, or third homicide. These cases are usually not referred to the FBI. Thus, the FBI experience base is rather skewed in the direction of the more difficult to apprehend organized offenders with multiple victims.

Some investigators (Godwin and Canter, 1997; Godwin, 2000; Rossmo, 2000) argue that the FBI approach to profiling is not "scientific" enough and relies too much on clinical experience rather than on empirical validation. These researchers have attempted to generate empirically driven profiles based, for example, on the geographic mobility of the offender. Their underlying theory of geographic profiling is based, in part, on the work of Felson and Clarke (1998), who found that unusual crimes (such as sexual murder) follow routine patterns. Thus, offenders victimize areas they know best. The further a person is from home, the less likely he is to commit a crime. But offenders also do not commit crimes exactly where they live; they provide themselves with a buffer zone. Given these patterns, "geographic profilers" argue that they can predict an offender's residence with a high degree of accuracy, sometimes within 5% of the total crime area.

Notwithstanding the lack of strong and consistent empirical validation of profiling, some researches (e.g., Ainsworth, 2001; Pinizzotto and Finkel, 1990) have demonstrated its accuracy, particularly when it is utilized by those who are experienced in the process. But for profiling to gain general scientific acceptability—so that its results, for example, can be admitted routinely in court—a higher level of empirical validation and general professional acceptance of the technique will eventually be necessary.

With almost any new approach or method, some individuals find it useful and some are critical of it. For example, O'Toole (1999) reviewed the basics of criminal profiling from the FBI perspective. She found that this type of behavioral analysis is "an investigative tool and its value is measured in terms of how much assistance it provides to the investigator" (p. 44). O'Toole emphasized that experience in investigation is critical to using the approach appropriately. Devery (2010), however, has been critical of the use of the FBI's behavioral profiling technique in investigations. He argues that "[it is] essentially educated guesses and wishful thinking" (p. 393). In fact, he states that behavioral analysis has not contributed to investigations and that, in many cases, the method has derailed investigations and has resulted in possible wrongful convictions. Kocsis' (2003) work on offender profiling was criticized by Bennell, Jones, Taylor, and Snook (2006), and then Kocsis (2006) criticized the critique. A review of offender profiling research by Fox and Farrington (2018) found considerable improvement in the recently published studies on the topic, with case-linkage analysis demonstrating moderate to strong accuracy rates.

Just like each individual research study, each critique must also be evaluated on its own merits. For example, Canter, Alison, Alison, and Wentink (2004) used the statistical technique of multidimensional scaling to assess the FBI's organized/disorganized typology of serial murder. They found a subset of organized features typical of most "serial killings," while they found disorganized features to be quite rare. Beauregard and Martineau (2016) and Mjanes, Beauregard, and Martineau (2017), however, revisited the organized/disorganized model and generally found support for the two distinct offender types, but with complexities noted in various behaviors such as organized offenders' ability to delay and avoid detection.

Canter et. al.'s (2004) use of an all-inclusive operational definition of serial murderers—individuals who commit a series of homicides—is an example of a significant problem. These researchers did not necessarily study serial sexual homicide (which is the primary basis of the FBI model). Such research is very much like an attempt to study mental illness by including in the sample individuals who are schizophrenic, depressed, anxious, and substance abusers. These disorders—all of which can be considered a mental illness by *DSM* standards—are quite different. If they are combined in one sample, the generalizability of the results is limited and, in the end, quite useless.

An important distinction can be made between academic researchers, who typically do not have much clinical experience, and those researchers who are practicing clinicians. For example, in the 1960s, a slew of studies supposedly demonstrated the lack of empirical support for the effectiveness of psychotherapy. As Brody (1972) stated, "There does not exist a body of research which would permit one to assert that psychotherapy in one or more of its several forms has been adequately shown to be effective" (p. 299). Yet, at the same time, patients treated with psychotherapy were getting better, more individuals were being treated, insurance companies were reimbursing for such treatment because of its obvious value, and psychotherapy's effectiveness had clearly stood the test of time. Academic research without the insight of individuals who practice is often filled with errors that are not recognized by the researchers because of their limited perspective. Some researchers incorrectly believe that scientific rigor is based primarily on the statistical techniques used—the more complex and esoteric the techniques, the more "scientific" the research. However, the level and type of quantification employed should be consistent with what is being studied. Premature quantification not only is often unhelpful but also can limit the development of our knowledge.

7.8 Comment

We have presented in this chapter illustrative cases of compulsive murderers not only from different times but also from different countries and different cultures. Despite their diverse backgrounds and criminal patterns, the common element in all such offenders is an internal drive to murder: an act which itself is sexually gratifying. This compulsion to kill was described by Krafft-Ebing at the end of the 19th century and is found as well in contemporary cases reported in the early years of the 21st century.

Although sexual homicide is not a new problem, relatively few scientists have studied this criminal behavior. Only a handful of psychiatrists and psychologists has evaluated and attempted to understand these offenders. While many important insights into the psychopathology and psychodynamics of such criminals have been gained, a few mental health professionals, shocked by the compulsive murderer's heinous conduct, have concluded (incorrectly) that the offenders must be psychotic. In fact, only a minority of compulsive murderers have psychotic symptoms (Meloy, 2000), and in those who do, the psychosis is not related to the underlying compulsion to kill (Revitch and Schlesinger, 1981, 1989). However, their mental illness can greatly affect the manner in which the homicide occurs.

Interest in the compulsive, repetitive offender by the FBI since the early 1980s not only has generated awareness in the general public but has reawakened interest in mental health and criminal justice professionals as well. A few empirical–descriptive studies have been carried out, but as pointed out in Chapter 1, empirical research on this population of offenders is extremely difficult, and perhaps in some respects, may even be premature. For example, Myers (2002) studied a group of 19 adolescents who committed sexual homicides. He used a broad definition of sexual murder, which resulted in grouping together those offenders whose murders were compulsive and sexually gratifying and those offenders who killed their victims to escape detection after committing a sexual offense. Because these are two different behavioral patterns—with different motives and dynamics—it is not clear how the two types of offenders differ on the important variables that were studied. But if the groups had been kept separate, Myers might not have had enough cases of adolescent compulsive murderers to study empirically.

Forensic issues with the compulsive murderer generally center on criminal responsibility and capital mitigation. Most of these offenders, beginning with Gilles de Rais, have been and continue to be found criminally responsible by juries (Myers, Reccoppa, Burton, and McElroy, 1993). Notwithstanding their level of psychological disturbance which is obvious, citizens have consistently decided (with only a few rare exceptions) that repetitive, sexually motivated murderers must take legal responsibility for their behavior. Brittain (1970) accurately summarized the sadistic murderer's level of understanding of the wrongfulness of his conduct: "Intellectually he *knows* that it is wrong to kill, but emotionally he does not *feel* this to apply in his case" (p. 200). In capital cases, juries often accept the various mitigating factors presented (e.g., some type of mental disorder, abusive backgrounds, and substance abuse) but decide that the aggravating factors, particularly multiple victims and the use of torture, outweigh the offender's problems. And some authorities, such as Revitch (1977), believe that semantic legal debates regarding sanity and competency should be secondary to the much larger problem of identifying potential offenders and deciding how to deal with them appropriately. Although the compulsive murderer has remained largely enigmatic, the public is demanding—and deserving of—further study of these individuals to provide incre\ased protection against a small number of offenders who can cause enormous tragedy.

Planned Compulsive Homicides

8

Compulsive murderers can be envisioned as falling on a hypothetical continuum. On one end are those who plan their crimes in exceptional detail and discharge their compulsion with such care that they often go undetected for long periods of time. On the other end are those individuals who also harbor an internal compulsion to kill but who act out in an unplanned, impulsive, spontaneous fashion, leaving a great deal of evidence at the crime scene; they are often apprehended after the first or second offense. In between these extremes, however, lie most compulsive offenders who exhibit a mixture of both planning and spontaneity in their criminal acts.

Despite the diverse clinical pictures of compulsive murderers—different MOs, different personalities, different types of victims, different crime-scene behaviors—Schlesinger (2000a), elaborating on Krafft-Ebing (1886), maintains that all these offenders have as part of their psychological makeup three interconnected components: sadism, fantasy, and a compulsion to kill (see Table 8.1). All three factors are present in each offender, but one element sometimes plays a dominant role. Thus, sadism is often pronounced in offenders who engage in torturous behavior, which masks both their inner drive to kill and their fantasies. In other cases, offenders' detailed and graphic writings depicting disturbed fantasies become the distinguishing feature. And, in yet other cases, offenders may not engage in excessive amounts of overtly sadistic behavior, nor is there evidence of elaborate and intricate fantasy; however, they may reveal or demonstrate an overpowering compulsion to act. In most cases, however, none of the three components is particularly dominant.

8.1 Sadism

The term *sadism* was coined by Krafft-Ebing (1886) after the French writer Donatien Alphonse Franscois, Comte de Sade, commonly known as the Marquis de Sade (1740–1814). De Sade graphically described individuals whose sexual gratification depended on the infliction of cruelty and pain. His works were labeled obscene and were generally banned until the 20th century. In fact, as a result of his beliefs, de Sade spent about a third of his life in prisons and institutions. Perhaps de Sade's view is best stated in an excerpt from one of his most well-known works *Philosophy in the Bedroom* (1795).

> Cruelty, very far from being a vice, is the first sentiment Nature injects in us all. The infant breaks his toy, bites his nurse's breast, strangles his canary long before he is able to reason; cruelty is stamped in animals, in whom Nature's laws are more emphatically to be read than in ourselves; cruelty exists amongst savages, so much nearer to Nature than civilized men are; [it is] absurd then to maintain cruelty is a consequence of depravity. ... Cruelty is simply the energy in a man civilization has not yet all together corrupted: Therefore, it is a virtue, not a vice. ... The debility to which Nature condemned women incontestably proves that her

Table 8.1 Components of Sexual Homicide Noted by Krafft-Ebing

Component	Quotes from Krafft-Ebing (1886)
Sadism (a desire for complete control over victims)	"I performed the act ... that she might feel the power I had over her") (p. 76). "She should feel that she is completely in his power" (p. 76). "The object of desire is seen to be capable of absolute subjugation" (p. 68).
Fantasy	"He would imagine that he carried out the sexual act with them and then killed them" (p. 69). "Bloody thoughts were constantly present, and induced lustful excitement" (p. 72). "Simple imagining representations of blood and scenes of blood. ... Without the assistance of this idea, no erection was possible" (p. 72).
Overpowering compulsion	"Then this impulse, with headaches and palpitations of the heart, became so powerful" (p. 70). "The impulse became constantly more powerful" (p. 74). "He could not resist his impulses" (p. 66). "Often he could scarcely overcome the impulse" (p. 71). "Amidst the greatest dangers and difficulties, he satisfied his impulse some fifteen times" (p. 70).

Source: From Schlesinger, L.B., *Serial Offenders: Current Thought, Recent Findings*, CRC Press, Boca Raton, FL, 2000, p. 10. With permission.

design is for man, who then more than ever enjoys his strength, to exercise it in all the violent forms that suit him best, by means of tortures, if he be so inclined, or worse.

Webster's *New Collegiate Dictionary* provides the common definition of sadism: "the infliction of pain as a means of obtaining sexual release." Despite the fact that many people regard sadism as a fairly straightforward behavior, it has been hard to define, and its causes and connection to sexual arousal are even more elusive. Krafft-Ebing (1886) defined sadism as involving sexual arousal through an essential feature: "the mastery and possessing [of] an absolutely defenseless human object, ... the desire for ... complete subjugation of the woman" (p. 68). Thus, Krafft-Ebing's view of sadism is somewhat different from the contemporary dictionary definition, which stresses the infliction of pain. Krafft-Ebing emphasized the total domination and subjugation of a victim—an act that itself becomes sexually arousing and eroticized.

8.1.1 Psychodynamic View of Sadism

Freud (1908) spoke of the innate connection between sex and aggression in sadistic acts. His psychosexual developmental stages included an oral erotic stage (sucking) and an oral sadistic stage (biting) in early infancy. He thought that the genesis of sadism lies in a fixation at the oral–sadistic stage, a view that he questioned later in his life (Freud, 1932). Freud (1908) also posited a connection between sadism and sex: children

adopt what may be called a sadistic view of coition. They see there is something that the stronger participant is forcibly inflicting on the weaker, and they (especially boys) compare it to the romping familiar to them from their childish experience—romping which, incidentally, is not without a dash of sexual excitation. ... They have interpreted the act of love as an act of violence, ... [in other words] a sadistic theory of coitus. (pp. 220–221)

In Stekel's (1953) text *Sadism and Masochism*, considered by many to be a classic, he elaborated on the psychoanalytic view of sadism and described 64 cases involving various forms of sadistic and sadomasochistic behaviors. He also concluded, as did Freud, that sado-masochism is a disturbance in the psychosexual development of the individual. Sadistic persons have a "retrospective" orientation: they relive certain conflict situations in their early lives by the use of symbols, projections, condensations, and role exchanges. But other psychoanalysts do not view sadism in these relatively straightforward terms; in fact, Hinsie and Campbell (1970) list nine different types of sadism, each with a slightly different psychodynamic etiology.

Fenichel (1945) provided perhaps the clearest psychoanalytic theory of the genesis of sadism. He viewed sadistic behavior as a reassurance against anxiety connected with the fear of castration. According to this view, sadism develops in several stages: (1) the individual derives a feeling of power from acts of cruelty, (2) he achieves sexual satisfaction from torturing other persons, and (3) feelings of power and satisfaction lead to a sense of security because the individual is able to inflict on others that which he would not like inflicted on himself. Thus, acts of self-protection become aggressive and eroticized.

The psychoanalytic view of the role of "the castration complex" in the genesis of sadism is illustrated by the case of Joseph Kallinger, reported by Arieti and Schreiber (1981) and Schreiber (1984). Adopted when he was 2½ years old, the offender was raised by parents who used corporal punishment, threatened to send him back to the orphanage for alleged disobedience, burned his fingers over a stove, isolated him from other children in preadolescence, did not allow him to go on class trips, and forced him to work long hours in his father's shoe-repair shop. The authors noted a pivotal experience in the offender's young life. When he was 6 years old, he had to have surgery. Prior to the hospitalization, the parents warned their young son that the doctor would use a knife to remove the devil living in his penis; his penis would therefore remain small, and he would never get into trouble because the devil does not stay in small penises.

As a preadolescent, Kallinger threatened a boy with a knife, ordered him to undress, and then attacked him. As an adult, he had to hold a knife during sexual relations in order to obtain an erection and ejaculation. He once burned his daughter's leg close to her genitals, rationalizing that she deserved it as punishment. The offender later killed two boys and then went on a spree of burglaries with one of his sons. Finally, before apprehension, Kallinger tied up seven people with the help of his son and ordered a woman to chew off the penis of a male victim. When she refused, he brutally killed her.

Fenichel's view that sadism is based on fear of castration seems obvious in this case. Fenichel (1945) stated,

> If a person is able to do to others what he fears may be done to him, he no longer has to be afraid. Thus, anything that tends to increase the subject's power or prestige can be used as a reassurance against anxieties. What might happen to the subject passively is done actively by him in anticipation of attack. ... The idea "before I can enjoy sexuality, I must convince myself that I am powerful" is, to be sure, not identical with "I get sexual pleasure through torturing other persons"; however, it is the starting point for sadistic development. (p. 354)

Not only does the Kallinger case illustrate the relationship between sadism and fear of castration, but it also illuminates the development of sadism from the stage of power and dominance to the eventual erotization of a destructive compulsion.

8.1.2 Other Views of Sadism

Psychoanalytic theory is not the only view of sadism. Rada (1978) reviewed the many, and often slightly contradictory, definitions of sadism that have been offered from different theoretical perspectives, including Siomopoulos and Goldsmith's (1976) five subtypes of the construct. Pallone (1996) describes the social-learning and neuropsychological theory of sadistic activity. He cites Bandura (1986) who, he believes, would have argued that sadism is learned through imitation and conditioning. Neuropsychologists, however, believe that certain forms of brain impairment cause sadistic behavior, a position that apparently has some empirical support (Pallone and Hennessey, 1993).

The Diagnostic and Statistical Manual of Mental Disorders (in all its various editions) approaches psychopathology from an atheoretical perspective, emphasizing description and classification rather than etiology. The most recent edition, *DSM-5* (2013), categorizes sadism as falling under the group of paraphilias, thus emphasizing the sexual element. In fact, the text refers to sadism as "sexual sadism disorder" and places it alongside other sexual deviations, such as exhibitionism, fetishism, frotteurism, and pedophilia. According to the *DSM-5*, sexual sadism involves "intense sexual arousal from the physical or psychological suffering of another person, as manifested by fantasies, urges, or behaviors ... the person has acted on these sexual urges with a nonconsenting person" (p. 695). Krueger's (2009) review of the empirical literature on sadism found not only support for the diagnosis but a need for dimensional and structured diagnostic instruments.

Interestingly, a prior edition of the manual, *DSM-III-R* (1987), included sadistic personality disorder, described not as a paraphilia and not emphasizing a sexual element. Individuals with sadistic personality disorder gain pleasure, although perhaps not sexual pleasure, from placing others, particularly subordinates, in a state of fear and dread. Such individuals are commonly found in bureaucratic organizations, where they demean, humiliate, or frighten others. Although not presently an affirmed diagnosis, the behavior and condition are very much present in murderers (Stone, A., 1998) as well as in noncriminal populations.

The *DSM*'s view of sexual sadism is a deviation from Krafft-Ebing's (1886) original concept of the disorder, in which power, domination, and control are more central than the suffering of the victim. Some contemporary researchers do not subscribe to the *DSM* view and find Krafft-Ebing's classic position to be more accurate. For example, MacCulloch, Snowden, Wood, and Mills (1983) note that it is

> precisely *the wish to control* [italics added] that is the primary motivating force in sadism, and because there is a range of degrees and kinds of control which can be applied by one person to another, sadism may manifest itself in a variety of ways. (p. 20)

Thus, these authors define sadism as

> the repeated practice of behaviour and fantasy which is characterized by a wish to control another person by domination, degradation *or* [emphasis added] inflicting pain, for the purpose of producing mental pleasure and sexual arousal (whether or not accompanied by orgasm) in the sadist. (p. 20)

Hazelwood, Dietz, and Warren (1999) are well aware of the different forms sadism can take, and they differentiate the sadistic personality disorder from sexual sadism (the paraphilia) and from yet other forms of sadism such as cruel actions that occur during the commission of various crimes; group behavior that involves cruelty—cruelty in war, in revenge killings, and sometimes in the interrogation of suspects. Knoll and Hazelwood (2009) discussed cases of sexual murderers who manifest elements of both sadism and masochism. In these cases "the offender assumes the identity of the victim that has been tortured to enhance his sexual gratification" (p. 106).

Although mental health and criminal-justice professionals have disagreed over the definition of sadism, one of Dietz, Hazelwood, and Warren's (1990) articulate and insightful subjects—a man who kidnapped, kept captive, raped, sodomized, audiotaped, photographed, and killed many victims—offered his definition of sadism, which is more in keeping with Krafft-Ebing's position than with that of the *DSM*.

> Sadism: The wish to inflict pain on others is *not* the essence of sadism. One essential impulse: *to have complete mastery over another person*, to make him/her a helpless object of our will, to become the absolute ruler over her, to become her god, to do with her as one pleases. To humiliate her, to enslave her, *are means to this end*, and the most important radical aim is to make her suffer since there is *no greater power over another person than that of inflicting pain on her* to force her to undergo suffering without her being able to defend herself. The pleasure in the complete domination over another person is the very essence of the sadistic drive [emphases in original]. (p. 165)

The World Health Organization's (2018) *International Classification of Diseases* includes sadomasochism, combining the infliction and receipt of pain. "A preference for sexual activity which involves the infliction of pain or humiliation, or bondage ... Often an individual obtains sexual excitement from both sadistic and masochistic activities" (p. 172). Interestingly, the actual prevalence of sadism in all its various forms is really unknown (Fedoroff, 2008).

8.1.3 Some Empirical Findings

Dietz et al. (1990) carried out a nonrandom descriptive study of 30 sexually sadistic criminals who intentionally tortured their victims in order to achieve arousal. The subjects planned their crimes carefully; they targeted and manipulated strangers in order to recruit them as victims; they then beat and restrained them and held them captive. The offenders typically forced the victims to engage in bondage, anal rape, fellatio, vaginal rape, and penetration with foreign objects. They often forced victims to speak in a degrading manner, and when a victim was murdered, manual strangulation was the most common method.

In a subsequent study, Warren, Hazelwood, and Dietz (1996) studied the personality characteristics and crime-scene behavior of 20 sadistic sexual murderers. The results confirmed the notion that the murders were well planned, involved preselected locations, and included captivity and a variety of painful sexual acts such as bondage and torture. Death was typically by manual strangulation (60%), sometimes by stabbing (30%). The primacy of strangulation in sexual homicide, previously reported by Revitch and Schlesinger (1989), occurs because the offender can *control* the length of time necessary to cause death and concomitantly increase his sexual gratification. Warren et al.'s (1996) subjects said their sexual arousal was a result of their victim's pain, fear, and especially their realization of their impending death. One subject breathed air into his dying victim, prolonging her life so that she could clearly realize that he was going to kill her. "This sense of being Godlike and in control of [the] life and death of another human being is reported by some of the men as one of the most exhilarating aspects of their sexual experiences and of their crimes" (p. 974).

Geberth and Turco (1997) studied 68 serial murderers and found that sadistic behaviors began in childhood and escalated and that sadism became an integral part of their murders as adults. The killings involved domination, control, and humiliation, as well as sadistic sexual violence. Myers, Chan, Vo, and Lazaron (2010) found sexual sadism in juvenile offenders to be predictive of recidivism. Other authors (Burgess, Hartman, Ressler, Douglas, and McCormak, 1986; Chan and Heide, 2009; Gratzer and Bradford, 1995; Ressler, Burgess, Douglas, Hartman, and D'Agostino, 1986) found a high incidence of childhood abuse in individuals who subsequently developed sadistic fantasies and then engaged in sadistic behavior. MacCulloch, Gray, and Watt (2000) concluded that when young children experience abuse, they also experience fear and anxiety; they then attempt to contain these negative feelings by acting out sadistically. Such findings are consistent with the psychoanalytic theory of sadism that had been espoused by Fenichel (1945) years earlier. Additional recent research has centered on various aspects of sadism such as the prominence of power (Cross and Matheson, 2006), rating crime scenes for sadism (Myers, Beauregard, and Menard, 2019) and the frequent under diagnosis of sadism in forensic populations (Nitschke, Blendl, Ottermann, Osterheider, and Mokros, 2009). In fact, Paulhus and Dutton (2016) believe various degrees of "soft sadism" is prevalent in modern culture.

In the following case a compulsive murderer plans his crimes; achieves sexual gratification by domination, control, humiliation, and degradation of his victims; and finally causes their deaths by strangulation.

Case 8.1: Overtly Sadistic Acts

A 30-year-old male (AA) was convicted of the murder of a 25-year-old woman and the subsequent murder of a 26-year-old woman and her two young children, ages six and eight. He also murdered two other women, ages 62 and 40, acts that he confessed off the record to his attorney but was never indicted for. Authorities also suspected the offender of committing a series of rapes prior to the murders but never charged him with them. He became a suspect in the murders of the first two women because he was acquainted with both. In fact, he had a sexual relationship with the first victim; the second victim dated a friend of his. The other two adult women were strangers but lived close to where he was residing at the time.

The offender killed all the victims by manual strangulation after torturing them. He hogtied the women, raped them anally and vaginally, made small knife cuts (to cause bleeding and pain) all over their bodies, beat them, and, then, after a significant time, killed them slowly by strangulation. He tied the women up with material found in their homes, although he brought with him a "murder kit," which contained various objects he believed he needed to carry out his crimes. AA explained that he did not include precut pieces of rope or duct tape in his murder kit because, if he had been stopped by the police, he would have had difficulty explaining these implements.

All the crime scenes had a common denominator: an absence of physical evidence. AA had read detective magazines and studied books on forensic psychology and investigation so that he could avoid detection by not leaving any evidence behind. Accordingly, he shaved his entire body of hair and entered the homes naked, except for sneakers with several socks pulled over them. He poured alcohol into the vaginas and rectums of the victims because he believed alcohol would remove any trace of DNA. AA said he got this idea from the movie *Presumed Innocent*, whose plot involved the use of a spermicide. AA reasoned that doctors used alcohol prior to giving injections in order to "get rid of the germs." Unbeknownst to AA, however, alcohol preserves—rather than destroys—semen, and a perfect DNA match was made.

Although AA could have told the police that the sex was consensual and that the women were killed by someone else, he did not. Instead, when confronted with DNA evidence, he confessed to four of the six murders. AA gave different versions of what occurred. For instance, he said he visited the first victim "just to have sex." Following sexual relations, he claimed that the victim tried to convince him to stay with her all night. When AA refused, she threatened to tell his girlfriend about their sexual relationship. He claimed that the victim tried to cut him with a knife, and he retaliated by starting to choke her. "I took her upstairs. I don't know why. I was still choking her. I asked her why she wanted to do this to me and expose everything. I left her on the bed, and I left and went home." This version was not consistent with the physical evidence, and he was unable to explain why the victim had been hogtied, strangled, cut all over, and her head smashed, or why he had entered her apartment wearing nothing but several layers of socks over his sneakers.

Six months after the first murder, AA killed the girlfriend of one of his friends. He gave a similar story, stating that he had had consensual sex with the victim and then got into an argument during which she also threatened to tell AA's girlfriend about their sexual encounter. He claimed that a fight ensued and he choked the victim, tied her up, and killed her. AA also killed this victim's two young children in a brutal manner. The 6-year-old boy received 25 stab wounds to the back and 4 to the chest and had a fractured skull. AA left him in the bathroom with an electrical cord wrapped around his neck, the same cord used to choke the mother. He killed the 8-year-old girl in a similar fashion but with fewer wounds. Investigators surmised that AA killed the children because they knew him and could have identified him. Following the murders, AA went to a local restaurant where he ate hamburgers and french fries and bought beer; he returned home and slept well that evening. He was a pallbearer at the victims' funerals.

AA denied achieving any powerful or sexually arousing feelings from the torture and killings.

> No. I am powerful in any way I need to be powerful. I get respect from everyone. I can conquer whatever I have to conquer. It is something I was born with. I do whatever it takes to overcome whoever it may be. When I tell you to do something, it's not intimidation or fear; either you do it or deal with me.

He also denied any underlying feelings of inadequacy, stating, "I have no fears or worries. People try to overcompensate when they fear something. I have no fear, none whatsoever."

In his early life, AA was fascinated with knives, occasionally used marijuana, and tortured and killed cats. His mother found a number of strangled cats dangling from her clothesline when AA was 8 or 9 years old. He graduated from high school and joined the military but was discharged because of intimidating, manipulating, and stealing from subordinates. He had no prior criminal arrests.

AA was remembered by his high school and military friends as popular but "tremendously self-centered." He had no difficulty attracting girlfriends and was living with one at the time of all the murders. He had one son (with one of his girlfriends) in whom he showed absolutely no interest. One of his friends remarked,

> His attitude was he is better than anybody. He knows all the answers. You don't know nothing. Everybody has to look at AA shoot basketball. Everybody has to see AA run football. AA can pull the girls, and AA can dress better.

Psychological testing revealed an individual with low average intelligence (Full Scale IQ = 93; Verbal IQ = 90; Performance IQ = 99). There was no evidence of any significant organicity on psychological and neurological testing. Rorschach perceptions showed significant characterological disturbance, with regressive and aggressive responses, illustrated by the following: "Blood, blotted and smudged on a piece of paper, running down a piece of paper." "Drops of blood. It's running." "Two boar hogs. Their heads have been cut off. Just their heads. Their heads have been severed. They are posted on a wall like a trophy." "Blood and guts. It looks like someone's back. The rib cage." "Blood. Dried blood. This part doesn't look wet." "A rabbit. It looks like he is bleeding out of his eyes. Blood, 'cause that would be the only thing. It's too much to be water or tears." "Blood, because of the texture. It looks thick to me." He produced one illogical Rorschach perception: "A human head. An artist's sketch. A cartoon thing. It looks like feet coming out of the mouth. An artist did it. I don't know what it is to depict." His perception "ovaries of a woman," given on the male Rorschach card, suggests a conflict in this area.

AA attempted to use the MMPI to present himself in a socially desirable way. Notwithstanding this test-taking attitude, there was a high elevation on Scale 4, indicating antisocial traits and thinking. The MMPI did not reflect depression, distorted thinking, or any psychotic symptoms. It did indicate a tendency toward suspiciousness, not an uncommon finding among criminal defendants awaiting prosecution. Projective figure drawings, displayed in Figure 8.1, were rather unremarkable given the complexity and dynamics of the case.

TAT stories were quite revealing of AA's inner thoughts, emotions, and dynamics, particularly his attitudes toward women and his narcissism.

- *Card 1.* "A music student … he is depressed. He wants to play better. He is doing well, but he is pressing himself to do better. He wants to be great, but he is impatient. He wants to reach his ultimate goal and to be a star in his field. That's the only thing he knows, and he wants to be great at it. He has some trouble reaching his goals because there are stumbling blocks in the way, like alcohol and drugs. He makes it. He becomes a world-renowned violinist."
- *Card 3BM.* "A woman. She is upset and depressed because her husband left her. It's her fault because she is not a pleasing wife. She is a nagging wife. They don't have trouble in the beginning, but he lost his high paying job and got a lower paying job, and that's when she changed. She started nagging him because there was less money. Eventually, he got a job, and they get back together."
- *Card 4.* "He had an argument. He is about to leave. He is tired of arguing. She was probably messing around. She enjoyed messing around. It's what she wanted to do, and now he is outraged. He wants to leave her. He is mad and upset because his wife had an affair. It's her nature. She has been doing it all along, and he didn't know it. It makes him angry. He leaves her. She stays with the guy she had an affair

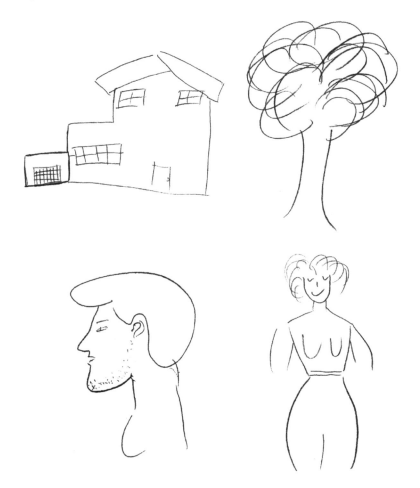

Figure 8.1 Drawings by a compulsive murderer whose planned acts were dominated by sadism.

with. She keeps the affair going. She dies of a disease, syphilis. She gets it from having so many affairs. She is a whore. She was born that way."

- *Card 3GF.* "A battered woman. She is leaving her room. She was just battered. Her husband did it. He is a drunk. He battered her for no reason. Maybe they had an argument. She was upset because he came in drunk. He didn't want to hear her. She stayed on his case. She provoked him, and he hit her. They get counseling. Life comes back together."
- *Card 8BM.* "Looks like someone getting ready to be cut. I don't know why there is a shotgun there. I don't know why they just don't shoot him instead of cutting him. I'd rather be shot than be cut. Looks like he is dead already. He's been shot, and they are cutting him open. This guy shot him. He had no reason, really. He was at the wrong place at the wrong time. He intended to shoot someone else. They disliked each other due to their competition. A lot more to it than just that. They just disliked each other. They had to prove something to each other. He spends the rest of his life in jail."
- *Card 18GF.* "A mother and her daughter. The daughter is on drugs. She is trying to comfort her. The mother is emotionally drained because of her daughter's actions. The daughter has no control over it. The drugs have control over her. She

is addicted. She wants to stop. She comes around in the end and straightens her life out."

- *Card 14.* "The guy is about to commit suicide. He is just sick of the world. He hasn't been able to get his life together, and he is giving up. His life has changed. He had it all, and now he lost it all. He is late for work and drinking and taking drugs. He just lost it. He kills himself. He jumps. He is dead."
- *Card 13MF.* "Looks like this guy killed his wife. She was sleeping around and she was unfaithful. He just couldn't take it any more, and he lost control of himself and killed her. Looks like he strangled her. He didn't want to do it. He didn't have control of himself. She just flaunted it. She flaunted the affair. She didn't hide it. He couldn't take it anymore. He didn't even think. He just did it. He calls the police, and he goes to jail. She made him into an animal because of her actions. When you love a woman, that's what they do to you. When you don't love a woman, she does what you want. She is honest and caring. But once she finds out that you love her, she changes and starts doing what she wants to do because she figures no matter what, you'll be there. You'll follow her. She figures she's got you—you are not going anywhere, so why not have an affair."

This case is an excellent illustration of a compulsive murderer whose acts were highly planned and dominated by sadism. He was narcissistic and antisocial; he demonstrated a need for power and control not only in his crimes but also in his general interpersonal relations. After making a confession, AA changed his story and told authorities that he had wanted to get caught; in this way he demonstrated his inability to be viewed as other than dominant, controlling, powerful, and in charge. The offender was raised in an intact family with apparent middle-class values, although a lot of the details about his background were unavailable. He was so untruthful regarding his upbringing, experiences, and the specifics of the crimes that much of the information he provided in this regard was useless. However, the crime-scene characteristics, which indicated a high degree of planning, and the use of torture, anal penetration, and strangulation are consistent with previously reported descriptions of sadistic compulsive offenders.

In the following case a compulsive murderer also planned his crimes and killed women in a manner that demonstrated power, domination, and control. However, his sadistic acts were less pronounced than those in Case 8.1.

Case 8.2: Planned Compulsive Murderer with Less Overt Sadistic Acts Involving Power and Domination

A 26-year-old male (BB) was arrested for choking an 80-year-old woman. He was a handyman and had worked in the woman's home several weeks earlier. BB stated:

I was drinking a little, and I was on my way home from work. I was going to pick up some soda. I was driving around and remembered the neighborhood because I worked there before. I drove in front of my customer's house. Then I drove around the block. I went to the door and told her my car broke down, that the radiator overheated. I asked her for some water. We both went to the garage. She picked the can up, and I shoved her. I jumped on top of her and started to choke her from behind, and she screamed. Because she screamed, I left.

The woman quickly recovered and called the police. That evening, BB was arrested and was also questioned regarding a double murder that had occurred 2 weeks earlier, about 10 miles away. Since the victims in both the homicide and the assault were choked and BB was a handyman at the homes of all the victims, he became a prime suspect.

BB initially denied killing the two women. Even after intensive police questioning, as well as an examination by an experienced hypnotist whom police often used, he continued to deny guilt. However, the cases were just too similar to ignore a possible link. As a last resort, the suspect was referred for psychiatric and psychological evaluation. Under the influence of sodium amytal, BB presented his "theory" of how the two women were murdered:

> The man would come in, take one woman at a time, choke each of them with his arms so that he would not leave fingerprints, and then hang them so that he could make it look like a suicide. It looks like they were murdered. I saw a lot of cowboy pictures on TV. Blood comes out of the mouth. They have seizures. You can grab them around the windpipe. I assume the guy was a sex fanatic, or he may be a homo who tried to fuck, and when he saw money, he took the money. I would say that the girls were strangled before they were hung. Strangled from behind. There are no marks if you use your arm.

Several days later, while in jail, BB confessed to the double murder. He said he had been working at the victims' home earlier in the day when the older woman (aged 45) and her 24-year-old pregnant daughter were present. That evening, BB returned to their home, knocked on the front door, explained that he left one of his tools there, and asked whether he could look for it. The younger woman let him in, and they walked around the house together.

> She was wearing a bikini. I grabbed her around the throat and started choking her. Both the mother and daughter had two-piece bikinis on. They were wearing bikinis during the day when I was working there too. I took her in the back and kept choking her. She passed out. I choked her some more, and I killed her. Then I took her to the storage bin downstairs.
>
> I moved my car. The mother came to the laundry room and asked where her daughter was. I grabbed her and choked her. She bit my finger. She took a big chunk of meat out too. I got the rope out of my car and hung her up on the dresser to make it look like a suicide. I brought the daughter [from] the basement and hung her up too. I carried her like a bride. It was like picking up a bride to carry her across the threshold to a new home or apartment. I pulled the tops off their bikinis and fondled their breasts. Then I took $81 and left.

BB explained that he choked both women slowly and reiterated that the hanging was to make the murders appear to be suicides. "I didn't even think about it after it happened. I didn't feel anything about killing the two women. I didn't lose a night's sleep."

Some interesting facts regarding these two victims came to light during the investigation. The daughter and her mother seemed to be "more like friends than mother and daughter," according to a family friend. On one occasion, while the mother was driving her daughter in the car, she stopped and asked a policeman to get help for her daughter, who apparently was hyperventilating because of anxiety. The daughter sat in the car without her skirt or underwear on, completely exposed. A neighbor revealed that the mother could not wait until her grandchild was born because she could then teach the baby his or her first word, which would be *fuck*. There were also reports of swimming in the nude and other instances of immodesty.

When examined at a later date, BB confessed to two similar murders that occurred several months prior to the double murder. The first victim was also a customer.

> I went to her house to do a job. I walked in and found out that no one was there, so I grabbed her and choked her. She was about 40 years old. She fell to the floor, and I choked her more. After I got done choking her and made sure she was dead, I dragged her in the bathroom, took her top half off and fondled her breasts. Then I put her head in the toilet. I went through the drawers, took some change, but no jewelry, and left. Then I went to a bar.

The next murder occurred similarly.

> I was in the neighborhood of an old customer, so I knocked on the door, and the housemaid answered. I asked her for a telephone to call the garage; ... since I told her my car broke. She left the front door open. We went to a little room where there was a toilet and a phone. I grabbed her and choked her. She broke free. I grabbed her again. She passed out after I kept choking her. I went to close the front door. I came back and choked her a little bit more because she wasn't dead. I took her top off, fondled her breasts, and then I pushed her head into the toilet too. I took two radios and left through the back door and went to another job. Then I went to my sister-in-law's house and went to another job.

The offender was raised in a lower-working-class family. His father was a disabled handyman, and his mother worked in a luncheonette. One sister died of cancer, and another lived in a common-law relationship with a man whom she subsequently killed (about 10 years after BB's conviction) with multiple stab wounds.

BB's home environment was described by a social worker: the house was

> untidy and an extremely dirty place. The father seemed to view BB as a rival in his own home and was constantly telling his wife to get rid of him as well as the other siblings. The mother was a person of limited intellectual resources and apparently unable to cope with her responsibilities. BB was persistently rejected and subject to corporal punishment without reason.

BB's school adjustment was also poor. He had trouble with peers, both boys and girls; he refused to follow the directions of teachers and school patrols and, on one occasion, broke 18 windows in the school. He frequently came to school unwashed and unkempt and had such violent temper outbursts that he injured other children. He sent abusive letters to a former teacher, stole money from his mother, and was finally expelled from school because of complaints from both children and parents.

During late childhood and early adolescence, BB was also described as emotionally unstable and aggressive. He had major difficulties with females; as an adolescent, he had no girlfriends because "I was afraid to ask them out." When he got his driver's license, he drove younger adolescents and their girlfriends around. "I'd look in the mirror to see what was going on, but it didn't bother me that I didn't have a girl." Several rejections by females "gave me a semi-relapse towards women."

BB was in and out of various youth correctional facilities and delinquency centers as a youngster. At age 10, he committed his first burglary, which was preceded by voyeurism.

He broke into the apartment of the woman who lived next door. For several months prior to the break-in, BB would peep into her window as she undressed.

> I knew exactly when this woman and other women would undress. When I did this break and enter (B & E), I first looked into the window and saw her in bed with her bra and panties on. There were no covers. I went in, looked more, and took $7.00 and started to leave. I went home. The woman found me and spoke to my mother. Her husband threatened to split my head. I returned the money.

After this episode, BB was sent to a child treatment center. He told the evaluating psychologist that he had stabbed two girls in a park when they called him a girl's first name instead of his correct name. A subsequent investigation failed to substantiate what was, at the time, considered a fantasy. He was later apprehended for two car thefts, a few assault and batteries on his father, failure to pay for a rented car, and an assault on another male with a baseball bat. The last offense he described is as follows.

> This was a few days after my sister died. Two guys hit me and split my head open. I took a baseball bat to find the guys who jumped me. When I got to the corner, no one was there. I saw a guy and hit him and broke his jaw. He spent two or three weeks in a hospital. His mouth was wired. I pled guilty because I felt sorry.

Additionally, BB had been charged with a rape and a threat to kill about a year prior to the homicides. "I was drinking. I was looking for a friend. I knocked at a girl's door. We were talking, stripped, and had sex. She later told her boyfriend, and he issued a warrant for my arrest. I didn't know why. Her boyfriend was my friend." However, BB gave another version of this event in which he went to visit a friend; the friend was not home, but the friend's girlfriend was there. After some conversation

> I pushed her on the bed. She was scared. I told her to take her clothes off. I took off my clothes. We had sex. I went to Mrs. W's apartment downstairs. She flipped. I told her who I was. I asked for her son. I asked if she could get in touch with him. For no apparent reason I choked her.

Both women claimed they were raped and threatened with a knife.

About 2 months prior to the first murder, BB married an obese woman reputed to be a prostitute. When he told coworkers and friends that he was going to marry her, "nobody believed me." He explained that he had one rule with his wife. "No men in the house unless I am there." He forbade his wife to see even her own brother or any male relatives when he was not there.

> If I came home and her brother was over, after he left, I'd nail her to the wall. When I met her, I knew she was a bar hopper, but she seemed to have emotions towards me. She had a 2-year-old child when we got married. I don't know if the baby is mine.

Psychological test findings revealed an individual of low average intelligence (Full Scale IQ = 90) with no evidence of significant organicity. The Rorschach was bland, with a little elaboration of perceptions (e.g., "couple of elephants," "high heeled shoes," "pair of boots," "rats without tails," "part of an arm," "looks like a shoe," "a pussy willow").

TAT stories were brief, with references to substance abuse, being arrested, suicide, and burglary. One TAT story involved choking, and one involved guilt over sex:

- *Card 18GF.* "Two women in battle. Mortal combat. The woman on top looks like she is trying to choke the other woman. Probably caught her in the house with her husband. From the angry look on her face, it looks like she will end up killing her. Then, again, she might let her go, just make her scared enough so that she doesn't come back any more. Something in her mind she will never forget. She got her on the verge of passing out."
- *Card 13MF.* "The way this one looks, it looks like a man and a woman in a room. The woman looks like a whore, and it looks like the fellow just got through with her and got dressed. The arm over his eyes looks like it might have been the first time. Like he is ashamed. She is lying there recuperating. He is fully dressed and going to leave. He feels ashamed, ashamed after having intercourse."

The offender demonstrated some degree of remorse as well as an interest in understanding his behavior. Just prior to the trial, BB telephoned the husband of one of his victims and said, "Mr. X, I did this to your wife and daughter. I am sorry, and I want to tell you this myself. I don't know why I did it." After the trial was over, he sent a letter to the examining psychiatrist with detailed drawings that "should give you a better understanding about what happened. I'm trying to put the pieces together but still have some holes in my memory" (see Figure 8.2).

This case lacks the progressive, slow infliction of pain described in Case 8.1. But it does involve death by manual strangulation, along with a distinct signature with the theme to denigrate the victims, as illustrated by hanging them with their breasts exposed and placing the heads of two women in the toilet. The offender used a clever MO, asking customers who knew him and felt comfortable with him to let him into their homes. With this ploy, he could also determine whether a male was home once he was inside. There are some interesting similarities between this case and that of Albert DeSalvo, the Boston Strangler (Chapter 7). Both offenders committed acts of voyeurism from an early age and then progressed to burglary, assault, rape, and sexual murder. They strangled the victims when they turned their backs, and both searched the homes, taking little of value. The fathers of both DeSalvo and BB were aggressive, and the offenders were much closer to their mothers. DeSalvo and BB had ambivalent feelings toward their wives; BB stated, "I love my wife so much, yet I hated her."

Case 8.3: Sadism as a Need to Control

A 36-year-old male (CC) was found guilty of the murders of two women. The first victim was an 18-year-old high school senior who worked at a local shopping mall. The offender stalked her for several weeks, and special security officers were put in place for her protection. The officers were released once the mall administration determined the threat was over, and CC abducted the young woman the next day. He drove her to a reservoir about 20 miles away and killed her with multiple stab wounds.

Several weeks later, CC forced a 24-year-old woman off the highway in his car. He took her into the woods at knifepoint and stabbed her multiple times. Assuming she was dead, the offender had anal intercourse with her, pulled her pants back up, and

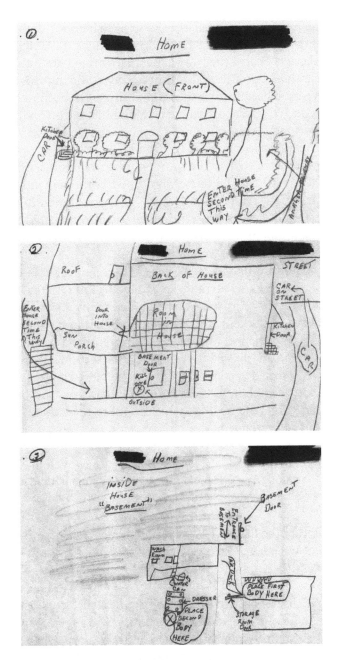

Figure 8.2 Drawings by an offender detailing the crime scene.

left. However, the woman had only passed out. When she awoke, she stumbled to the roadway, a trucker who was driving by stopped to assist. She said, "He didn't try to rape me; he tried to kill me." The woman then lost consciousness and died at the hospital several hours later.

The medical examiner concluded that both killings were not sexual murders, primarily on the basis of lack of evidence of sexual assault with the first victim and the second victim's dying declaration. The authorities assumed that the semen found in the rectums of both women was a result of their promiscuous conduct prior to their deaths.

Several weeks later, CC was arrested after he went to a police station and claimed that he was assaulted while driving his car. He said he thought the culprit might have been the unknown offender who killed the two women. He immediately aroused the suspicion of the police because the wound he claimed he received during the assault appeared to be self-inflicted. He was subsequently arrested and linked to both murders by hair, fiber, and tire-track evidence. CC had an extensive criminal history involving assault and three other murders, one of which was of a fellow prison inmate. He had served time in a Florida prison where he befriended the infamous Ted Bundy.

Although CC never admitted to the murders directly, he did offer his theory as to what happened. He claimed that he knew who killed both women and that "it was the same person." The first victim was killed because "she took something [drugs] that didn't belong to her." The second victim "was a mistake." He also reported that a third woman was abducted from the shopping mall and killed at a nearby reservoir in the same manner. He did not reveal the identity of the "true murderer."

When CC elaborated on his theory, he referred to the fact that the first victim was Asian, stating, "It was a Vietnam veteran who wanted to kill Orientals." He reported that he had met Vietnam veterans in prison who had killed many Asians and cut their ears off and fashioned necklaces from them. This was his explanation for the first victim's having had part of her ear cut off. "She was killed with a bayonet that a soldier might use."

When asked why the Vietnam veteran killed the second victim, a Caucasian, the offender stated, "Mr. X testified in court that his daughter looked Oriental at night. Possibly the killer, driving a car at night and looking into her car, mistook her for an Oriental." When asked why "the killer" did not stop when he got to the car and discovered that the victim was Caucasian, he responded:

> The adrenaline was pumping. He was in too deep. She may have seen the license-plate number. You could get in trouble. So it's possible he just went through with it. How would the guy explain it to the police if he drove the car off and let her go? He could go to jail for it.

He explained further that the first victim was killed in a vicious manner, "really butchered all up with a bayonet," whereas the second victim "only had four stab wounds." Therefore, he theorized that the killer had more anger toward the first victim because she was Asian than toward the second victim.

CC described his obsession with Asian women; he had a collection of pornographic pictures of Asians, and he said he had over 50 pen pals who were Asians. He corresponded with them while in prison, having obtained their addresses from the back pages of pornographic magazines. He also said that he was a member of the Ku Klux Klan (KKK) and the National Association for the Advancement of White People. He spoke of his fascination with Vietnam atrocities, which he had learned about in prison. He was involved with neo-Nazism and corresponded with David Duke, then Grand Wizard of the KKK.

CC was fairly articulate and had extensive courtroom experience; he handled himself quite well when cross-examined. For example, to one of the prosecuting attorney's questions, he replied,

> Sir, that's your opinion. I have a different opinion. You and I can both read the Bible and form different opinions. Your opinion isn't necessarily the correct one. It's just an opinion. I view this much differently.

During the evaluation, CC was pleasant and fairly cooperative, with no symptoms of significant overt mental disturbance. He was superficially friendly, joked and laughed at times, and complained that the evaluation was a "waste of time because my life's not worth saving." Although he did not see the point of the evaluation, he cooperated on his attorney's advice. He indicated that he did not drink or take drugs and that he was definitely "not crazy." His intelligence was average (Full Scale IQ = 96) with no evidence of organicity.

On the Rorschach, CC produced many primitive responses, which indicated much internal disorganization and characterological disturbance, as illustrated by the following: "A bug that somebody stepped on. A squashed bug. The worst thing is to see the blood. I don't see any blood, although it does look like there is blood on it. Yeah, it looks like blood." "Explosion." "A cancerous growth." "A slide under a microscope. A specimen of tissue. Living tissue because of the color."

> It looks like someone could have hemorrhoids, and this is a piece of toilet paper because of the color. It's what that person was eating to make him shit like that. I don't know what he ate. The green is spinach. The yellow is corn not digested.

"Somebody vomited because of the color, the way it's all splattered out." He responded on the TAT in a fairly guarded fashion as the purpose of this test was apparent to him. He produced only innocuous stories, attempting to project an image of normalcy. For example, on Card 13MF, which typically elicits themes of violence, sex, and aggression, the offender said,

> This guy got up early in the morning with a hangover, and that's it. Or it could be a woman asleep while her husband is getting ready to go to work. Two married people. Or it doesn't look like a man with a prostitute. She is naked in bed. I don't know what it is.

CC's sadism was manifested by his need for control over the victims, which is well illustrated by this statement: "When I kill people I want to see them die. I want to watch them shit and piss for the last time. I want to watch them die the slimy bastards." The offender was also a necrophiliac. He had anal intercourse with the victims after their deaths so that he could completely control and dominate their lifeless, nonthreatening bodies. Although the second victim passed out from shock and had no realization of having been raped, CC thought that she was dead (if he had known she was still alive, he never would have left her). Although the offender did not directly admit that he committed the murders, it is hard to believe that he was not talking about himself when he presented his theoretical description of the events. He certainly would not have admitted to having fantasies or an underlying compulsion to kill, but both these elements can be easily inferred from his conduct and his statements during evaluation.

8.2 Fantasy

Beres (1960) has defined fantasy as a "group of symbols synthesized into a unified story by the secondary processes; ... it may be a substitute for action or it may prepare the way for later action" (p. 328). Fantasy is an imaginative process that is not always a direct response to an external stimulus; more often the stimulus is internal. The content of fantasies can be about anything—typically money, revenge, fame, and sex. Sexual fantasy specifically involves thoughts and images of a sexually arousing or erotic nature. In their comprehensive review of the literature on sexual fantasy, Leitenberg and Henning (1995) note that sexual fantasies are commonly experienced by both men and women and fall into four general categories: conventional heterosexual imagery; scenes involving sexual power and irresistibility; images of varied settings, practices, and positions; and images of submission or dominance, in which some level of physical force is involved or implied.

8.2.1 Sexually Aggressive Fantasies

Sexual fantasies, particularly deviant sexual fantasies involving force, play a significant role in a number of sex crimes. Not everyone who has deviant fantasies commits sexual crimes; in fact, a sizeable portion of the noncriminal and nonpsychiatric ("normal") population also reports deviant sexual fantasies, as well as homicidal fantasies (Kendrick and Sheets, 1993; Crabb, 2000 Maniglio, 2010), but do not act them out. For example, Grendliner and Byrne (1987) found that 54% of men who never committed a sexual assault fantasized about forcing sex on a partner. Similarly, Briere and Runtz (1989) found that 21% of male undergraduate students acknowledged sexual attraction to children, and 9% admitted to having had specific sexual fantasies about children. All these individuals, however, denied acting on their fantasies. Crepault and Couture (1980) report that 61% of their nonoffender adult male samples had fantasies in which they "sexually initiated a young girl"; 33% fantasized raping a woman; 12% fantasized being humiliated; and 5% fantasized having sex with an animal. In a plethysmographic study Barbaree and Marshall (1989) also found that about 20% of their nonoffender control subjects were aroused by the imagery of prepubescent children.

Although not all individuals who have deviant sexual fantasies act out, many do. A number of investigators (Abel and Blanchard, 1974; Finkelhor and Araji, 1986; Groth, 1979; Malamuth, 1986; Marshall, Laws, and Barbaree, 1990) have found that sexual crimes such as rape and child molestation are a result of multiple factors including deviant sexual fantasy. MacCulloch et al. (1983) explored the relationship between sadistic fantasy and criminally sadistic behavior. In their study, 13 out of 16 subjects (81%) committed sadistic crimes as an outgrowth of repetitive, sadistic masturbatory fantasies. These authors note the importance of deviant fantasy in the compulsive offender while also recognizing that not all individuals who harbor such fantasies act out. They also acknowledge their inability to distinguish the critical features differentiating these two groups.

Reinhardt (1957) noted the important role of fantasy in the genesis of sexual murder:

> These sadistic [fantasies] seem always to have preceded the brutal act of lust murder. These fantasies take all sorts of grotesque and cruel forms. The pervert, on this level of degeneracy, may resort to pornographic pictures, grotesque and cruel literary episodes, out of which he weaves fantasies. On these, his imagination dwells until he loses all contact with reality, only to find himself suddenly impelled to carry out his fantasies [in] the world of actuality. This is done, apparently, by drawing human objects into the fantasy. (pp. 208, 209)

Burgess et al. (1986) found that about 80% of men who had been convicted of a sexual murder had masturbatory fantasies relating to sexually assaultive conduct. Prentky, Burgess, Rokous, Lee, Hartman, Ressler, and Douglas (1989) found that about 86% of serial sexual murderers reported violent sexual fantasies, while 23% of offenders who committed a single sexual murder had such imaginings. Accordingly, these researchers postulated a clear relationship between fantasy and sexual homicide, particularly in the repetitive sexual murderer. Carabellese, Maniglio, Greco, and Catanesi (2011) found fantasy to play multiple roles in sexual offending including planning, victim selection, stimulation, arousal, mood regulation, and escape from reality.

The importance of fantasy in the investigation of sexual crimes was stressed by Hazelwood and Warren (1995) who concluded that "fantasy is the link between the underlying motivations for sexual assaults and the behavior exhibited during the crime" (p. 137). In an empirical study of the role of fantasy and cognition in the premeditation of criminal behavior, Deu (1998) used Schlesinger and Kutash's (1981) "Criminal Fantasy Technique" to measure subjects' fantasies. Deu found that cognitive flexibility and impulsivity interacted in the offender's use of fantasy for planning and organizing violent crimes.

Bartholomew, Milte, and Galabally (1975) reported the case of a 23-year-old male whose murder of a 12-year-old girl was a direct outgrowth of his deviant fantasies. The offender had an IQ within the superior range and experienced an essentially normal upbringing but was somewhat isolated. From age 18, he had written down bizarre, aggressive sexual fantasies. A few months prior to the homicide, the young man removed the underwear of two female children about 3 and 5 years old in order to inspect their genitals. The night before the murder, the offender slept in his car, dressed in several pairs of plastic pants. He defecated into his pants and drove around sitting in his excreta, which provided him with sexual arousal.

While driving, the offender spotted a 12-year-old girl, a stranger to him, whom he abducted. He made the girl eat biscuits saturated in urine, undressed her, smeared her with feces, played with her genitals, gagged her, tied her up, cut her throat, and slit her abdomen, but never attempted intercourse with her. He disposed of the body behind some bushes. When examined, he showed no evidence either clinically or on testing of any type of psychotic process. An example from this offender's diary provides insight into his detailed sadistic fantasies:

> Get 2 boys (6–10) and 2 girls (6–14) or boy (6) & girl (6–14) and take them out to place. When I get there blindfold them and strip them, and have a good look & feel. Tie them to trees with ropes coming from behind, under armpits, around behind neck & under other arm, and around tree. Nail a stick to the tree & tape their heads to it. Put a pr. of plastics on each of them & tie string around legs, so they won't leak. Put deep cut into cunt/cock on each of them so they won't leak. Unblindfold them. Bite nipples off tits. Give them each a box of licorice & tell them to eat it within 5 mins or else; for each piece they don't eat, cut a cross on their chest. Make them skull a can of beer. Untie elder girl and blindfold her. Ask her if she knows diff. between boy & girl. If so, tell her to find a boy & a girl with her tongue. I carry her to each one with hand in cunt & arse & around body. When she finds each one they piss in her face. If she doesn't know difference tell her to put her hand under pants. Guide her to cunt. Tell her to use her tongue to find boy. When she does he puts cock in her mouth and piss, then she bites the cock. Take her to others and make them piss in her face while she licks cunt/cock. Tell them facts of life and rude terms for things. Name them cunt, cock, shit & piss & carve names on them. I root girls and poufter boys. Then make boys root girls or poufter each other. Make girls suck boys' cocks & eat each other out. Don't give [them] anything to eat or drink until they are hungry enough to eat anything. If they say yes tell them what will happen if they refuse, i.e. put cracker in cunt & arse/arse & around cock and light them simultaneously. Get

youngest one and lead to eldest, put his/her head in other's pants & make him/her eat till it is dry. The[n] swap them around. Make other pair do same. Dig hole about 18″ deep, 7″ long and 41″ with light depression in centre, line it with plastic so it won't leak. On first night take them into it one at a time, lay them on top of me and take their pants off so shit & piss runs on me. Spread it on them too. Then I lay on them too. Then I lay on them & root &/or poufter them. Repeat with others. In morning dress them in a pr. fancy undies & nappy (or 2 pr thick undies), pr. plain plastics, pr. thick undies, pr. fancy plastics. Tie string around legs of fancy plastics so they won't leak. Set them low on hips so there is plenty of room for shit. etc. Put dresses on all of them. Cut all hair off (incl. eyebrows, lashes) Give them big feed, with plenty of laxettes & beer. At night clothes are left in hole, and wrung out & put back in the morning. Make them spew into each others pants & in bed. I wear pr. fancy undies, 2 pr. thick undies, pr. plain plastics, pr. thick undies, pr. fancy plastics. Try to breed maggots to put in their pants and make them eat. If there is a kid under 3 it stays in the bed & eats & drinks normally, with a laxette and a glass of beer every hour. It wears a pr. of plain plastics with legs & top tied so they won't leak. Its leg is tied to a rope going over top of pit. After a couple of days don't give it anything to drink. Wait a couple of days more, then strip it, and if girl skin the inside of piss flaps, then sew them together. If boy, cut cock & balls off & block up piss tube. Tie girls legs together at top. After a week or so make them drink lots of beer and water and see if they leak. If they don't, keep on giving them piss & water until their piss bags bust. * If they leak, give them a big feed with plenty of shit & piss to flatten them. * At night boys root & poufter girls and girls give boys love bites & eat out their arse & other girls' cunts. They all have hands tied & one leg tied to rope. Each night I have oppo. girl and root her. Other boys root & poufter other girl and poufter mine. * After a few days make a barbeque pit with rotating spit on each end. Make sure baby is full of piss & shit, gag it, and tie to spit, hands one end, feet the other. Make kids get on each end & turn & cook baby alive. When properly cooked, put it in shit pit & make others start eating it. If boy, give cock & eyes to eldest girl. They eat it & drink beer till only bones left. (quoted in Bartholomew et al., 1975, p. 150)

In the following case a young man killed a 12-year-old girl after fantasizing about the act for over 15 years. When he was no longer able to contain the compulsion, he carried out "the plan."

Case 8.4: Carrying Out a Homicidal "Plan" after 15 Years of Fantasy

A 33-year-old male (DD), a college graduate with superior intelligence, entertained a detailed sadistic fantasy for over 15 years. During some of this time, he saw a psychiatrist but never revealed the fantasy to him. He was raised in a middle-class, professional family and had no history of prior juvenile or criminal offenses. DD's work record was spotty, and because he had little income, he lived with his parents. He was withdrawn, rarely dated, experienced periodic depression (sometimes with a mild paranoid tinge to thinking), and entertained many grandiose ideas.

DD's long-standing, detailed fantasy, which he referred to as "the plan," involved abducting a female at gunpoint, raping and then murdering her. For years, he did not act on the fantasy because he feared that instead of his overpowering the woman, the victim would overpower him. After a woman whom he intermittently dated ended the relationship, DD decided to "put the plan into action." He traveled to another state, where he believed the gun laws were lenient. However, when he got there, he learned that only residents could purchase guns. Instead, he bought a gun from a stranger on the street. DD rented a car and drove around for several days fantasizing about a victim. He did not want to harm a child because "a child was not guilty for my suffering"; rather, he targeted female college students. He viewed the planned murder as some type of revenge killing against women in general.

For several days, he fantasized about committing a series of rape-murders, each one involving torture and an "ingenious plan" for escape.

> I have had very violent fantasies, but I don't like violence. I fantasized that I would find beautiful women, college students, kidnap them, and have my way with them, and then kill them in a clever way which would look like an accident.

DD picked up some of these sadistic ideas from television programs.

DD was not sure whether his plan consisted of rape alone or rape-murder, but he was certain it would end in violence, perhaps even suicide. He added, "I did not really believe I would do it"; in fact, when examined following the homicide, he was not completely sure if the murder had occurred or whether it was still a fantasy.

> What happened was a horrible nightmare version of the plan. All Monday night I looked for victims. I really believed it could not and would not happen. When there was an opportunity, I hesitated. Then I returned to the motel, watched TV, and slept poorly. Tuesday morning I was very frightened. All day long, I looked around. It was an acting out of a fantasy, but I did not think I would do it. Oh my God!

The offender eventually saw a young girl with blond hair, dressed in a blue suit, "the epitome of the object of my fantasies."

> God damn, the plan started and would not stop. I pulled the gun. I drove up and asked her for the way to the city. I knew if I hesitated I would fail again. It just kept happening, and I couldn't stop. I asked her, "Can a person run faster than a bullet?" It was in my plan. At the same time, I realized she was younger than I thought. She was too young, but I could not think. She was pretty. A nice person. That was not the type of person I wanted in my plan, but there was nothing I could do. I told her not to worry. That was in the plan. Unfortunately, she did not give me time to think. I tried to think how I could let her out of my car, but I could not because this was not in the plan. Then, tears on her cheek. I said, "My God, how old are you?" She said, "Twelve years old." I was mistaken. I wanted to let her out, but for this I would have to formulate a different plan. I tried to force myself to let her out, but this confused me. We got out of the car, and we walked to the woods.

DD attempted intercourse but was unable to get an erection. He penetrated her vagina with his finger, and she bled. The offender continued with "the plan because I could not deviate from it. If I stopped to think, I would get upset." He then gave her a tissue to clean herself. "From that point on, I tried to stop, but I could not change direction. I tried to stall. All the time I was trying to stall, I was thinking of an alternative. Every time I stopped, she would get so frightened."

DD tied the child's hands behind her back and pushed her into a shallow pond. "She screamed. I sat on top of her in the pond. Why do I feel sorry for myself? My mind went one way, but my body continued the plan." He described how he slowly drowned her and sat on her body for what he thought was 10 minutes. After she died, "she was no longer a person. I thought maybe I could revive her, but again I had no time to think. Then I thought to revive her and to drown her again because the plan called for it."

The offender went back to his motel and had a fleeting suicidal thought. He cut his shoes and clothes into small pieces and put them in various bags, all part of the fantasy. The next day, he took a train back to his home state because he did not believe he would be allowed on an airplane with a gun.

Throughout the evaluation interview, DD was interested in the "moral aspects" of his behavior more than in his legal predicament. When the examination was finished, the only question he had was, "What's my IQ? Is it superior or higher?" Psychological testing revealed a Full Scale IQ of 134. The Rorschach was disorganized with illogical perceptions ("a horse's head together with a human skeleton because there's no flesh on it") and aggressive content ("two elephants with blood dripping down from their nose, where they fought"). Figure drawings were elaborate, detailed, but not that revealing. TAT stories involved themes of depression, violence, and impotency. ("He is getting up from bed with a woman; he's impotent. She is lying there thinking how can I get rid of him. He realizes he is not good sexually.")

Long-standing sadistic fantasies preceding the murder dominate this case. Sadism, power, and control were certainly components, as well as the compulsion to kill, but his fantasy ("the plan") was the dominant feature. Feelings of inferiority, particularly male inadequacy, a need for revenge against women, and some grandiose ideas are additional factors. DD plead guilty and received a life sentence.

Case 8.5: Long-Standing Fantasy Finally Acted on

This case was initially reported by Revitch (1957, 1965) and is described here with further detail. A 40-year-old male (EE) was charged with assault. The prosecutor and the judge were uninterested in the underlying sexual aspects and motivation, which clearly stood out during the evaluation. The assault stemmed from a fantasy to "tie women's legs," which began when EE was 9 years old. While playing with a girl, he tied her legs together; he received a "peculiar thrill" from the victim's screaming and kicking. EE forgot about the incident for several years, but the memory resurfaced when he saw a movie involving a woman tied up by jungle inhabitants. This image gave him a similar "thrill," and he then developed a fantasy of "tying female legs" that went on for about 30 years. The offender reported several homosexual experiences as a child involving forced fellatio and also described strong feelings of sexual inadequacy and fear of women. He did not date many women, rationalizing that he did not have a good job and had to support his mother.

In addition to the fantasy, EE developed a strong urge to rob a woman and tie her legs. He prepared for carrying out the compulsion by turning the license plate on his car upside down so it would be difficult to recognize. He then grabbed a blackjack from the back seat and waited in his car. He hit the first young woman who walked by, pulling her into the car. The victim screamed, and a passerby ran to her assistance. Frightened, EE quickly left the scene but was arrested within several hours. During the search, the police found a blackjack, noose, rifle, knife, pornographic pictures, and a copy of Krafft-Ebing's *Psychopathia Sexualis* (1886) in the trunk of his car. EE said he bought the book to find an explanation for his fantasies.

Under the influence of sodium amytal, EE stated:

When I tie girls' legs, I do not want them to feel pain. I tie legs because I want to feel that she is my own, that she is close to me. I don't want to hurt people. During the robbery, I wanted to hit a girl's head, and, at the same time, I wanted to soften the hitting since I didn't want to hurt her. I didn't want to do it. I tried to hold my own hand. I was scared. I was afraid that I'd hurt her. She told me to let her go, and I said, "Keep quiet." She kept screaming. When the man approached, I told him she had a convulsion. I didn't want him to know that something was wrong. I was afraid. I thought people would kill me. Later, I found her gloves and her shoes, and I threw them in the backyard. When I went home, I changed my clothes and washed my hands. It was raining that day. I walked and walked and walked. I was afraid of people. I wanted to give myself up, but I was afraid to give myself up since I felt people would kill me.

EE's fantasy was not as complex or as involved as the fantasy in the preceding case, but it was present for many years prior to the act. It is not completely clear why the compulsion to act became overpowering after EE was able to contain it for so long, but he did describe feeling particularly depressed and lonely. If EE had not been apprehended, he said he would have attempted to act out his fantasy again.

8.2.2 Fantasy and the Ritualistic Offender

Compulsive murderers who plan their crimes often engage in repetitive, ritualistic behavior at the crime scene, referred to as *personation* or *signature* (Douglas, Burgess, Burgess, and Ressler, 1992). "The offender often invests intimate meaning into the [crime] scene in the form of body positioning, mutilation, items left, or other symbolic gestures" (p. 354). These repetitive ritualistic acts, which serve as the offender's "calling card" (Keppel, 1997, 2000), have little to do with the perpetration of the crime itself. Instead, they are an outgrowth of the offender's long-standing deviant fantasies. The purpose is to provide psychosexual gratification which the murder alone does not allow the individual to achieve.

The importance of fantasy can be seen in these ritualistic activities. The distinct behavior of one individual is seen in Figure 8.3. Here, a young woman was killed by manual strangulation. Following her death, the offender carefully cut out her vagina and reproductive system. This was not an impulsive act; rather, the offender probably fantasized about this activity for years and finally carried it out. The suspect in this case was found guilty of killing several other women but was never charged with the murder of the woman shown in Figure 8.3. At his home, investigators found several briefcases (which contained rope, duct tape, and surgical scalpels), along with a collection of detective magazines. It is important to emphasize, however, that not everyone with deviant sexual fantasies acts out; in fact, most do not (Leitenberg and Henning, 1995; Maniglio, 2009).

Hazelwood and Warren (2000) have differentiated the ritualistic offender from the impulsive offender. The ritualistic murderer is characterized by "a pervasive and defining fantasy life, and a carefully developed and executed set of crime scene behaviors" (p. 267) that are an outgrowth of his imaginings. The authors note that the impulsive offender, unlike the ritualistic offender, may be unaware that sexual fantasy underlies his criminal behavior. The ritualistic offender, however, will "invest a great amount of time in the pursuit of his fantasies" (p. 272). There have also been several cases of offenders videotaping or photographing their murders in order to create their own pornography.

Hazelwood and Warren (1995) have identified five elements of the ritualistic offender's fantasy life: relational, paraphiliac, demographic, situational, and self-perceptual. "For example, a rope may have a relational component (i.e., date, sexual slave), a paraphiliac component (bondage, sadism, fetishism), a situational component (war, arrest), a

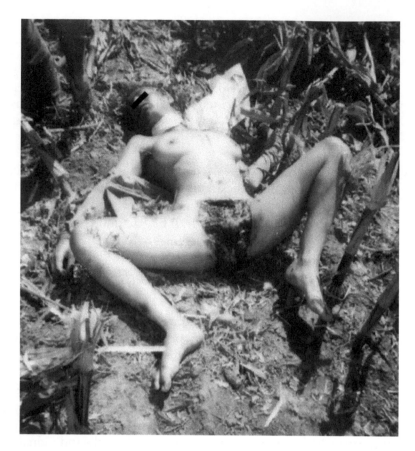

Figure 8.3 Crime-scene photo of a woman whose vagina and reproductive system were carefully removed.

self-perceptual component (powerful, God-like), and a demographic component (victim characteristics)" (p. 129). Many times one aspect of the fantasy is dominant. For example, the authors report the case of a 42-year-old male whose sexual fantasies were dominated by his perceived relationship with his victim. This man abducted a 13-year-old female, kept her captive for 6 days, during which time he cut her hair off, tortured, raped, costumed, and photographed her in various stages of undress; he then bound her with silver-colored chains and eventually strangled her with wire. Following the murder, he called the victim's grandmother and said, "Wendy is in a barn with her hair cut off." When arrested, he had another victim in his trunk. A subsequent search of his home revealed detective magazines and lengths of silver-colored chain.

In a number of well-known cases the offender's fantasy life is distinctly observable. For example, John Sweeney (Balmer, 2017) was dubbed the Sketchbook Killer because of his numerous drawings, which provide a clear glimpse into his inner life and fantasies. They depict axes, knives, torture, abuse, and dismemberment. He created over 300 pieces of artwork, most reflecting his hatred of women and preoccupation with dismemberment. In a sense he drew his own pornography, a practice that had been reported years earlier by Krafft-Ebing (1886): "Among his effects were found objects of art and obscene pictures painted by himself" (p. 73). Sweeney acted out his fantasies including the dismemberment of his victims. Another case in which an individual's fantasy life and ritualistic killing are distinctive is that of Charles Albright (Matthews and Wicker, 1996), who was fixated on eyes; he skillfully removed the eyeballs of victims. As a child, Albright removed the eyes of stuffed animals and replaced them with buttons. Serial sexual murderer Peter Tobin (Wilson and Harrison, 2010) had an obsession with women menstruating, captivity, and burying people alive. He masked much of his pathology by using his affiliation with various churches in order to appear as an upstanding citizen. And serial killer Robert Napper (Levi, 2019) targeted women with children, an obsession that also seemed to be an outgrowth of his long-standing fantasies.

The following case involves an individual who had a specific fantasy of stabbing women in the neck with a sharp object and watching them die slowly while sexually abusing them. Because of his background and comfort in committing crimes, he did not resist acting the fantasy out, and he did so in a ritualistic manner.

Case 8.6: A Ritualistic Murderer

A 30-year-old male (FF) pled guilty to the murder of a 37-year-old woman who was his neighbor. He entered the victim's home at knifepoint, forced her into the basement, and stabbed her in the neck with a piece of metal (a knife or a pair of scissors). After her death, he removed her clothes, ejaculated near (but not on) the body, and wrapped her in draperies and clothing. He put the body in the victim's car and dumped it in a neighboring town where he used to live.

At the time of his plea agreement, he also admitted to killing his 16-year-old cousin 2 years earlier. This victim was found dead lying face up in the backyard, unclothed, with a sock stuffed down her throat. Although he was considered a suspect in her suffocation death, he was not charged. FF was also a suspect in five other homicides that occurred within a 2-year period in the same vicinity and in a neighboring state where his mother resided and where he used to visit. All these victims were killed by what seemed to be knife or scissor wounds in their necks. Their bodies were similarly discovered unclothed, wrapped in fabric or sheets, and dumped in a location different from the murder site.

FF had an extensive juvenile and adult record. As an adolescent, he was arrested 14 times during a 4-year period for a variety of different crimes including burglary, aggravated assault, robbery, and receiving stolen property. As an adult, he was arrested for possession of narcotics, assault, robbery, and the rape of a 9-year-old girl. The rape was downgraded to endangering the welfare of a minor, and he was released from the county jail after serving less than a year.

When arrested for the last in what seemed to be a series of homicides, FF was uncooperative, but he did "nod yes" when the detectives asked him whether he needed help to stop from hurting women. At first, he refused to give a statement but admitted to all the killings without supplying details. Some of the details he later supplied turned out to be fabricated, as is often the case with such offenders.

FF was raised by his mother, whom he was close to; in fact, he referred to himself as "a mama's boy." He developed drug dependence problems as an adolescent and dropped out of high school in the ninth grade. He held various jobs, including construction worker, truck driver, cook, and factory worker. He was also a Golden Gloves boxer in his youth and won some important matches. At the time of his arrest, FF was living with a woman. He had two children with another woman and claimed he kept in touch with them.

The offender had average intelligence (Full Scale IQ = 94) with no organicity detected. The Rorschach revealed significant characterological disturbance evidenced by a number of regressive and aggressive responses, such as the following: "Looks like something of a pit bull with his ears bleeding. His nose is bleeding and red eyes. The ears are clipped. They are bleeding." There were no signs of a thinking disorder, and reality testing was good. Conflict with females and lack of empathic capacity were also noted on the Rorschach; these characteristics are illustrated, respectively, by his inability to offer a single response to the female card and his total absence of any human perceptions. Figure drawings were not that remarkable.

Responses on the TAT included a number of stories with aggressive themes involving strangulation ("She is trying to grab the person around the neck to strangle the person"), as well as the following interesting production: "He just killed her, or they finished having sex. He is dressed. She is lying there. He broke in her home. She cheated on him with another woman or man. He is just crazy. He went in her house and killed her. He doesn't have a key. It could be his wife and he caught her in bed with a woman or a man. He caught her and killed her. Or he could have broken in the house. He broke in to rape her. He can't believe it."

FF pleaded guilty to aggravated manslaughter and received a relatively light sentence considering his long criminal record, prior homicide of an adolescent, and him being a strong suspect in five other murders. The lack of physical evidence at the crime scene, as well as his refusal to give a detailed statement, led the prosecutors believe they would have a difficult time getting a conviction for (first-degree) murder, and they feared the possibility of a not guilty verdict. Although FF refused to discuss any of his inner life, it was obvious that his behavior was directed by fantasy, especially the ritualistic stabbing of victims in the neck.

Schlesinger, Kassen, Mesa, and Pinizzoto (2010) conducted the first empirical study—which included 38 offenders and 162 victims—of ritual and signature in serial sexual homicide. Ritual was operationally defined as a repetitive crime-scene behavior above and beyond what is necessary to kill the victim; signature was operationalized as simply a unique ritual among the sample. The results showed that offenders did not engage in the exact rituals or leave unique signatures at the scene of every crime that they had previously been suspected of committing. Instead, the crime-scene behavior of these serial sexual murderers was complex and varied. Offenders' ritualistic behavior was not always exactly the same, but it involved consistent themes across victims; additionally, in about half of the cases, there was a distinct evolution or elaboration of the ritual as the murders continued. For example, several offenders engaged in increasingly elaborate torture rituals with subsequent victims; another offender began with genital mutilation, which progressed to dismemberment; and another offender's ritual evolved from eye-puncturing with the first victim to enucleation of the eyes with later victims in the series. The authors also studied whether ritualistic behavior could legitimately be considered signature (i.e., unique). They found that unique crime-scene behavior occurred in about 18% of the cases in their sample. Most notably, the researchers also found that about 70% of the serial sexual murderers did something unique at one crime scene that they had not done with other victims in their series, indicating that they had "experimented" with one victim in a totally different way. Accordingly, from an investigative perspective, when one victim in a series looks different from the others, it does not mean that the crime was necessarily the work of another offender.

Koeppel et al. (2019) studied foreign object insertions in sexual homicide. The foreign object insertion prevalence rate for sexual homicide was about 19%. Of the 260 sexual homicide cases (207 nonserial and 53 serial) studied, nonserial offenders engaged in foreign object insertion at about the same rate (21.7%) as serial offenders (18.8%). Moreover, the findings do not support the previously held notion, based mainly on case reports, that offenders who engage in foreign object insertion are psychotic and that the insertions occur only post-mortem. In fact, the insertion behavior of the nonserial sexual murderers reflects a level of sadism and deviancy comparable with that of serial murderers.

8.3 Compulsion to Kill

In order to understand compulsive murderers, it is necessary to consider the role of sadism and fantasy in their lives. However, these components are not sufficient explanations for offenders' drive to act out their fantasies. As previously noted, most individuals who harbor sadistic, sexually oriented fantasies do not act on their imaginings (Crepault and Couture, 1980; Templeman and Stinnett, 1991, Maniglio, 2009). Schlesinger and Revitch (1997b) examined numerous individuals—many of whom had committed nonsexually motivated crimes or no crimes at all—who reported elaborate sadistic fantasies but never felt the desire to act them out. For example, Figure 8.4 contains drawings by a man who was briefly incarcerated for the theft of a watch, an act that seemed impulsive and spontaneous. Although he had never been involved in any sexually motivated crimes, he wrote about and drew pictures of men who cut off female breasts, stabbed women, chained them, scraped the skin off their bodies, whipped them, and introduced swords and rods into their vaginas. Many of his sketches depicted medieval dungeons and executions. He claimed that his creations were a mere pastime. His actual life seemed more masochistic than sadistic. The following is a sample of his writing:

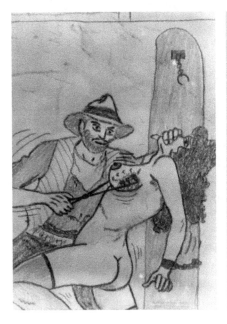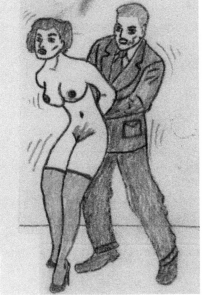

Figure 8.4 Sketches by a man who denied having a desire to engage in any sadistic acts; he considered his drawings a mere pastime.

He heard the howling grow louder now, which meant more victims. He looked out and gasped. A naked man hung swinging and writhing by his genitals. Next to him hung a plump woman who had cords threaded through her breasts and she was hanging by them. The weight of her body pulled them up by her face. It was a pitiful sight, and she writhed and squirmed. The mob was jabbing sticks at her buttocks and vagina while she hung there writhing. The man was being jabbed about the thighs, chest, and buttocks; and over by the wall hung two naked girls. The men were inserting objects into their vaginas while others were scraping the skin off their arms and breasts with little steel rakes. Men ran around with parts of bodies, women's breasts and legs, also men's genitals.

Why do some individuals act on their violent and sadistic fantasies, and others do not? Revitch and Schlesinger (1981, 1989) concluded that those individuals who act out these fantasies do so because of a compulsion. In many cases, the compulsion is so strong that an attempt to resist it results in anxiety and various somatic manifestations. For example, Krafft-Ebing (1886) cited the case of a 21-year-old man who attacked and stabbed girls in the genitals during broad daylight. "For a while he succeeded in mastering his morbid craving, but this produced feelings of anxiety and a copious perspiration would break out from his entire body" (p. 74).

Vincenz Verzeni, described by Krafft-Ebing and reported on in Chapter 7, recognized the strength of his compulsion to kill. "Verzeni said, himself, that it would be a good thing if he were to be kept in prison, because with freedom he could not resist his impulses" (Krafft-Ebing, 1886, p. 66). In fact, most compulsive murderers recognize the strength of their compulsion to act; as Brittain (1970) notes, "Given the opportunity the [compulsive] murderer is likely to murder again and he knows it" (p. 205). Perhaps William Heirens best explained the strength of this compulsion by writing on his victims' mirrors his infamous plea for help: "Catch me before I kill more, I cannot control myself" (quoted in Kennedy, Hoffman, and Haines, 1947, p. 120).

An offender can describe his fantasies simply by reporting his thoughts. But a compulsion is more abstract and difficult to explain. Offenders, therefore, often do not attempt a description, and many examiners also overlook the importance of the underlying compulsion when they evaluate such individuals. Those offenders who do describe—and attempt to explain—their strong urge to act report that a feeling of tension drives their behavior. A 25-year-old compulsive murderer spoke of "a feeling that comes into my head; a sharp pain in the back of my head, an angry overwhelming feeling to kill," in explaining his urge to act. People who report sadistic fantasies but do not act out lack a corresponding state of tension. Thus, the release of the tension seems to be directly linked to the underlying compulsion. The acting out liberates compulsive murderers from this pronounced inner tension (see Figure 8.5); they achieve a sense of satisfaction and then return to their prior state. As one individual said, "After I kill, I am out of the zone and back to myself." After a time, however, the inner tension builds again, and the urge to act out resurfaces; thus the repetitive nature of compulsive murderers' actions.

Some offenders describe "another personality taking over" in an attempt to explain— or concretize—the compulsion. These statements are sometimes thought to be an attempt

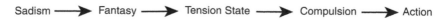

Figure 8.5 Fantasy grows out of sadism and creates a state of tension that leads to a compulsion to act out the fantasy and gain relief.

to create a legal defense, such as multiple personality disorder or "irresistible impulse." But compulsive offenders know exactly what they are doing, and they can, to a large extent, control their actions. They usually choose not to exercise restraint because they seek gratification as well as relief from the building inner tension. Such a tension state is totally different from the tension state found in individuals who commit catathymic homicides. The catathymic offender is driven not by fantasy or a compulsion but by a change in the thinking associated with a released sexual conflict. Catathymic homicides are rarely repeated, except when there is also an underlying compulsive aspect (as reported in Case 6.4).

Meloy (2000) attempted to determine "the factors that contribute to the behavioral acting out of the fantasy: the most important predictive data in sexual homicide cases" (p. 9). He proposed a "structuring" of sexual fantasy that provides the offender with "certain positive reinforcements prior to, or between his sexual homicides. … If a sexual homicide is committed this mechanism would reset, but the high arousal of the actual sexual violence would have less propensity to extinguish over time" (p. 9). Perhaps Meloy's model explains the "reinforcing" quality of the compulsion once a homicide is committed.

In addition to a behavioral component, a physiological ingredient is also quite likely in the compulsion to kill. In fact, a neurobiological substrate underlying sexual murder was first theorized by Krafft-Ebing and was supported years later by MacLean (1962), who pointed to an anatomical interconnection between sex and aggression. More recently, Miller (2000) has contended that an abnormality in the temporal lobe–limbic mechanism is the foundation for the "driven quality" of the compulsive murderer's urge to kill: "He won't stop and doesn't want to, because nothing in life could possibly replace the thrill of dominating and destroying another human being" (p. 158).

The following case of a 16-year-old who prayed at bedtime not to wake up so that he would not have to carry out his crimes clearly illustrates the strength of his compulsion.

Case 8.7: Overpowering Compulsion to Kill

A 16-year-old male (GG) was arrested for two murders, attempted murder, voyeuristic acts, and a series of burglaries. Because of the numerous burglaries which had occurred prior to the homicides, the police department had set up an investigative task force to apprehend the unknown offender. The investigators obtained one fingerprint, but because of GG's lack of a prior criminal record, they were unable to make a match. The offender was finally caught when he was spotted leaving a home after an attempted burglary. Unfortunately, GG was not apprehended until after two women were killed and a third was seriously assaulted. He was linked to the murders and the burglaries by his fingerprints.

During the evaluation, GG spoke in a bland, matter-of-fact way, without displaying any emotion. He did not seem upset by the homicides, burglaries, or his legal predicament. He stated repeatedly that he could not control the urge to peep into houses, break inside, or kill. The offender first explained the burglaries:

> I started breaking into homes. I don't know why I did it. I just started when I was sleeping one night. Something woke me up. I heard some kind of voice inside my head that told me to go out and rob a house. I sent away for a gun. It cost 14 dollars. I used to send away for a lot of things.

GG also obtained burglary tools, which he kept hidden in his room. He said that he burglarized mostly when it rained, about once a week. Around 9 or 10 o'clock at night, after his parents thought he was asleep, he would sneak out of the house with his burglary tools and either peep into other people's homes or burglarize them for money, "which I didn't need." At one point, he broke into his school and vandalized it, an act he could not fully explain.

I was looking for money. I don't really know why because I didn't need it. After a while, it was just to get into the houses. It was a drive to get into the houses. I think it was looking for money, but the drive was really, really strong.

About 18 months after the burglaries began, GG committed his first murder. He woke up around midnight, laid out his burglar tools on a table, and climbed out his bedroom window, which was on the second floor of his one-family house. He began looking for a home to burglarize. He wound up at the home of his math teacher, a house that he had been to in the previous week to get an award.

GG entered through the basement window after cutting the phone lines. He went directly to his 36-year-old teacher's bedroom. When she awoke, "I told her to stay there. I won't hurt you. I just want your money." The victim began to scream, which prompted GG to strangle her. As he ran out of the house, he bumped into the woman's daughter, whom he pushed away. Following the homicide, GG went back home and slept well. When questioned regarding the strangling of the victim, he said that he did not want to do it. "I just wanted to leave, but I couldn't go until I finished it. I had to kill her."

The next day, a Saturday, a girl from school told GG about the murder when she ran into him in front of his house. He questioned the classmate as to how it happened, and the girl answered, "She was strangled." GG stated, "I didn't think about it. I felt sorry for her. Then I went back outside and continued to wash the car. I never thought about it at all." He said he liked the victim very much. "She was a nice lady and the nicest teacher in the school. That was my best class. I got A's in her class. My best subject was math."

About 3 weeks later, the offender broke into another home, where he came upon a 43-year-old woman sleeping in her bedroom. He gagged and hogtied her and forced her into her car after brutally sexually assaulting her, twisting her breasts, and inserting objects into her vagina, including a toothbrush. He drove the victim around, torturing her for several hours. GG dumped her in an unconscious state in a park, returned home, went to sleep, and "didn't think about it." Miraculously, the woman did not die.

Following this attempted murder, he continued his voyeurism and burglaries. Several weeks later, he laid out his burglar tools, left his home in the same ritualistic manner, and broke into another house in the surrounding area. Since no one was home, GG waited, watched television, and ate some of the occupant's food. When the 60-year-old woman entered her house, she became terrified at the sight of GG lying on the couch. She begged, "Don't kill me." GG reassured her, "I just want your money." He then gagged her, hogtied her, dragged her upstairs to the bedroom in a brutal manner, and abused her sexually by twisting her breasts and inserting various objects into her vagina. He then filled the bathtub with water and drowned her; he compared this incident with drowning a dog years earlier.

Something made me go back and pour the water in the bathtub. I was on my way out. I grabbed her and put her in the bathtub when she was tied up and gagged. I pushed her in. Pushed her down and left.

GG then went home, slept well that evening, and continued his uncontrolled acts of voyeurism and burglary until his arrest.

The offender was raised in a middle-class family; his father was an accountant, and his mother worked in business. His mother had pulled a knife on him once; he was frightened of her, yet protective as well, and he thought she was "sexy." He had an abusive relationship with his father and once thought that his father would kill him. GG had a history of bed-wetting, cruel behavior toward animals (including killing dogs and birds), and no friendships with males or females. He admitted to having sadistic and grandiose fantasies but did not elaborate on them except under the influence of sodium amytal when he revealed ideas about being "the king and ruler." GG explained that he first got the urge to peep after making a hole in the wall separating his room from his parents; he watched them having sex, which stimulated and also frightened him. He claimed he had a girlfriend (although his family and classmates knew nothing about her), and he also claimed that he had had sex with her on one occasion, but this assertion seemed doubtful.

The Rorschach elicited many primitive and aggressive responses: "A spider ready to attack." "A dead bird." "A bull. He is going to stab somebody. He is lying down because his head is pointing down." "A man with a bow tie, being shot." "A monster ready to attack. They are trying to kill it and it's bleeding. An army is trying to kill it. His hands are tied behind his back." "A man and a firing squad, he's been shot. The blood's coming out of his chest too. Blood is splattering out on the wall." "A jet shooting a rocket, attacking another plane." "Explosion. An atomic explosion." "Two spiders fighting. There is a couple of bodies in the middle," etc.

The TAT reflected themes of loneliness, isolation, and abandonment. On Card 14, he gave the following production:

A man and a dog were looking out and feeling all alone. Nobody to love him. Since he was a child, he was abandoned and grew up in an orphanage. He had no education. He is not too smart. He is in his early thirties now and figures he can make it in the world, but no one will give him a chance. He spends time with himself in his room. He doesn't eat or drink much. He is thinking why nobody will help him.

On Card 13BM, GG said,

somebody is behind him telling him to look. His wife was killed. He has to identify her. He sees blood, and he is scared to look. There is blood. He is afraid it will be his wife. The person behind him is a detective. It's his wife. She is dead. He breaks out crying and says "why." The detective tells him a robber did it. They catch the guy who did it.

Further insight into some of the psychodynamics of GG's conduct is gained through his TAT story to Card 13MF:

A lady is dying in the bed. She is dead. He just killed her. He is crying, saying he is sorry. But it's too late. He calls the cops and turns himself in. He knows he'd done wrong. If he lets it go for the night, he might do more. He wanted to go to bed with her; she didn't want to, so he killed her. He thought that she would come over to help him with his homework and hoped she liked him a lot, enough to go to bed with him. He just couldn't have her. He was real hurt so he tried to take it out on her. He strangled her and felt sorry. He might see another girl he liked and she'd say no, and he might end up killing her or somebody else. There is too much anger after the person says no. He can't stop himself. He has to turn himself in.

Although GG was unable to articulate his motivation for the break-ins and homicides, he could describe the powerful compulsion that drove him to these actions. He referred to his compulsion as "a drive" that he could not explain. In fact, he stated that he would "pray at bedtime, so that I would not have to wake up and commit these crimes again"—an indication of the force of the compulsion. GG told several examiners that if he did not get help, he would kill again because "the drive is too strong."

The compulsion to kill, rather than the number of victims, distinguishes the compulsive murderer from other offenders. However, some cases are complex and may involve a mixture of motives. For example, doctors (or nurses) who kill their patients may be driven by compulsion or they may be motivated by money, other incentives, or a combination. The case of physician Marcel Petiot (Grombach, 1982) is illustrative. Petiot killed many people during World War II, primarily for money. Most of his victims were wealthy Jews fleeing the Nazis. The doctor gave them a "typhoid inoculation," which caused their death; he then took their money and valuables. Although monetary compensation seemed to be the primary motive, he observed their "death agonies through a peephole" (Schechter and Everitt, 1996, p. 221)—behavior that perhaps reflects an underlying compulsive element as well. The strange case of nurse Beverely Allitt (Askill and Sharpe, 1993), who killed four children, attempted to kill three others and caused severe harm to six others who had mixed and unclear motives. Some argued that she had Münchausen by proxy (Feldman, 2004), but clarity was never achieved. Since the crime scene in a hospital homicide is quickly sterilized, the investigation is made more difficult.

Although serial sexual murderers have a strong compulsion to act out, the temporal patterns (i.e., the time periods between murders) of their homicides have hardly been examined. Anecdotal case reports have described serial sexual murderers as committing homicides in a methodical manner, taking a substantial period of time between homicides in order to plan their next attack and to avoid law enforcement. But a study by Schlesinger, Ramirez, Tusa, Jarvis, and Erdberg (2017) found that many serial sexual murderers behave in a rapid-sequence fashion. Slightly over half their sample (44 serial sexual murderers and their 201 victims) killed with longer than a 14-day period between homicides; however, just under half (43.2%) committed homicides in rapid-sequence fashion, with fewer than 14 days between all or some of the murders. In fact, six offenders (13.6%) killed all of their victims in one rapid-sequence, spree-like episode, with homicides just days apart, or they sometimes committed two murders on the same day at different times and in different locations. And 13 offenders (29.5%) killed in one or two rapid-sequence clusters (i.e., with more than one murder in a 14-day period), as well as committing additional homicides with greater than 14 days between each. The authors argue that mental disorders with rapidly occurring symptom patterns, or perhaps atypical mania or mood dysregulation, could serve as exemplars for understanding this previously unrecognized group of offenders.

8.4 Murderous Partners and Murderers' Romantic Partners

8.4.1 Killer Partners

Most compulsive murderers who plan their crimes function by themselves; however, a small minority operates with a partner. In most of these cases, a dominant partner, perhaps the only one with an underlying compulsion to kill, typically recruits or teams up with a more submissive, passive individual (Furio, 2001). The partner may have sadistic proclivities that erupt only when that person is under the influence of the more dominant offender. Revitch and Schlesinger (1989) argued that the prestige of the stronger figure, as well as mental contagion, often plays a primary role in group assaults and homicides. Crimes such as group rape are greatly influenced by the sense of security that having another dominant person brings (Brownmiller, 1976), as well as diffusion of responsibility. Freud (1921) agreed with the French sociologist Gustave LeBon (1910) who contended that the individual loses his or her uniqueness in a group and unconscious forces frequently take over. In fact, there is some experimental research (Kogan and Wallach, 1967) that found groups of individuals are more likely to act in risky ways when the group supports such behavior.

Revitch and Schlesinger (1989) reported the case of a 23-year-old who, along with a friend, broke into a house and viciously killed a 76-year-old woman, thrusting a broomstick into her vagina prior to her death. The weaker partner described the stronger one as "a big wheel and a leader of the neighborhood. He was a good fighter, not afraid to beat up the kids." He admired his companion and was proud to be associated with him. The follower had aggressive fantasies that were hidden behind a weak, frightened, and submissive exterior.

In some cases, a dominant male works with a submissive girlfriend who helps in the commission of the crimes. Men who kill with their wives or girlfriends are a somewhat rare, but not a new, phenomenon. The Marquis de Sade's wife participated and assisted her husband in many of his sexually sadistic exploits (Du Plessix-Gray, 1998). Sinnamon and Petherick (2017) argue that although rare, there are cases of women who commit planned compulsive murders on their own. The Moors murders (Williams, 1967), committed by Ian Brady and his girlfriend, Myra Hindley, illustrate the effect of a dominant male on a female follower. For several years in the mid-1960s the couple abducted and killed at least four children. Hindley would lure the victims into the car, but Brady took the active role in the killing. One murder was tape-recorded, and on the tape one could hear a 10-year-old child's pleas, screams, and cries prior to and during her death. The couple was finally arrested after Brady tried to enlist another young man as an assistant. The would-be recruit became horrified after observing Brady kill a person and called the police. Brady and Hindley were tried and sentenced to life in prison.

Brady was raised in a foster home and had a long criminal record of arrests and imprisonments. He tortured cats, admired the Marquis de Sade and Adolf Hitler, and showed clear sadistic tendencies throughout his life. His girlfriend said after her arrest, "I loved him and I still love him." Those who evaluated the pair felt that Hindley would do anything that Brady wanted her to do. Before she met Brady, Hindley had been a friendly individual and a reliable babysitter who showed no inclination toward sadism or homicide. Johnson (1967) concluded that Hindley would not have committed the atrocities if she had not met Brady.

In some more recent cases, the same pattern of a dominant male and a more submissive female is also found. Paul Bernardo and his wife, Karla Homolka, together killed at least three women (Vronsky, 2015). Bernardo was a sadist and serial rapist who enjoyed humiliating and beating women. Karla seemed to encourage his sadistic acts and, in many ways, was more than just a willing accomplice. She even drugged her younger sister so that Bernardo could assault and kill her. The couple created their own pornography by videotaping some of the offenses. Following their arrest, Karla testified against Bernardo, claiming that he severely beat her.

Douglas Clark and his girlfriend, Carol M. Bundy, were another killer couple (Becker and Veysey, 2018). Clark was a psychopathic and narcissistic individual, smooth and manipulative, while Bundy was an unattractive woman who was abused her whole life and would have done anything for male attention. In a sense, Clark essentially groomed Bundy to help him obtain victims. Two of the victims were prostitutes, and the crime involved necrophilia on the part of Clark. In one case, Bundy put makeup on a dead woman's head, which was kept in their refrigerator. She also killed a former boyfriend and brought his decapitated head to Clark, believing it would please him. At trial, Clark represented himself and put on a show, displaying his arrogance, narcissism, and sadism.

Another interesting case of a killer couple is that of Gerald and Charlene Gallego (Flowers, 1996). Charlene was instrumental in helping to get her husband female victims, whom he kept as sex slaves. Most of the victims, young women or teenagers, were abducted from shopping malls. As in the cases of Bernardo-Homolka and Clark-Bundy, Charlene testified against her husband. And like Douglas Clark, Gerald Gallego acted as his own lawyer, putting on a show in court and gaining sadistic gratification by personally cross-examining victims' family members.

Less common cases involve two male partners, both of whom have underlying compulsions to kill. The cases of Henry Lee Lucas and Otis Toole (Norris, 1991) and of Leonard Lake and Charles Ng (Douglas and Olshaker, 1995) are examples. Lucas had a terribly brutal background which involved sex with animals, animal torture, murder, rape, strangulation, and numerous prison and psychiatric incarcerations. He claimed to have killed over 100 people while traveling around the U.S. In 1975 he met Toole, also a compulsive killer. The two roamed the country, murdering untold victims. Similarly, after Lake and Ng, both of whom were compelled to kill, joined forces, they abducted three women and kept them captive in an underground bunker on Lake's farm. They videotaped the victims being sexually tortured and finally murdered. The interpersonal dynamics between such partners, as well as the distinguishing characteristics of the dominant and subservient offenders, remain unresearched and unknown.

The case of Angelo Buono and his cousin Kenneth Bianchi (Crisp, 2002) involved a more dominant male figure (Buono) and Bianchi, who was essentially his assistant. They targeted prostitutes, used ligatures to torture the victims sadistically, and were eventually apprehended after killing ten individuals. At trial, Bianchi turned on Buono, and both were convicted. David Gore and Fred Waterfield (Ward, 1994) were also cousins who killed together. Gore, an auxiliary police officer, stalked his victims and then abducted them in a fairly sophisticated way. Even when under police suspicion and surveillance, Gore could not control his compulsion to kill and continued to act, demonstrating the enormous sexual gratification he gained from his murders. As in the other cases of killer couples, Gore turned on Waterfield. He said that Waterfield was the mastermind, while Waterfield insisted on his innocence. Both men were convicted.

8.4.2 Killers' Romantic Partners

Krafft-Ebing (1886) first observed that many sexual murderers had wives and girlfriends whom they did not harm. In fact, the offenders remarked that the sexual pleasure they gained through violence was more pleasurable than traditional sexual relations with their romantic partners. Compulsive murderers' wives or girlfriends typically claim they knew their partner was sexually disturbed but had no knowledge of his homicidal behavior.

Whether this is an attempt to distance themselves from involvement in criminal conduct or represents a true lack of awareness is hard to determine and may differ depending upon the case. Nevertheless, some credibility to romantic partners' lack of knowledge of their companions' murders must be given since this has been widely reported at different times, different countries, and different cultures.

There has been very little research or study of wives and girlfriends of such offenders. Bastani and Kentsmith (1980) reported three cases of wives of sexual offenders (two pedophiles and one exhibitionist). These authors found that the wives were aware of their husbands' sexual deviancy, but they tended to deny, rationalize, and minimize the problem and were reluctant to discuss it. The women also demonstrated difficulty empathizing with their husband's victims. The authors found that the wives defied the preconceived view of such women fitting a stereotype of being cold and sexually unresponsive.

Isenberg (1991) studied 13 women who were romantically involved with and in some cases even married men who committed homicide. She was able to draw a nonscientific profile of the women who typically came from dysfunctional families and were victims of abuse by dictatorial fathers. "Their relationships with [the murderer] mimic[ed] the one they had with their fathers. Married young, their first husbands were often violent, alcoholic, sexually and/or emotionally abusive" (p. 223).

Many of the women Isenberg studied maintained fantasies that their boyfriends or husbands would somehow be released from prison; they also intermingled their own suffering and pain—as a result of their disturbed relationships with the murderers—with their "romantic passion." The author concluded that the women did not love "real men," but rather loved "an illusion that is based on denial" (p. 225). Women who fell in love with serial or high profile murderers seemed to gain a vicarious sense of fame from being closely connected with a notorious criminal. Thus, the offender provided the woman, who had low self-esteem and emptiness, with a sense of importance.

It is important to draw a distinction between a woman who has had a prior relationship with a husband or boyfriend who had become incarcerated and a woman who first met an inmate while he was in prison. The phenomenon of women who meet and become romantically involved with incarcerated men has never been systematically studied. Some of the women explain that having an incarcerated boyfriend lets them know exactly where he is, as well as giving them a feeling of being needed. The relationship, in a way, organizes their life and gives them a sense of purpose. Many of these women are fairly substantial, are well educated (sometimes with advanced degrees), and often give money to the inmate to pay for attorneys and the like. It also seems that some of these women achieve vicarious status by being associated with a notorious offender in whom there is some degree of media interest. Other women seem to gain a sense of arousal from being connected to a notorious offender, a syndrome sometimes referred to as a hybristophilia. And almost every prison has had female employees who have become involved sexually and romantically with inmates. Interestingly, recent research by Vicary and Fraley (2010) found women—much more than men—are drawn to true crime books and stories involving rape, murder, and serial killers.

In a slightly different phenomenon, Hazelwood, Warren, and Dietz (1993) studied several women who became romantically involved with sexual sadists and had even willingly endured much of their abuse. In addition to describing the physical, sexual, and psychological torment the victims were subjected to, the authors discussed the transformation of these women from independent individuals to "compliant appendages of their criminally active partners" (p. 474). Interestingly, many of the personality characteristics of Hazelwood et al.'s subjects were not that different from the profile painted by Isenberg, specifically the women's backgrounds of abuse and their strong feelings of low self-esteem.

8.5 Comment

Although in many homicides the dominant feature is sadism, fantasy, or a compulsion to kill, as illustrated throughout this chapter, many others, perhaps most offenses, have no such outstanding characteristic. A review of some of the more well-known cases leaves the incorrect impression that all compulsive murderers have rich fantasy lives, behave in markedly sadistic ways, or have such an overpowering compulsion that they are out of control. This view is gained because usually extraordinary and dramatic cases receive the most interest and notoriety. They are not only the ones covered by the media but are often the ones reported in the scientific literature as well. However, most cases are not all that dramatic. And our notions of how these offenders behave – based on media reports or fictional characters – is very often inaccurate, as illustrated by several empirical studies reported in this chapter.

Unplanned Compulsive Homicides 9

Sexually motivated compulsive homicides are fueled by a combination of sadism, fantasy, and a compulsion to kill. These elements, to one degree or another, are present in both compulsive murderers who plan their crimes and those who act in an unplanned, impulsive, and spontaneous manner. Whether the murder is planned or spontaneous, however, is not a result of the compulsion or various sadistic fantasies; rather, it is a result primarily of the offender's personality makeup. Thus, the individual's personality is an intervening variable between the three elements and the way the crime is committed.

9.1 Personality as an Intervening Variable

Behavior is shaped largely by personality. People who have reasonably intact personalities with minimal overt disturbance carry out their lives in an orderly and thoughtful manner. When such people commit crimes, they are likely to do so in a logical, methodical fashion. If individuals have a compulsion to kill, they are likely to plan the murder in a manner consistent with their personality. Compulsive offenders who commit planned sexual murders typically have psychopathic, sociopathic, narcissistic, antisocial, and other personality disorders that do not disorganize their thinking and conduct. They are manipulative and deceptive, but they are not distracted by interfering with overt psychopathological symptoms (such as hallucinations and delusions).

Conversely, compulsive murderers who act in an unplanned, spontaneous fashion do so not because of different underlying motivating elements but because they have more overt psychopathological disturbances, which usually fall within the borderline, schizotypal, or schizoid spectrum of personality disorders. Their resulting disorganized personalities prohibit thought and careful planning.

Individuals with these types of personality disorders do not necessarily have a predilection to act out spontaneously; however, they do lack, to a large extent, the controls and defenses necessary to contain their behavior. Thus, if their fantasies build to a point where the compulsion becomes overbearing, they may act out—in a high-risk manner that is likely to get them apprehended—in order to release the inner tension the compulsion creates. These offenders are distracted by their psychopathology, and they lack the inner resources necessary to plan much of their behavior in general, including their criminal behavior.

Individuals with borderline, schizoid, or schizotypal personalities can potentially experience brief psychotic-like episodes. Although as a rule they do not become psychotic, they are chronically unstable or stable in their instability. For example, the borderline engages in intense, emotional, interpersonal relationships along with a lot of destructive or self-destructive behavior. The person with a schizoid personality is withdrawn and isolative; he has never had many friends and does not want friends. The schizotypal individual is somewhat more disturbed than the borderline or schizoid personality; he is heavily involved in daydreams, difficult to relate to, and often isolated, and he appears odd, eccentric, and unusual. In fact, the schizotypal personality was referred to as latent schizophrenia in the first and second editions of the *DSM*. This clinical condition is now placed among the personality disorders primarily because of the absence of overt symptoms indicative of schizophrenia such as hallucinations or formed delusions. Recently, many individuals with similar symptoms have been considered to fall on the autistic spectrum using *DSM*-5 criteria.

Sometimes the compulsive murderer who does not plan is profoundly mentally ill, suffering from schizophrenia. The diagnostic criteria for schizophrenia have changed over the years as a result of the influence of several theorists who emphasized different sets of symptoms and behaviors. For instance, Bleuler (1951) stressed the rather subtle symptoms of associative loosening, blunted affect, autistic withdrawal, and ambivalent thinking. Schneider (1959) emphasized a different diagnostic pattern that required an overt symptom picture of auditory hallucinations and bizarre ideation. Other practitioners, such as Mayer-Gross, Stater, and Roth (1969) and Langfeldt (1969), attempted to integrate the work of Bleuler and Schneider, but their synthesis has been less well-received than the original theories. Prior to the *DSM-3* (1980), the Bleulerian conception of schizophrenia was predominant in the U.S. However, since then, a Schneiderian view of the illness has been used. Thus, the current diagnostic criteria for schizophrenia include a constellation of overt symptoms such as hallucinations, delusions, disorganized behavior, and disorganized speech, as well as negative symptoms such as emotional flattening and lack of motivation. The subtypes of schizophrenia, which have been time-honored, have been eliminated in the *DSM-5*, a decision which has been somewhat controversial.

Schizophrenia is generally considered to be a progressive illness with onset typically in the early 20s, followed by a general deterioration, including disturbances not only in thought but in mood and behavior as well. New pharmaceuticals have been successful in reducing the symptoms in many schizophrenic patients (Rasmussen, 1997). However, a subgroup of individuals stops taking the medication (because they find the side effects irritating or because they believe they are not ill) and continues to remain symptomatic, often functioning in an ambulatory psychotic manner. In another subgroup, medication only has minimal effect on symptom reduction. When these people have an underlying compulsion to kill, they act on the drive in a disorganized, spontaneous fashion primarily because the severe symptoms of their mental disorder make planning impossible for them.

There are, however, exceptions to the notions that severe psychopathology results in unplanned crimes and that the absence of severe psychopathology results in planned crimes. Two severe forms of mental disturbance—paranoid personality disorder and the paranoid form of schizophrenia—do not disorganize the underlying character structure. Paranoid personality disorder is malignant. However, the behavior of individuals with this type of personality is often highly organized, systematized, and thoughtful. Consequently, if they have a compulsion to kill, they have the ability to plan the murders. The paranoid form of schizophrenia also leads to functioning in an organized, systematized, thoughtful fashion. If people with schizophrenia involving paranoid symptoms have a compulsion to kill, they, too, are able to plan their actions despite the primary psychiatric diagnosis.

Individuals with intact personalities can act in an impulsive manner if they are angry or if they have an impulse-control disorder or are intoxicated. An impulse-control disorder can limit the ability to resist drives or temptations. If a compulsion to kill is present,

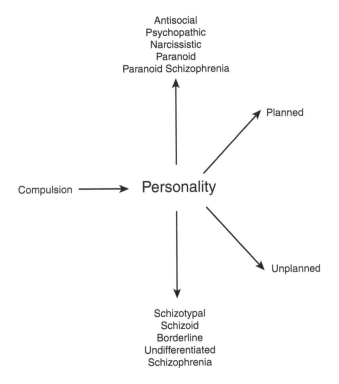

Figure 9.1 Personality as an intervening variable guiding how a compulsion is released and a murder is carried out.

offenders may respond impulsively when a victim crosses their path. Substance abuse, specifically intoxication, can also weaken inhibitory controls. Therefore, individuals with a compulsion may act spontaneously when their controls are compromised because of the effects of various substances.

Offenders' personalities (antisocial, narcissistic, borderline, schizotypal) or underlying mental illnesses (schizophrenia) do not directly cause them to kill. The drive to kill is a result of inner compulsion. The underlying personality (or psychopathology) simply shapes and influences how the compulsion is carried out (see Figure 9.1). Since planning is often necessary to elude law enforcement, it is easy to understand why compulsive murderers with multiple victims (serial murderers) usually do not have a major psychiatric illness that results in disorganized thinking (Karakasi, Vasilikos, Voultsos, Vlachaki, and Pavlidis, 2017). Compulsive murderers with a mental disorder that results in thought disorganization are unable to plan their crimes; their apprehension is thus much easier and quicker, and, as a result, they have fewer victims. As noted in Chapter 2, a major mistake in understanding criminal behavior in general, and homicide in particular, is overreliance on the diagnosis. Behavioral analysis of the offense must be primary.

9.2 Descriptions of Compulsive Murderers Who Do Not Plan

Many cases of unplanned, disorganized compulsive homicides are reported in the literature. These crimes usually do not receive the same level of notoriety as those committed by offenders who plan. Those who plan, especially those who use intricate, clever, and sophisticated MOs that enable them to elude law enforcement and kill a large number of victims, are considered by many people to be more intriguing than their counterparts who do not plan their crimes. However, since the earliest times many individuals have committed compulsive homicides in an unplanned, spontaneous fashion.

Joseph Vacher, for example, impulsively killed 11 people (of both sexes) by stabbing, strangling, mutilating, biting, and disemboweling them (Schechter and Everitt, 1996). His actions earned him the title the "French Ripper." Vacher was born into a poor family, the last of 15 children. When he was 19 years old, he attempted to rape a young boy. At age 21, he joined the army, and he cut his throat when he was not promoted. He attempted suicide several years later after he was rejected by a woman. Vacher shot the woman and then shot himself in the face, sustaining a number of injuries including paralysis of the right eye, "which was reduced to a raw, suppurating hole … that leaked a steady stream of pus" (p. 297). Although his geographic mobility impaired apprehension, Vacher was eventually caught and executed after unsuccessfully attempting a psychiatric defense.

Compulsive murderer Jesse Pomeroy (Schechter and Everitt, 1996) also abducted and killed multiple victims in an unplanned, disorganized fashion; he engaged in postmortem mutilation and left a great deal of forensic evidence at the crime scenes. Pomeroy began attacking and abducting little boys when he was 11. After binding them, he tortured the children and beat them severely. Following his arrest, Pomeroy was sent to a reformatory for a number of years. When released, he kidnapped a 10-year-old female and mutilated and killed her. A month later, he abducted a 4-year-old male and cut him savagely with a pocket knife, almost to the point of decapitation. When the offender was arrested, he had the bloody weapon in his pocket and mud on his boots; he quickly confessed.

Peter Sutcliffe, commonly known as the "Yorkshire Ripper" (Yallop, 1980), killed about 13 women (mostly prostitutes) in an unplanned, impulsive, disorganized manner. He was a withdrawn, angry person, married and employed as a truck driver. As a young man, Sutcliffe worked as a mortuary attendant and spent hours in a wax museum, observing the effects of venereal disease on the human body. He killed prostitutes, typically by hitting them on the backs of their heads. Sometimes he would mutilate the victims' genitalia after their death, using knives, chisels, and screwdrivers. His final four victims were three female college students and a young working woman. The offender was arrested by accident after a police officer found him in a stolen car with a prostitute. Sutcliffe claimed that he heard voices, but he was found sane and was sentenced to life in prison.

Serial Killer Patrick MacKay (Clark, 1976) killed 11 people, mostly elderly, including a priest, during a robbery. The murders were impulsive and very sadistic. William Devin Howell (Howard, 2018) is proud of being considered Connecticut's most prolific serial killer. He killed women in his van, many drug abusers, and did so as soon as a victim was available to him.

Various authors who have studied such spontaneous compulsive murderers have described their characteristics and categorized these offenders as disorganized, impulsive, and, frequently, young. In fact, recent research (Schlesinger, et al., 2017) found that almost half of serial sexual murderers kill in rapid-sequence fashion, some killing more than one victim at the same day and at different locations. This type of impulsive killing suggests very little planning. In addition, those evaluating such offenders often do not recognize the sexual nature of some of their crimes.

9.2.1 The "Disorganized" Murderer

Ressler, Burgess, and Douglas (1988) describe the personality profile of a "disorganized" murderer who kills in an unplanned, impulsive, spontaneous manner:

> The disorganized offender is socially inadequate. Often he has never married, lives alone or with a parental figure, and lives in close proximity to the crime scene. This offender is fearful of people and may have developed a well defined delusional system. He acts impulsively under stress, finding a victim usually within his own geographic area. The offender is also sexually incompetent, often never having achieved any level of sexual intimacy with a peer. … There is a clear suggestion that the disorganized offender is ignorant of sex and often may have sexual aversions. (p. 130)

Table 9.1 lists a number of characteristics of Ressler et al.'s disorganized murderer. In addition, these offenders may also look disorganized (unkempt, dirty, and with poor hygiene) and be almost oblivious to how the world sees them.

Douglas, Burgess, Burgess, and Ressler (1992) report the case of an unplanned sexual homicide committed by a disorganized offender. A 12-year-old girl with a physical handicap was looking for a missing bicycle fairly close to her home. While briefly separated from her sister, who was also looking for the bike, the girl was abducted. Her body was found the next day in a nearby creek. She was left nude from the waist down, except for her socks, and her clothing was scattered about. The assault, death, and body recovery all occurred at the same location. The physical evidence indicated that the offender had attacked her "blitz-style" (her face had been badly beaten) and had then strangled her. There were also deep postmortem cuts on her wrists and forearms, in addition to other cuts that were believed to have been "exploratory in nature reflecting the offender's curiosity" (p. 132). As is characteristic of crimes committed by disorganized offenders, a lot of evidence was recovered, including footprints and semen (in the victim's vagina).

Table 9.1 Profile Characteristics of the Disorganized Murderer

- Average intelligence
- Socially immature
- Poor work history
- Sexually incompetent
- Minimal birth-order status
- Father's work unstable
- Harsh discipline in childhood
- Anxious mood during a crime
- Minimal use of alcohol
- Minimal situational stress
- Living alone
- Lives/works near the crime scene
- Minimal interest in news media
- Minimal change in lifestyle following the homicide

Source: Adapted from Ressler, R.K., Burgess, A.W., and Douglas, J.E., *Sexual Homicide: Patterns and Motives*, The Free Press, New York, 1988, p. 122.

A 17-year-old unemployed high school dropout was quickly apprehended. At the time of the arrest he was living with his 16-year-old girlfriend. The offender had some prior contact with the victim and even spoke with her several nights before the attack. When he saw her alone—with little ability to defend herself—he spontaneously attacked and killed her in a manner typical of his personality and lifestyle.

9.2.2 Hazelwood and Warren's Impulsive Offender

Hazelwood and Warren (2000) draw a distinction between the "ritualistic offender" who carefully plans his criminal actions and the "impulsive offender" who is like the disorganized offender. The impulsive offender

> invests little or no planning in his crimes. Instead, he acts impulsively, takes little or no measures to protect his identity, and is seemingly oblivious to the risk involved in committing crimes. Both informal and systematic assessment of his modus operandi ... suggests a criminally unsophisticated reactive offender. (p. 270)

As an example of the impulsive offender, these authors report the case of a 24-year-old male who, while walking through a parking lot, spotted a 37-year-old woman loading groceries into her car. He walked over to her, struck her in the face with his fist, threw her into the rear seat, ripped off the clothes from the lower part of her body, and vaginally raped her. After knocking her unconscious, he left her in the rear seat and casually walked away. He was subsequently arrested and convicted of 18 similar impulsive, unplanned crimes.

Hazelwood and Warren find the impulsive offender's fantasies, sadism, and inner compulsion to kill to be undifferentiated. Such an offender is generally unaware of the fantasies underlying his actions. And if he does describe fantasies, they are typically simplistic and concrete, usually involving simple victim characteristics and demographics.

Impulsive offenders do not seek out a particular type of victim; any victim will do. If this type of offender has a pornography collection, it usually lacks a specific theme; his fantasies are as undifferentiated as the pornography he reads. Postmortem paraphiliac behavior is often absent because such acting out is chiefly fantasy-driven and the impulsive offender lacks the differentiated fantasies that might direct such conduct. They often impulsively victimize their spouses and, occasionally, prostitutes because these women are easily accessible. Their actions are so spontaneous that they may attack a stranger while they are committing another crime simply because the victim is around. They rarely preselect victims through stalking or voyeurism.

These crimes often involve a great deal of physical cruelty, as displayed in the cases of Vacher, Pomeroy, and Sutcliffe; such cruelty is distinct from intricate forms of sadism. Because they lack criminal sophistication, impulsive offenders resort to immediate violence (usually excessive and brutal) in order to control the victim. Also, such offenders often have diverse arrest records involving multiple offenses with no specific theme. They almost always travel short distances to offend, and because of their unsophisticated spontaneity, the men usually make little effort to elude law enforcement. James and Proulx (2016) found nonserial sexual murderers are "impulsive and extremely violent, and use sexual murder to diminish their internal tension" (p. 200). Recent empirical research (Koeppel et al., 2019; Park, Schlesinger, Pinizzotto, and Davis, 2008) supports these clinical findings that single-victim offenders display as much brutality in their offenses as the serial offenders.

9.2.3 Adolescent Offenders

Adolescents and very young adults whose development is not yet complete typically commit crimes, including homicides, in a spontaneous, unplanned, or poorly planned fashion. Myers and Blashfield (1997), Myers, Burgess, and Nelson (1998), and Myers (2002) conducted extensive studies of adolescents who committed sexual murders. These researchers found that adolescents were typically disorganized offenders in that their crimes were impulsive, unplanned or poorly planned, and occurred in their own neighborhoods. In fact, most adolescent offenders knew the (typically older) victims to some extent.

Woods (1961) reports an interesting case of a 15-year-old who committed an unplanned sexual homicide. The young man impulsively killed his middle-aged cousin by hitting her on the head with a pipe and then stabbing her. He said the attack was triggered by her nagging him about his dirty shirt.

> I wanted to stop [from killing her], but her eye was blinking and I couldn't control myself. I hit her again and again. Her eyes wouldn't close and I tried to choke her. Three more times I hit her. I couldn't stop. I took the knife then and stabbed her. (p. 529)

When evaluated, he revealed that since he was 13 he had had an overpowering drive to kill. The offender admitted to voyeurism, homicidal and rape fantasies, and two prior vicious attacks on women for which he was not apprehended. He said he was unable to achieve sexual gratification except through fantasies of rape, murder, and violence. Stabbing in the genital area was part of his fantasy.

In a study of young adults who committed sexual assaults and murders, Drvota and Student (1975) also found that when a young person committed such a murder, it was sudden and brutal and stemmed from the inability of the offender to contain a breakthrough of sadistic fantasies that had been ongoing—a result of his lack of adequate controls. These young subjects also fit the disorganized-offender pattern: they were intellectually weak, not well-educated, unstable, and impulsive. Frequently employed as unskilled laborers, they drank and had histories of criminality.

9.3 Nonrecognition of the Sexual Aspect of Crimes

Banay (1969) found that a lot of criminal behavior which on the surface seems nonsexual is actually sexually inspired and due to a compulsion. Assaults, stabbings, and shootings are all crimes that are sometimes driven by a hidden sexual compulsion. The author noted that when impulsive individuals commit such crimes, they are often unaware of their own sexual dynamics and may believe that their behavior (which sometimes seems nonsexual on the surface) could be sexually motivated.

In the following two cases, those who were evaluating the offenders also failed to recognize the sexual nature of some of the offenders' crimes.

Case 9.1: Evaluators Ignore Facts Pointing to a Dangerous Compulsion

A 42-year-old male (AA) was arrested and confessed to killing a 17-year-old girl (A) 10 years earlier. A, who was AA's former girlfriend, was physically handicapped and also had a learning and speech disability. The offender was grossly overweight, was uncomfortable with females, had no friends, rarely worked, and lived with his mother. He was exceptionally possessive of A; in fact, when the victim's foster mother came to see her, AA hid her so that no one else could speak with her.

When interviewed, the offender explained the homicide as follows:

> I went to the store with A. We were walking and talking and began to argue. I pushed her down by the railroad tracks. I lost my temper and struck her with a pipe, not intentionally; I lost control. I got scared and covered her body up and left. I went home and went to bed.

When asked what precipitated the argument, he said, "She told me she had an abortion. She said the baby might be mine, and I said it wasn't. I got angry and upset because she was saying things about me. I lost control. It was an accident." A was pregnant and had told others that AA was not the child's father. Thus, a more likely trigger for the murder was AA's anger and humiliation when A told him she had become pregnant by another man. His anger was obvious; he used a nail for joining railroad ties to make 25 puncture wounds in A's skull. The body was not found for several months and was skeletonized by that time. The victim's skirt was pulled up, and her underwear was taken. AA had covered the body with several railroad ties and some branches.

Although AA was a suspect at the time of the homicide (because he had a relationship with the victim), he denied guilt, and no physical evidence linked him to the murder. His name resurfaced 10 years later because of other sex offenses. When the detectives visited AA, ostensibly to advise him of the Megan's Law community notification program, he quickly confessed.

AA had a history of various offenses typical of the impulsive, disorganized offender, including burglary, car theft, and multiple municipal charges such as failure to give a good account, damage to property, and setting off a false alarm. However, he also had been convicted of sexual assault on his 6-year-old niece. While the child was sleeping, AA got in bed with her, pulled down her underwear, and touched her vagina with his fingers. The niece and her 8-year-old brother reported this incident, along with some other sexual behavior that AA engaged in, and the offender was arrested. When interviewed at a state diagnostic facility at the time of this arrest, he denied committing the offense but said he pled guilty "because these cases are hard to beat." He then admitted, "I did touch her legs and vagina." In addition, he had been arrested for abducting a 9-year-old girl in the neighborhood. He brought the child to his house; however, before any type of sexual activity could occur, AA's mother came home. She quickly brought the girl back to her home and later convinced the child's parents to drop the charges. AA was also arrested several years later for another sexual assault, although, for reasons that were never made clear, he was not indicted.

One other event should have been a red flag indicating the presence of an underlying dangerous compulsion. During an apparent mugging which occurred several years before the homicide, AA grabbed a woman, knocked her to the ground, kicked her in the head and body, and said, "If you don't stop fighting me, I'm gonna kill you." He was sent to prison for this assault, but evaluators completely missed the underlying sexual dynamics. Not only was his behavior not typical of muggers who try to grab a pocketbook and flee the scene quickly to avoid detection, but the amount of force used far exceeded that necessary for a mugging. In this case, evaluators ignored important facts in the offender's background and thus failed to recognize the underlying sexually driven compulsion, which indicated a high potential for repetition.

In the following case, an underlying compulsion was also missed by several mental health examiners who focused entirely on the legal issues and did not link prior behavior to the current offense.

Case 9.2: Examiners Miss Underlying Sexual Compulsion

A 22-year-old male (BB) was arrested and confessed to the murder of a 15-year-old girl. The victim (B) was a family friend with whom BB had a long-standing "brother–sister" relationship. The offender told the police that while he was visiting B, they had a consensual sexual encounter. During intercourse in the bathtub, he accidentally held B's head under water and caused her death. He became frightened, put the body in a closet, and left. B was missing for 5 days; her mother finally discovered the body in the closet. BB became a suspect because he not only had contact with the victim but was conspicuously absent following B's disappearance and did not even attend her funeral.

The offender had an IQ of 73 with mild organicity, a finding consistent with a long-standing learning disability. This IQ level was determined to be an underestimation because some of BB's projective test responses seemed relatively sophisticated. For example, on the Rorschach, he responded: "It's like a sword inside a rock. A big stone from King Arthur. They took a sword out of the rock. It's an Excalibur. The sides come out, and there is the handle." "It looks like three lizards, chameleons. They are touching something else and touching a color. Their color changes, and that's why they are called chameleons. When they touch this chameleon, his color changes." "These are puppets. It looks like they had a mask on from China, like a Chinese parade with dragon heads, a big nose, and a horn." TAT stories were also well done with simple themes that suggested conflicts with women. Projective figure drawings were simplistic and not revealing.

BB was evaluated by a defense-retained psychologist who found him incompetent to have waived his *Miranda* rights; this conclusion was based on BB's low intelligence and supposed passive personality, which rendered him unduly influenced by the police. Although the presenting legal issue structured the psychologist's evaluation, BB's past conduct did not raise a red flag with this examiner who seemed more interested in the narrow competency issue than in fully understanding the case. For instance, BB had previously pled guilty to assaulting a prostitute. The prostitute claimed that the offender severely beat her "for no reason"; BB said that the assault was a misunderstanding and that the prostitute had threatened him. In the same year, BB also seriously assaulted his sister, seemingly without provocation. This offender's dangerous compulsion to attack women finally culminated in the impulsive sexual murder of the adolescent. The offender was also under suspicion of killing two other women, including a prostitute who lived in his mother's neighborhood.

In addition, BB was involved in an unusual case of assault, sexual assault, and criminal restraint servitude. BB and his then-girlfriend held the girl's mother captive (in her apartment) for 3 days. He undressed the mother, beat her, and sexually abused and raped her continuously. BB also shoved a screwdriver up the victim's rectum, causing damage. He assaulted her in this manner several times during the period of captivity. BB took the doorknob off and nailed the windows shut so that the victim would be unable to leave. But while BB and his girlfriend were out shopping, the victim managed to escape. After giving a detailed statement to the police, she decided not to cooperate with the authorities, fearing BB would kill her.

9.4 Compulsion Spontaneously Released by Circumstances

In some individuals, the compulsion to kill is often released only in certain circumstances, with a certain type of (often slight) stimulation, or under the influence of various substances. In these cases, if it were not for the particular set of conditions—the mere presence of a victim, comments made by a victim, or some other situation such as the commission of a common crime—the homicide would not have occurred. The presence of such a compulsion can be detected by the excessive amount of force used in committing a crime, force that is out of proportion to what would seem necessary. The use of excessive force reveals a deeper dynamic fueling the extreme aggression. The subject in the following case entertained undifferentiated violent fantasies for years that were released only during the commission of a robbery.

Case 9.3: Compulsion Released During Robbery

A 25-year-old male (CC), along with an associate, brutally murdered a storekeeper during a robbery in which a small amount of money was taken from the cash register. They beat the victim to death with a club and hit him in the face with a bottle—both objects found in the store.

CC was the youngest of nine siblings who lived in severe poverty. All his brothers had some criminal involvement, including vandalism and aggression. His father was an abusive alcoholic who abandoned the family after serving a short jail term for nonsupport. As an adolescent, CC committed acts of violence that necessitated multiple appearances in juvenile court. A school report described him as "an antisocial troublemaker without close friends." He skipped school frequently and sometimes just walked out of class. On one occasion he pulled out a knife and was sent home. CC stole from stores, businesses, and other adolescents and was involved in bullying behavior as well. For several years, he set fires, sometimes to relieve anger and at other times because he felt euphoric when he watched the flames.

CC looked dejected and much older than his age. He passively cooperated in the evaluation but lacked emotion and seemed indifferent. He did not appear to be upset about his legal situation or the outcome of his trial. He seemed interested only when he told the examiner stories of violence and distrust of people and when he described his bizarre fantasies. He was proud of pulling a knife on a teacher at age 9 or 10, and he seemed preoccupied with knives and guns.

The evaluator easily elicited intense fantasies of murder and torture. "In a fight I try to kill the guy. I always want to kill." He found it relaxing to fantasize about murdering people, burning their eyes out, cutting out their tongues, and cutting the tendons of their arms and legs so that they would be helpless. He distrusted people and felt others were sneaky. CC hoped to be executed, stating, "I will come back in this form and prove that God is wrong."

The extent of CC's aggressive fantasies (with pronounced sadistic content, including a preoccupation with weapons and repetitive fire setting) indicates that the murder was not incidental but rather an outgrowth of an underlying compulsion that would be expressed only under the right circumstances. In this case, the compulsion was masked by the robbery. Social isolation, preoccupation with bizarre and aggressive fantasies, flat affect, friendlessness, and the perception of him by others as being eccentric and strange mark CC as having a schizotypal personality disorder.

The next case illustrates an offender who harbored a dangerous hidden compulsion to kill that was released situationally.

Case 9.4: Compulsion Released by Fetish Stimulation

A 26-year-old male (DD) killed a 45-year-old woman known in the local bars and described as a "common slut." The death was caused by manual strangulation and smashing her head with a hammer following intercourse with her in his car. DD gave two slightly different versions of the homicide. He told the police that he met the victim at a bar and had sex with her in his car and that the murder was triggered when she asked him whether he had a venereal disease. He said he strangled her while saying, "Go and die there, bitch." After she died, DD smoked a cigarette, cleaned her fingernails to get rid of any trace evidence, and then smashed her skull with a hammer so it would appear "like a sex maniac killed her." He went home, slept well, and then turned himself into the police on the urging of a friend to whom he confessed the crime. The police officer who arrested DD said, "It was incongruous that he, throughout the lengthy recantation, was completely calm, that he at no time displayed any remorse or other emotion, and that he at times made smirking, sly remarks for the benefit of a female stenographer present."

When interviewed under the influence of sodium amytal, however, DD gave a somewhat different story in which he revealed a long-standing fetish for female underwear, which played an important role in the attack. He said that he touched the victim's underwear in the bar when he met her, and doing so excited him sexually. While in the car, he wanted her underwear, which apparently upset her and led to a struggle that also excited him sexually. DD said he killed her in order to "cover up his secret" (i.e., the fetish for female underwear) which the victim had discovered.

The offender's fetish involved stealing. "I read about someone who collected 65 pairs of panties, but I stole 185 pairs, and I beat the guy." He had been arrested both as an adolescent and a young adult for stealing female underwear. As a child, he and his brother used to dress in their mother's clothes. DD referred to women as "bitches and whores." He claimed he had a girlfriend whom he never met (as she lived in a distant state) and whom he had contact with only through a lonely hearts' correspondence. The offender's fantasies included being "king of the world, a powerful wizard, and a master of the whorehouse." He also had repetitive dreams of chasing women up a tree. DD received a dishonorable discharge from the Marines (which he joined right after high school) for engaging in some type of black-market activity in a foreign country.

This case is marked by the offender's overt hostility and denigration of women, fetishism, ambivalent feelings toward his mother, and fantasies of power over women, which he revealed prominently and rather crudely. He also had a long-standing compulsion to hurt and humiliate women, which was expressed in his fantasies and dreams and was finally released in the unplanned sexual murder. It took a special situation, however, to disrupt his controls enough for him to commit the act. His affect was flat, and there were some grandiose paranoid features, but from a diagnostic perspective he would fall within the schizotypal spectrum.

The following two cases involve a compulsion to kill which was impulsively triggered by the victims' conduct; their behavior aroused feelings of anger and humiliation in the offenders.

Case 9.5: Compulsion Released by Victim's Promiscuous Behavior

A 23-year-old male (EE) met a 17-year-old female (C) at an amusement park. After speaking with her briefly, he took her for a ride in his truck. C told him that she had a boyfriend and was concerned about the boyfriend's finding out that she had left with EE. He took her home but dropped her off about 00 yards from her parents' house so her parents would not know that she had been out with him. They planned to meet the following evening at the amusement park.

When they met the next day, EE suggested they immediately go to a motel; C thought that was "a good idea." At the motel they quickly got undressed and had intercourse and oral sex. The offender stated:

> I couldn't stand it that she would have sex with me without even knowing me. I was real angry now, so I grabbed her by the neck and put her on the floor. I was real angry, man. I put my belt around her neck, and it broke. She passed out and didn't die. She was dizzy. I helped her get dressed. She kept saying, "Let's go back to my girlfriend's and get high." Actually, I didn't think I did anything wrong.

After assaulting her in the motel room, EE drove C to a remote area because

> I wanted to hurt her again. I was really angry. It had nothing to do with her; it was my whole life, so I beat her up. I kicked her. I left her. Nothing affected me at this time. I had no feelings at the time for nobody.

Following the homicide, EE went to a gas station where "I saw blood on my pants." He then drove to a bar and got cleaned up and went to his girlfriend's house where he was staying. He had a conversation with his girlfriend but lied to her regarding the sexual encounter and homicide. "I made up a story about cocaine because if I told her the truth, there could have been another body." EE had trouble sleeping that night because he was thinking about what had happened.

The next day, EE went back to the crime scene "because I was curious. I covered her when I found her because I didn't want to move her." He then told his girlfriend that he had killed a young woman, "but I didn't tell her we had sex. I told her I left her there. I didn't get rid of her. If I didn't say nothing, I wouldn't be arrested. I'd be out there doing it again." The girlfriend called the police, and EE was arrested.

During the interview the offender revealed a tremendous amount of anger toward his biological mother whom he viewed as promiscuous. He was also angry at various foster parents, particularly one family who "got rid of me because I wet the bed." EE described anger toward women in general but especially toward women who acted promiscuously and "engaged in sex without knowing the person." "I wanted to teach her [the victim] a lesson for having sex with an individual that she did not know on the first time." The offender had a history of two prior attacks on women—one a prostitute and the other a girl whom he casually met. He had served fairly brief sentences for both crimes, but the underlying sexual compulsion which fueled the assaults went unrecognized at that time.

EE had low-average intelligence with a Full Scale IQ of 80. However, his IQ was considered an underestimation of his potential level; the verbal scores were thought to be low because of poor academic achievement. The MMPI profile was consistent with an antisocial personality disorder, along with bizarre thinking and paranoid ideation, which reflected borderline traits that were noted both clinically and on the Rorschach. On the Rorschach the borderline traits were illustrated by the following regressive perceptions: "Some thing split in half. It was killed. Bleeding or something. I don't know what. There is a head here." "Blood." "Lungs, the shape and color; vital organs." The Rorschach also showed conflict in relationships with females and conflict in the sexual area, as noted by the offender's inability to offer a single response to the cards with stimulus pull in these areas. Projective figure drawings were meager and empty, consistent with his below-average intellect; they are illustrated in Figure 2.2 (Chapter 2).

TAT stories were surprisingly rich and rather revealing of some important dynamics motivating this crime. For example, on Card 4, EE produced the following story of an unfaithful woman:

> Looks like he is leaving her, and she didn't want him to go. She is holding him. He is ignoring her because he doesn't like her. She used him. She was with someone else. She didn't like to be with just one guy. He didn't take it that way. He takes it hard. He is hurt. He treated her good and she didn't care.

EE's response on Card 14 reveals the extent of his inner emptiness and anger at the world, family, and friends.

> A guy looking out a window, looking up at the sky. He is looking out on how messed up the world is. The world is so rotten, the way they treat him. He doesn't like the world. He is waiting for something to happen. He'll commit suicide and jump out. He's got a problem. Something hurt him in the past, and he can't handle it, and he can't talk to anybody. He closed his mind. No one cares about him. He'll take care of his life or conquer other people to show them that things are bad and people don't care. Something bad happened. Maybe he lost a friend, maybe a divorce, or maybe something with his parents. His parents were no good. They mistreated him. They didn't care about him. They ignored him. His mother is not a caring person. He grew up feeling hate and anger for being ignored. His mother was rotten. She left him. He started fighting with people who would hurt him. He was used by a friend, maybe a girlfriend. His girlfriend competed against him. She wanted to be in control, wanted to make him feel rotten. He couldn't handle it.

On Card 8BM, EE further revealed his attitude toward friends and relationships.

He got shot. Looks like he did it. It was an argument over something. Maybe over a girl. He went with his girlfriend, and he found out and shot the guy due to anger. It made him feel angry. He wanted to kill him. Relationships are strong, and sometimes you kill people because they are so strong. He didn't care about the person. He is nothing to him. He kills him so he can have that girl to himself.

His response on Card 13MF describes the homicide:

> Something happened to the woman in bed. She is dead. Something happened. He killed her. She used him. All he was good for was to go to bed with. He went off and killed her without a weapon. He choked her to death. It was emotional hurt and anger. He was being treated bad. She didn't care. Most women don't care. When it comes to relationships, when you love someone, you don't get it back. You get hurt and offended by it. He put all his feelings into another girl. She hurt him. He wanted to go out and do something to another girl. He loved the other one too much. He would hurt her, but he didn't care. He didn't plan it. He was just so angry.

It all built up, and it came out on the wrong person. It was a one-night stand. He met her in a bar. He didn't want to hurt the one he loved, but he wanted to show her how hurt and angry he was. He is only human, and he can only take so much. His girlfriend didn't treat him with respect. She had a jealousy problem. He takes off and leaves her.

In addition to antisocial and borderline personality traits, as well as tremendous anger toward everyone, EE also had an impulse-control disorder that appeared under certain circumstances. He said he initially did not have any thought of killing the victim but wanted only to have a sexual encounter with her: "But I lost it. My temper was always a problem." EE was unwilling to articulate any fantasies. "I don't really want to discuss it." As an adolescent he attempted to discuss his disturbing fantasies with several therapists, but "the doctors never took any notes. They never wrote anything down."

The unplanned, disorganized, rather brutal nature of the offense is typical of the offender whose compulsion is released by a situation. Here, the trigger was the victim's eagerness to have sex with someone she did not know. EE stated quite clearly that if he were released from prison, he would definitely kill again if a similar situation presented itself.

9.5 Breakthrough of Compulsion with Just Slight Stimulation

Sometimes an underlying compulsion breaks through spontaneously when only slightly aroused. Eisler (1953) described a rather strange case of an unplanned sexual murder committed by a well-respected, middle-aged scientist. While taking a walk, the offender was stimulated by sexually aggressive feelings and fantasies involving women he knew or had seen. When he noticed an elderly woman carrying a basket, he suddenly grabbed, raped, and choked her to death. He was shocked that he could have committed such an act. He told the court he wanted no leniency and deserved to be executed. Here, the latent compulsion broke through with the stimulation of sexually aggressive fantasies and the presence of a vulnerable victim.

In the next case, a sexual murder resulted from a sudden breakthrough of a compulsion after just slight stimulation.

Case 9.6: Compulsion Breaks through after Spotting a Vulnerable Victim

A 20-year-old male drifter (FF) abducted an 8-year-old female, brought her to a vacant apartment, raped and killed her, and then threw the body in a closet. FF spotted the victim playing with a friend in the hallway of their apartment building. He took her by the hand and led her to the vacant apartment where he was staying. As soon as the victim entered the dwelling with the offender, the victim's playmate heard "a banging noise" and her friend yelling "stop, stop."

The victim was missing for a day before the playmate told her parents what she had witnessed. The police went to the apartment and quickly noticed a child's body in a closet under a pile of dirty clothes. The body was lying in a fetal position with her underwear around her ankles and body fluids emanating from her nose. A search of the apartment uncovered the child's clothing as well as the clothing of another missing child whose body had never been recovered. The police found child pornography there as well. The autopsy revealed massive trauma to the victim's vagina and anus. The cause of death was listed as mechanical asphyxiation, along with vaginal and anal sexual assault.

FF gave two statements to the police. He first denied sexually assaulting and killing the youngster and said he did not know how the child's body got in the closet. Eventually he admitted to sexually assaulting and killing her but claimed that he was drunk at the time. The offender's background included arrests for various minor drug-related offenses, several assaults, and an attempted abduction of a child (although the charges were eventually dismissed for unclear reasons).

In this case, FF's compulsion to kill erupted spontaneously when he spotted the victim. Only seconds after he entered the apartment he brutally assaulted the child, and he probably killed her within an hour or less. Lack of planning is evident in his actions; he did not remove the dead body from the apartment, nor did he leave the apartment. His intelligence was in the low-average range. He had a schizotypal personality with deep feelings of inadequacy and was addicted to alcohol and cocaine. FF was possibly under the influence of alcohol at the time of the abduction and homicide—although there was no corroborating evidence—and his drinking could have weakened his controls further.

9.6 Compulsion Released by Substances

Some individuals struggling with an underlying compulsion to act do so only under the influence of various substances, primarily alcohol. The disinhibiting effects of alcohol, as well as other drugs, are well-known (Powers and Kutash, 1978; Mayfield, 1976). Alcohol, which is involved in many homicides (Wolfgang, 1958), is a cerebral depressant that reduces the discriminatory functions of the psyche and frees repressed or suppressed fantasies, feelings, and drives. Most aggression occurs at blood alcohol levels ranging from 0.1% to 0.35%; at higher levels the individual is too stuporous to attack anyone, and at lower levels there is no disinhibiting effect.

Bradford, Greenberg, and Motayne (1992) reviewed the relationship between alcohol and various types of criminal behavior. Pernanen (1976) provides an interesting discussion of alcohol's direct physiological disinhibiting effects and their relationship to criminal behavior. The author also notes that in addition to disinhibition, alcohol and criminal behavior may be related indirectly, as (1) symptoms of another psychological disorder such as antisocial personality, (2) a result of increased frustration because of substance use, or (3) a result of some intervening variable, such as sleep disturbance from chronic alcohol use. The overwhelming consensus is that many violent crimes, including murder, occur when individuals are intoxicated; in many cases, if it were not for the intoxication, the criminal acts may not have been committed.

In the following case, a young man's long-standing compulsion to sadistically injure other men was acted on only when he was intoxicated. In fact, he stated that "I could not bring myself to do it unless I was drunk."

Case 9.7: Compulsion to Kill Released by Alcohol

A 24-year-old male (GG) was arrested for the murders of two men which occurred within days of each other. The first victim (D) was a 17-year-old hitchhiker. When D got into the offender's car, GG grabbed him, threatened him with a knife, and drove to a remote area. He made D undress, fondled his genitals, and made him perform oral sex. He then took a cigarette and burned the victim on the stomach. He next burned D's hair with the cigarette while holding a knife to his neck. GG subsequently forced D out of the car and, with his cigarette lighter, set D's hair on fire. While the victim was screaming, GG stabbed him repeatedly; he eventually drove off when it became apparent D was dead.

The second victim E, a 19-year-old male, was killed by strangulation. GG was "driving around looking for hitchhikers" and eventually picked up E.

> I found him walking along the street. I wanted him to be with me. He was nice looking, about six inches taller than me. At first, I drove by and said to myself, "No." I thought instead I would go, and I passed him again. I stopped and asked directions to some street. I then asked him to come [with me to] show me where the street was, and he agreed. I pulled over, and then I started to strangle him. He got out of the car, but I took my knife and pulled him over to me again and told him that if he did as he was told, he wouldn't get hurt. I just wanted him to do as he was told. The boy said, "Okay, okay, don't hurt me." The guy was bigger than me. I am just a little guy that people push around.

GG then tied E's hands together and made him lie down. He ran his hand over E's arms and head and said he felt embarrassed doing this.

> I then drove to a dark place. He was crying and whining. I told him to stop that. Nothing he said could stop me now. I opened the boy's shirt and pulled up his undershirt. I had him take off his shirt, his undershirt, shoes, socks, and pants. He looked scared. I was embarrassed and told him not to look at me. I know I should be a man, not a woman. How nice he looked. I touched him and kissed his eyes. He opened one eye, and I said I would cut his eye out if he didn't keep it closed. Then I thought to myself, how many new cars are like mine in the area. I am going to get caught. Maybe I should kill him with the knife. I told him I thought I should kill him because the police would catch me. The boy said, "I promise you I won't tell."
>
> I started touching the boy's neck again. I thought that he had a nice neck. I then put my legs around the boy's body and laid alongside him, touching his face. I thought to myself; this is a nice kid. I then had the desire to see what would happen if I squeezed his neck. I squeezed and the boy squirmed. I was afraid of getting caught. That's why I thought of killing him. It was all in my power to let him go or to kill him. It was up to me. I let him know that. I often have the thought of punching people in the mouth. I thought of setting him on fire, but I just squeezed his neck until he died and threw him out of the car and left.

The offender acknowledged that he had vague fantasies of hurting other men following homosexual encounters and that he preferred boys 16–17 years old. He said he had fantasies and "impulses" on many occasions when he was not intoxicated, but then he could contain the compulsion to hurt his partner. He could only act out homosexually or carry out the compulsion to kill when intoxicated.

> I couldn't do it unless I was feeling high. I had to be feeling good with alcohol to get the nerve up to do it. I would drink, get to feeling real woozy, and then drive my car around, looking to pick someone up. I would be driving along in the car. I would have nothing to do. I would just drive. When I saw young guys, I would stop and pick them up. I never wanted to hurt them, but yet I did. I always carry a knife in my car. I do it to scare some if I have to.
>
> When I drink, I go out to look for someone. It is just a need. I want to be close to somebody, somebody that is more or less mine. It is not to hurt but to scare, but I guess to hurt too. I only killed two people, but I hurt a lot of others. I once burned a few boys when I was a kid, and I also strangled some kids but didn't kill them. I put my hands around their necks, and

I stopped. I pressed, but then I let them go. I once put a handkerchief around this kid's neck and then I tried to strangle him. There was no anger while I tried to do it.

GG was raised in a middle-class family. His father was a dentist who died when the offender was six. His mother remarried a brutal person with a lower intellectual level who worked as the superintendent of a building. GG managed to maintain a marginal, but reasonably stable, life; he held a job (as a store clerk) and was able to have relationships with others. He reported a relationship with a girlfriend that ended just prior to the first murder, a rather typical aspect of compulsive-murder cases. After the relationship broke up, GG felt isolated, depressed, frustrated, and angry. "It upset me. I guess you could say I got depressed. I don't know why we broke up. I still haven't figured it out." These feelings, plus the disinhibiting effects of alcohol, released the compulsion to assault young men, which resulted in the unplanned and spontaneous murders and other sadistic acts that GG committed while intoxicated.

When interviewed under the influence of sodium amytal, GG elaborated on the emotions that went along with his sadistic fantasies, sadistic acts, and the two homicides. He explained that it made him "feel superior" when he controlled others. He described long-standing feelings of loneliness and nervousness around people. He had also had a preoccupation with fire since childhood. As he said on another occasion, "It was a sudden impulse when I did this. I don't know. It's something strange. I don't know where it came from. It's not revenge, but I felt strong when I did it. By burning people I felt happy."

9.7 Unplanned Ritualistic Murders

Although most ritualistic murders (where the offender engages in repetitive behavior at the crime scene) are highly planned, individuals sometimes commit unplanned sexual murders that involve elements of ritualistic activity (Schlesinger et al., 2010). These cases are relatively rare and are an important exception to the general finding that the vast majority of ritualistic murders are thought out in detail because they flow from intricate fantasies. The following two cases illustrate this important exception.

Case 9.8: Unplanned Compulsive Homicide Triggered by Fetish Stimulation

At the time of the homicide, HH was 20 years old and receiving psychotherapy for a series of bizarre solo burglaries. He broke into many homes in order to obtain black leather objects that the female occupants had either worn or handled. If he could not find black leather, the offender stole an object of insignificance such as toothpaste or several pencils. He was handsome and well-liked, had won a high school athletic scholarship, and was described by teachers and classmates as an all-American boy. HH was neat and well-groomed, and he had superior intellect and exceptional verbal fluency.

One afternoon while driving his car, HH noticed a woman in another car wearing black leather gloves. The offender followed her for about 30 miles and watched her enter her residence. After a while, he knocked on the door, pushed his way in, and forced the victim to the back of the home. He said, "Whose bedroom is this?" She responded, "It's my daughter's. She is away at college." He then killed her by inflicting about 40 stab wounds and took her black leather gloves. At the time of this homicide, police suspected that HH had committed a number of other murders that occurred under similar circumstances. He was never indicted for any of the other murders, but he revealed his guilt years later.

HH was a model prisoner during his 20 years of incarceration. He obtained a college degree and was eventually granted a furlough to earn a master's degree. While attending courses at a nearby college, HH again began burglarizing homes to steal black leather objects, particularly gloves. During a 10-day period, he spontaneously assaulted seven women walking outside their homes; miraculously, none of them died. He hit the women over the head with pipes, sticks, and rocks. After assaulting them, he grabbed a black leather object (typically gloves, but sometimes shoes or handbags) that they were carrying or wearing. On one occasion, he assaulted a woman, took off her black leather shoes, and then gave them back to her. He was eventually arrested for trying to break into a home where he was again looking for black leather apparel.

The offender was returned to prison and served about 10 more years. Once again, he was paroled and began to break into homes in an attempt to steal black leather objects. After several break-ins, he seriously assaulted and almost killed a women occupant. About a week later, he was arrested while attempting to burglarize yet another home.

This case is marked by an unusual fetish for black leather, which triggered the unplanned assaults. Significant disorganizing characterological disturbance was not found with this offender. He was rather rigid and controlled, not at all impulsive, except when he observed a woman wearing black leather. He said that under these conditions he had an impulse "so overpowering" it disrupted his otherwise intact defenses. Not only does this case show the unusual association of fetishism with unplanned attacks, but it is also an example of an offender whose otherwise controlled personality was not capable of initiating any level of planning when stimulated by the object of his fetish.

Case 9.9: Unplanned Compulsive Murder with a Distinct Signature

A 32-year-old male (II) was arrested after he brutally attacked and almost killed a woman who came to his assistance after his car broke down on a highway. When the victim entered II's car, he suddenly attacked her, hitting her in the nose and eyes multiple times. He then shoved his fingers up her rectum while strangling her and, at the same time, bit her on her chin and then on her left breast. After the assault, the offender threw her out of his moving car and assumed that she had died. The woman did not die and the offender, who had committed the crime in a rather public place, was quickly apprehended. Following his arrest, the authorities recognized the unusual manner in which this woman was assaulted, particularly the bite marks, and quickly linked II to an unsolved homicide in a distant state that was committed in the same ritualistic manner.

In this previous case, II killed the victim after he met her walking home from a convenience store on a busy highway. He grabbed her and dragged her inside a construction area on the side of the road. II shoved his fingers up her rectum while strangling her and biting her on the chin and then the left breast. He told a fellow inmate that the reason for the chin biting was so that he could "look in the victim's eyes while I was killing her and watch her die slowly." Although II denied guilt in court, he was convicted of both crimes.

II's history included serving several years in prison for killing a friend during an argument, as well as chronic behavior problems, school expulsion, and an allegation of being sexually abused. He had worked sporadically as a handyman but was never steadily employed. Over the years, II had many girlfriends whom he physically assaulted, but he never engaged in any of the ritualistic behaviors with them. Psychological testing revealed average intelligence, pronounced antisocial and impulsive traits, an impulse-control disorder, and some substance abuse. Interestingly, he was nicknamed "Cat Man" as an adolescent because he had killed several cats after engaging in some type of sexual activity with them.

This individual acted in a specific ritualistic manner but did not have the personality characteristics or crime scene behaviors typical of the ritualistic offender, as described, for example, by Hazelwood and Warren (2000). Most compulsive murderers who have a ritualistic aspect to their behavior are much less impulsive than II. Because of his pronounced impulsivity, II was unable to contain the compulsion when a victim of opportunity crossed his path. He never planned any of his crimes, sexual or otherwise. The compulsion to kill and the need to commit the ritual were present, but the way the crime occurred was a direct result of his underlying personality.

9.8 Differential Diagnosis: Catathymic vs. Compulsive Homicides

The differential diagnosis of catathymic and compulsive homicides is sometimes problematic. Both catathymic and compulsive homicides have a basis in underlying sexual conflict. However, the nature of sexual conflict is quite different. Catathymic homicides are (usually) single explosions triggered by some type of challenge to the individual's sense of sexual competence. Compulsive homicides, on the other hand, stem from a long-standing and developing urge to kill, which itself is eroticized. Catathymic homicides typically stem from feelings of inadequacy extending into the sexual area, while compulsive homicides involve a fusion of sexual and aggressive drives. Meloy (2000) lists some additional differentiating characteristics in Table 9.2.

9.8.1 Acute Catathymic and Unplanned Compulsive Homicides

Acute catathymic homicides may be confused with unplanned compulsive murders since both involve a sudden attack. However, they have a number of distinguishing characteristics (see Table 9.3). Individuals who commit acute catathymic homicides have no preexisting compulsion to kill or prior sadistic fantasies. They do not harbor an underlying urge to act out but rather explode when victims trigger poorly defended sexual conflicts that the

Table 9.2 **Meloy's Distinctions between Compulsive and Catathymic Homicides**

Characteristics	Compulsive	Catathymic
Nature of sexual homicide	Organized	Disorganized
Axis I diagnosis	Sexual sadism	Mood disorder
Axis II diagnosis	Antisocial/narcissistic personality disorder	Various traits and personality disorders
Psychopathy	Severe (primary)	Mild–moderate
Attachment pathology	Chronically detached	Attachment hunger
Autonomic nervous system	Hyporeactive	Hyperreactive
Early trauma	Often absent	Often present

Source: From Meloy, J.R., *Aggression and Violent Behavior*, 5, pp. 1–22, 2000. With permission.

Table 9.3 Differentiating Characteristics of Acute Catathymic and Unplanned Compulsive Homicides

Characteristics	Acute Catathymic	Unplanned Compulsive
Compulsion to kill	Not present	Present for years
Sadistic fantasy	Not present	Present in simple, undifferentiated form
Motive	Sexual; stemming from feelings of inadequacy extending into the sexual area	Sexual; involving a fusion of sex and aggression
Victim	Often a stranger who triggers underlying conflict	Often known; the victim does not trigger conflicts, but her vulnerability provides an opportunity for the offender to kill
Warning signs	Threat to explode sometimes made and often ignored	No threats, but many ominous signs in the offender's background
Sexual activity at the time of the crime	Necrophilia or dismemberment is common	Insertion of objects into orifices; sometimes sexual assault
Postcrime behavior	Offender does not try to elude authorities for long	Offender attempts to elude authorities but typically is unsuccessful

offenders have been secretly struggling with. On the contrary, compulsive offenders who act out spontaneously have been harboring sadistic fantasies, usually in simple, undifferentiated form, for years. Although they have had an urge to kill for quite some time, they do so only when an opportunity presents itself.

The victim of the acute catathymic perpetrator is often a stranger, while the individual who commits an unplanned compulsive homicide (especially his first murder) typically kills someone whom he has had a connection with. Threats to explode, usually ignored, are sometimes made by the individual destined to commit an acute catathymic murder. The compulsive offender rarely threatens to kill. However, he may exhibit various ominous signs (Schlesinger, 2001b). Postcrime behavior is also different. The acute catathymic offender typically does not try to elude authorities for long, if at all. The individual who commits an unplanned compulsive homicide does attempt to elude authorities, but he is usually unsuccessful due to the physical evidence he leaves at the crime scene.

The following case of an unplanned compulsive murder may be incorrectly viewed as an acute catathymic murder because of the spontaneity of the attack.

Case 9.10: Sudden Sexual Attack on Vulnerable Victim

A 19-year-old male (JJ) abducted and killed a 14-year-old female (F) who was walking home from school at dusk after having missed the last school bus. The offender became preoccupied with the attractive teenager while he was working at a local gas station—a job from which he had recently been fired. An observer noted that JJ once tripped over a hose as his eyes followed the future victim's passage. Although JJ never spoke with F directly, he saw her on many occasions when she went to the gas station with her father.

When JJ saw the victim walking alone, he followed her, took out a knife that he always carried in his boot, and forced her into the woods where passersby would be unable to see them. He tied F's hands with the strap from her purse, tore her clothes off, and shoved her underwear in her mouth. He apparently let the victim get partially dressed, but as she started to run away, JJ attacked her and stabbed her 26 times with his knife, causing her death. He also engaged in vaginal and anal rape (probably before the murder). The knife was found near the crime scene; F's partially clothed body was found 2 days later in a shallow ditch close to where the assault and murder took place.

Several days after the body was discovered, the police interviewed the offender because he was suspected of having stolen tools from the gas station where he had been working. The police noted anxiety in JJ, and he quickly implicated himself in the murder. But, after going to the county jail, he retracted his confession, following the advice of other inmates.

JJ was a tall, thin individual who looked younger than his age. He combed his hair straight down in front of his face in an attempt to cover his eyes; one of his eyes was crossed, and that bothered him. His affect was flat, and he looked away from the examiner. JJ answered only direct questions and frequently mumbled when he did so. When discussing specifics regarding the crime, he had periodic outbursts of hostility, but he managed to maintain control. The examiner found no evidence of bizarre or grossly inappropriate behavior or thought content, and his overall attitude was adequate.

JJ achieved a Full Scale IQ of 80, which was consistent with his poor school performance. Some mild organicity was indicative of a learning disability. The offender had dropped out of school in the 11th grade because of persistent failure and social problems, including being teased by his classmates. The Rorschach was sparse, with unelaborated responses and a few indicative of borderline traits (e.g., "coffee spilled," "a cat that's been run over, flattened out"). The MMPI suggested borderline/schizotypal traits with scale elevations indicating suspiciousness, social alienation, withdrawal, and depression.

TAT stories reveal strong feelings of inadequacy, rejection, and hostility:

- *Card 1.* "He wants to learn how to play, but he is upset because nobody will teach him. He is sad and depressed. Nobody will help him. He feels bad about himself. His father could play it, and he can't. He thinks if he can't play it, his father won't like him."
- *Card 3BM.* "He is upset. All his friends are bothering him. He is not as smart as them. They make fun of him and call him names. They call him stupid and stuff like that. His parents get him a special teacher to help him learn. At the end, he turns out smarter than his friends."
- *Card 3GF.* "She is upset because her grandfather died. He was the only one she could talk to. She thought nobody else understood her. Both her parents never had the time to listen to her. They were always working."
- *Card 7GF.* "The girl thinks her mother doesn't love her anymore 'cause she has a new baby. The mother pays a lot of attention to the baby, and she thinks she doesn't get attention. She is all upset."
- *Card 14.* "Going to jump out a window. Maybe his wife left him. He wants to kill himself. He is so upset. He was drunk."
- *Card 13MF.* "She got shot. He shot her. He was robbing her house and she found him when she came home. He didn't know who she was. He was scared. He gets out of there and goes to a bar and drinks. He takes the money he stole and mails it back to her so her husband can have the money back. He didn't want to kill her. He wanted to scare her so she wouldn't tell nobody. It was an accident. He didn't feel good. He feels bad. He dies. He drove his car off a bridge. It was an accident."

Projective figure drawings (in Figure 9.2) illustrate inadequacy and emptiness; note the male figure's incomplete facial features.

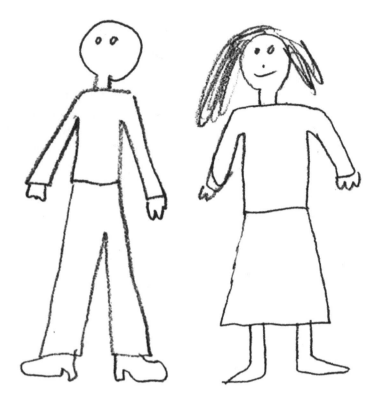

Figure 9.2 Drawings by a compulsive murderer who committed an unplanned sexual homicide.

Although JJ gave a fairly detailed statement to the police which he eventually retracted, insight into the criminal psychodynamics was revealed when he offered his theory of the crime:

> She walked by the woods, going home, and he followed her from the back. It had to be one of two things: Robbery or rape. ... Maybe [it was rape because] she did something that scared him. She said she'd go to the police. That would be when he killed her. She said it before and after the rape. She was afraid. Maybe he threatened her with a knife. He raped her before he killed her—before, because after there would have been blood on him and he would have been easy to find. ... [She may have] acted stuck up because of the way she walked.

When questioned as to what the victim might have said to anger the offender, JJ responded,

> The guy asked for sex. She said, 'Fuck you, you are a pervert,' she might have said. After the rape, she could have given the police a description, and they could draw a picture; possibly she knew him or saw him around.

As to why there were multiple stab wounds, JJ responded, "The person was fucked up." When asked why the victim's underwear had been stuffed in her mouth, he responded, "So she wouldn't scream, I guess." He explained that the entire incident took about an hour. The offender admitted to prior fantasies about raping women in general but denied any particular rape or murder fantasy regarding the victim. He explained that he was angry at women because of persistent rejection. The offender said he had a girlfriend but would not say who she was; those who knew JJ—including family, friends, and former co-workers—were doubtful.

JJ's description of vague, undifferentiated rape fantasies points to a compulsive process. The murder itself was unplanned and occurred when he spotted a vulnerable victim alone at dusk. Multiple stab wounds revealed the depth of his anger toward women, which was displaced onto this victim. Using the victim's underwear to contain her potential screaming and tying her hands with the strap from her purse point to the unplanned nature of the crime. JJ's personality was replete with feelings of inadequacy, emotional detachment, and borderline/schizotypal traits. He was found guilty of murder but was spared the death penalty primarily because of his young age.

9.8.2 Chronic Catathymic and Planned Compulsive Homicides

Differentiating a chronic catathymic homicide from a planned compulsive murder is also sometimes problematic, but important differentiating characteristics are present here as well (see Table 9.4). For example, the chronic catathymic murderer does not harbor a compulsion that has been building for many years; instead, he experiences a build-up of tension, along with deep-rooted feelings of helplessness and inadequacy extending into the sexual area. The compulsive offender's motivation stems from a long-standing drive to kill, which involves a fusion of sex and aggression. This drive is discharged initially through elaborate sadistic fantasies. The chronic catathymic offender does not have sadistic fantasies; instead, he develops obsessive thoughts to kill a particular victim. To the catathymic offender, killing seems to be a solution to a problem, not a way to achieve sexual gratification. The victim in a chronic catathymic homicide is usually an intimate or former intimate partner or is sometimes (but rarely) a stranger with whom the offender has become obsessed. The individual who commits a planned compulsive homicide typically targets

Table 9.4 Differentiating Characteristics of Chronic Catathymic and Planned Compulsive Homicides

Characteristics	Chronic Catathymic	Planned Compulsive
Compulsion to kill	Not present	Present and building for years
Sadistic fantasy	Not present; instead, obsessive thoughts to kill a particular victim; murder is seen as a solution to a problem	Present in elaborate form; not in reference to a particular victim, almost any (with certain characteristics) victim will do
Motive	Build-up of tension and feelings of helplessness and inadequacy extending to the sexual area	Fusion of sex and aggression
Victim	Intimate or former intimate partner; or stranger with whom the offender becomes obsessed	Often a stranger; sometimes an acquaintance, but almost never an intimate or former intimate partner
Warning signs	Tells confidant of ego-dystonic ideas that are developing	Rarely warns others, but many ominous behavioral signs in the offender's background
Sexual activity at the crime scene	Rare	Common
Postcrime behavior	Does not try to elude authorities; sometimes makes a suicide attempt following the murder	Tries hard to elude authorities and, because of the planning, is often successful; as a result, there are multiple victims

strangers; he may begin a series of killings with an acquaintance-victim, but he almost never kills an intimate or former intimate partner.

The chronic catathymic offender might confide in another person and reveal the ego-dystonic ideas that are building. The individual who commits planned compulsive homicides rarely warns others, but, like his nonplanning counterpart, he exhibits many ominous signs. Following the murder, the chronic catathymic offender does not try to elude authorities; in fact, he may make a suicide attempt. The individual who commits a planned compulsive homicide tries hard to elude authorities, and his success in doing so results in him having a series of victims. At the time of the murder, sexual activity is rare for the chronic catathymic offender. However, the individual who commits a planned compulsive homicide commonly rapes, sodomizes, or tortures the victim before killing her.

The following case of a planned compulsive homicide may be mistaken for a chronic catathymic murder because of the offender's obsession with the future victim.

Case 9.11: Planned Compulsive Murder Preceded by an Obsession with the Victim

A 22-year-old male drug dealer (KK) became obsessed with (G) one of his attractive female customers. In addition to following her, he asked G several times for dates and was turned down on each occasion. One night, after watching G for several hours, he observed her enter her apartment building. He broke in through a window and stabbed G many times with a knife after having choked her with a cord. He also sexually assaulted G vaginally and anally. Following the murder, he went into the bedroom of the victim's two young children (ages 5 and 9), who possibly could have recognized the offender from the neighborhood, and stabbed them repeatedly. Miraculously, the children lived despite their severe injuries. They were able to give a fairly detailed statement about the event, which was in complete contrast to the offender's statements to the police and during his psychological examination.

When evaluated, KK was reasonably pleasant and tried to be friendly. But his account of events was totally inconsistent with witness statements—given by those who knew both the victim and the offender—as well as with other forensic findings. He said,

> She invited me into her apartment. She propositioned me. I wasn't prepared for that. Sex for a fee, but I was reluctant. I didn't want to give her no money. Eventually, we had sex. I thought she'd leave me alone when she got the money, 10 to 20 dollars. I was lying there in her bedroom. She went to another room and got high. She started propositioning me again for sex. I really didn't want to get involved. She kept on and on. She took her clothes off to arouse me. She said stuff and did stuff, trying to arouse me. She touched herself.
>
> The next thing I know, I was at my cousin's house. He asked me what happened. I said I don't know. I had a wound, so I knew something was the matter. I didn't remember at all what happened. I thought maybe she attacked me with a knife. I told the police that but it was a lie.

He denied attempting to kill the children.

"I wouldn't do that to them kids. They didn't have nothing to do with it. If I intended to kill G or the kids, I would have went about it in a much different way." When asked why he tied a cord around the victim's neck, the offender had no answer.

KK had a background of antisocial and violent behavior that began in adolescence. He quit school at 16 after severe behavior problems. He was incarcerated in juvenile facilities about five different times for various forms of violence, and he was arrested for violent acts several times as an adult. The offender also had been arrested when his mother filed a domestic-violence complaint.

> She [his mother] was trying to show me she had some power. She wanted to liberate herself. She told the police we used to fight, and we had an argument that night. That's all. My mother said I stabbed her with a pen. She showed me the marks here and there. Two or three little marks. That's all.

Even while in jail (for the current charges) KK was involved in three episodes of violence. In one of them he tried to break another inmate's neck because "he kept talking and talking, and chewed gum too loud."

Testing and clinical evaluation revealed both antisocial and borderline traits. The Rorschach included regressive perceptions such as the following: "Two people fighting over something. Head, the arms, and objects, the legs. They are ripping it in half." "Blood on the top, because of the red." The MMPI also showed significant elevations on scales 4, 6, 8, and 9, scores that indicate both antisocial and borderline traits. Projective figure drawings (Figure 9.3) were meager and empty, done without much effort.

TAT stories were reasonably rich, revealing an angry, violent, and sadistic individual. The following TAT excerpts provide considerable insight into some of KK's inner thoughts and emotions.

- *Card 1.* "He is mad because he can't play. He feels like breaking this thing. He never wanted to play it anyhow. He winds up killing himself because people try to manipulate him. His parents broke his will. People take advantage of him. They use him. They try to get things out of him. He kills himself with a gun."

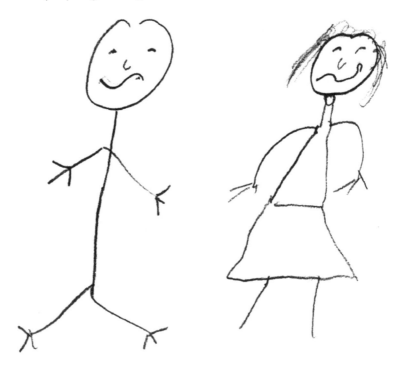

Figure 9.3 Figure drawings by a man who committed a planned compulsive homicide.

- *Card 3BM.* "Her husband beat her up. She approached him, and she verbally talked back to him. She protested to him, and he protested to her by physically assaulting her. He assaulted her because she protested and spoke out against him. He doesn't have any feelings. He liquidated the situation. He resolved it the way he saw fit. He beat her up. She is hurting inside so she shuts down. He disregards everybody else but himself. He doesn't really care. He sees things the way he sees it. The situation goes on and on and on. There is no ending. She loses her will. He just doesn't care. He is a very cruel person. He doesn't know why he is like that. I've been asking myself that for a long time."
- *Card 4.* "Things are going to get hectic. She is trying to corner him, and he is going to come out fighting against her because she is the predator at that point. He comes out fighting."
- *Card 18GF.* "It looks like a mother abusing her child. The mother is trying to kill the child. The child hates his mother. He tries to do things his way. He just hates her. He has nasty feelings when he thinks of her. As far as he is concerned, she doesn't exist. He finds it hard to understand women. He is suspicious of women because of his mother. He is aware that women can act like his mom. They can become really confused. They can get kind of evil."

This offender was not only filled with anger and hatred toward just about everybody but was also quite sadistic. In fact, he was proud of his sadistic acts, which were directed at men and women alike. His lack of truthfulness makes complete understanding difficult. Notwithstanding his obsession with the victim—as reported by numerous individuals who knew them both—this is not a catathymic homicide. KK did not kill the victim as a solution to an underlying conflict that broke into consciousness. Rather, he was a sadistic man who evidenced an underlying compulsion to kill. He carried out the murder in a planned manner after observing the victim's behavior for several months.

9.9 Theories of the Compulsive Murderer

There is no shortage of theories or explanations to account for individuals who have committed compulsive, repetitive, and sexually motivated homicides. In general, theories can be divided into three groups: social, psychological, and biological. Although all the theories are heuristic, none has yet gained anything close to general acceptance.

9.9.1 Social Theories

Most practitioners and researchers favor a psychological etiology to account for the compulsive murderer's behavior; however, some authors have commented on social factors as well. Since all behavior takes place within a social context, social determinants always exert some degree of influence on behavior, particularly criminal behavior. Holmes and DeBurger (1985), for example, believe social and cultural elements in American society have a causal impact on serial murder. They cite media violence, the use of aggression as a way of dealing with problems, increased anonymity in an increasingly urban society, and even the mobility of Americans as factors that in some way contribute to such crimes. Newton (1992) claims that serial murder is a recent phenomenon in the U.S., presumably because various social factors have now become widespread. This position is echoed by Norris (1998), who argues that 75% of the world's serial murderers are from the U.S. and fears that "as the influence of American culture spreads to the less developed countries, ... the disease of serial murder will spread as well" (p. 19).

Even Ressler et al. (1988) and Ressler and Schachtman (1997), who primarily support a psychogenic explanation of the sexual murderer, believe that social factors play a large role. Compulsive, repetitive sexual murder "is connected to the increasing complexity of our society, to our interconnectedness via the media, and to the alienation many of us feel. ... Wherever people become alienated from society, wherever neighbors hardly know one another, wherever families do not keep in very close touch, wherever runaway teenagers roam dangerous streets, wherever violence is made to seem a viable response to troubles, an upsurge in serial murder would be one troubling response" (Ressler and Schachtman, 1997, pp. 51–52). And Hazelwood and Michaud (2001) also refer to various social and cultural changes (the relaxed behavior code, increased mobility, and overt hostility to women and technology) that can affect an increase in such crimes.

However, Meloy (2000) offers two cogent criticisms of Ressler et al.'s (1988) discussion of the social antecedents of sexual homicide, particularly the authors' emphasis on the offenders' troubled family backgrounds, including the high prevalence of alcoholism, psychiatric illness, and abuse. First, no comparison group was used; therefore, these background characteristics do not necessarily predict sexual murder. For instance, it is highly likely that the backgrounds of most nonsexual murderers would also include many of these negative social experiences. Second, and perhaps more important, Meloy notes that most of Ressler et al.'s sample did not experience such negative social problems. And socially deviant backgrounds were also conspicuously absent in the sexual sadists studied by Dietz, Hazelwood, and Warren (1990), a finding supported by Gratzer and Bradford (1995).

More recently, Chan, Heide, and Beauregard (2011) proposed a theory of sexual murder integrating social learning and routine activities theory. However, a strictly social theory—even when adding on routine activities theory—of the compulsive murderer leaves more questions unanswered than answered. Often cited sociogenic causes of crime—poverty, overcrowding, and broken homes—do not differentiate sexual murderers from other types of criminals. Neither does examination of their routine behavior and travel patterns. Because social factors play a role in just about all behavior, they probably play some role in compulsive murder too, but a specific etiological contribution has not yet been demonstrated.

9.9.2 Psychological Theories

The most widely held view of the etiology of compulsive murder involves some type of psychological or psychodynamic explanation. One of the earliest of these theories was the notion expounded by Revitch (1957, 1965) and later by Revitch and Schlesinger (1978, 1981, 1989) that the compulsive murderer is committing a displaced matricide. According to this theory, the compulsive offender kills women as a result of an unhealthy emotional involvement with his own mother: "repressed incestuous feelings seem to be the main stimulus to gynocide" (Revitch and Schlesinger, 1981, p. 174); by killing other women, the sex murderer is symbolically killing his own mother.

Support is fairly widespread for the general notion that some men emotionally split women into sexual objects they view as bad and nonsexual objects they view as good or pure. For example, Freud (1910) described a need in some men to degrade women in order to experience sexual arousal: "pure" women, whom they do not degrade, reflect the image of a mother and create in these men sexual inhibitions and anxiety associated with incest. Mathis (1971) reported some extreme cases of this phenomenon, which he referred to as the "Madonna-prostitute" syndrome. Here, a man who loses potency after marriage—or after his wife gives birth to a child—frequently insists that his spouse utter profanities during intercourse or admit to or describe details of other sexual encounters and indiscretions. If she does, the man is able to become aroused. The perceived "purity" of the wife (or new mother) generates too much incest anxiety. Revitch and Schlesinger (1981) postulated that in the compulsive murderer "the bad mother is either eliminated in totality, or she is split into a good mother (in the fantasy life) and a bad mother, or mother-prostitute, that deserves to be eliminated. ... This elimination, assault, or murder is eroticized" (p. 175). In such cases there is a psychogenic fusion of sex and aggression, similar to that observed by Freud (1905), who found that the sexual instinct can form various perversions as a result of a fusion of the two basic drives.

Meloy (2000) also supports a displaced-matricide theory of the compulsive murderer, but he adds a classical conditioning paradigm that combines a psychodynamic model and a behavioral model. Specifically, Meloy finds in many cases of sexual murder "a classical pairing of sexual arousal and extreme violence towards women" (p. 13). The author cites a number of cases of children who achieved some level of sexual arousal at the same time they experienced violence. For example, he described a 21-year-old perpetrator of a sexual homicide whose mother "would soothe him as a child by stroking his penis after his father would physically assault him, homogenizing his feelings of fear, rage, and sexual arousal" (p. 13).

Meloy and his colleagues (Gacono, 1992a,b; Meloy, Gacono, and Kenney, 1994) have delineated important traits of the compulsive sexual murderer that add to their overall theory. These traits are based largely on the Rorschach perceptions of a sample of 38 sexual murderers that were contrasted with a control group of nonsexually offending psychopaths and pedophiles. Six characteristics differentiated the sexual murderers. They were more chronically angry, obsessional, and narcissistic; they had abnormal bonding patterns, displayed impaired reality testing (usually on a borderline level), and evidenced illogical reasoning, specifically in regard to sexuality.

In addition to the displaced-matricide theory, several rather straightforward psychological theories attempt to explain the conduct of the compulsive murderer. Several researchers (e.g., Ansevics and Doweiko, 1991; Hickey, 1991; Liebert, 1985; Pollock, 1995; Stone, M.H., 1998) argue that this type of offender simply has a personality disorder—or perhaps a subtype of a traditional personality disorder—such as borderline, narcissistic, or antisocial. Or, perhaps, the offender experienced a horrible childhood event (McKenzie, 1995) such as severe humiliation or embarrassment (Hale, 1994). Notwithstanding the virtues of parsimony, these notions are just too simplistic and do not even begin to explain the fact that most people who have such personality disorders or who have experienced unpleasant events do not become sexual murderers or even criminals. Arrigo and Purcell (2001) take a slightly different approach, calling sexual murder simply another paraphilia. However, although correct, such labeling does not explain the behavior.

In contrast to these overly simplistic views, Burgess, Hartman, Ressler, Douglas, and McCormack (1986) provide a rather complex theoretical model of the sexual murderer. These researchers present a motivational model of causation divided into five stages:

1. *Ineffective social environment.* The future offender fails to bond as a child because of his abusive upbringing.
2. *Formative events.* The future offender's thinking becomes fixated on traumas he has experienced, particularly abuse. He feels helpless and, as a result, develops compensatory fantasies of domination and control.
3. *Patterned responses.* The future offender becomes socially isolated, engages in auto-erotic activities, and develops an antisocial/hostile view of the world. The feelings of others are not important to him.
4. *Actions toward others.* The future offender's behavior toward other people is based on achieving a feeling of domination. At this stage, he may be cruel to animals, set fires, steal, and destroy property. As he gets older, his actions become increasingly violent: assault, burglary, nonsexual murder, and finally sexual murder involving torture, mutilation, and necrophilia.
5. *Feedback filter.* The murderer is proud of his violent behavior, and he justifies it to himself.

Meloy (2000) notes the heuristic value of this model, but he also stresses its limitations. Specifically, Meloy believes the theory could have been enhanced if psychological test results were added. And as in the Ressler et al. (1988) research project out of which this theory grew, no control or comparison group was used. Thus, whether the model is specific to sexual murder or to sexual aggression in general remains unknown.

9.9.3 Biological Theories

The first theory of sexual murder, proposed by Krafft-Ebing (1886), was based on a biological/evolutionary perspective. Krafft-Ebing considered sexual murder to be atavistic, in that it is a throwback to behavior that was common at an earlier time in the evolutionary cycle.

> The conquest over women takes place today in the social form of courting, in seduction and deception. From the history of civilization and anthropology we know that there have been times, as there are savages today that practice it, where brutal force, robbery, or even blows that made a woman powerless, were made use of to obtain love's desire. (p. 60)

The author reasoned that primitive men would force themselves on women in an effort to propagate the species. "In the intercourse of the sexes, the active or aggressive role belongs to man; woman remains passive, defensive. It affords a man great pleasure to win a woman, to conquer her" (p. 59). Thus, contemporary sexual murderers have a pathological reservoir of aggression that has become "excessively developed, and express[es] itself in an impulse to subdue absolutely the object of desire, even to destroy or kill it" (p. 60).

MacLean (1962) offered a different biological/evolutionary theory involving the development of the psychosexual functions of the human brain. This researcher referred to the "animalistic" or lower brain centers, which involve "the primitive interplay of oral, aggressive and sexual behavior" (p. 289). This oldest or most primitive part of the brain (sometimes called the R-complex or the reptilian brain) and also the slightly more developed limbic structures of the brain (amygdala) are areas that control fear and aggression. These centers are closely connected to other limbic structures governing sexual functions (septum, hippocampus). MacLean referred to male squirrel monkeys' natural display of their genitals during a fight as an example of this brain-behavior fusion occurring naturally in less advanced species. Such observations in the animal kingdom "appear to shed some light on psychiatric observations that the acts of mastering, devouring and procreating seem to be inextricably tied to one another" (p. 299). Thus, sexual murderers may have an anatomical connection between sex and aggression—in other words, a biological, rather than a psychogenic, fusion of these instincts.

Money (1990) supports a neurobiological explanation for all sexual aggression; in fact, he thinks all sexual offenders suffer from some type of nonspecific "brain disease." This author agrees with MacLean that the problem most likely lies in the older centers of the brain, including the limbic system:

> The limbic region of the brain is responsible … for predation and attack in defense of both the self and the species. In the disease of sexual sadism, the brain becomes pathologically activated to transmit messages of attack simultaneously with messages of sexual arousal and mating behavior. This pathological mix up of these messages in the brain is brought into being by faulty functioning of the brain's own chemistry. Faulty functioning may be triggered by something as grossly identifiable as brain damage resulting from the growth of a tumor, or from an open or closed head injury. Alternately, the trigger may be submicroscopic and too subtle to be easily identified on the basis of current brain scanning technology. (pp. 28–29)

Money also stresses the contribution of genetics, abnormal hormonal functioning, pathological relationships, sexual abuse, and the overlap of traditional psychiatric disorders.

Building on prior research and theory, Miller (2000) offers a neuropsycho-dynamic model of the compulsive murderer. He also contends that the problem lies in hyperactive temporal lobe/limbic mechanisms, which result from a combination of factors including biology and experience. "The predatory serial killer is literally a limbically kindled 'engine of destruction.' He won't stop and doesn't want to, because nothing in life could possibly replace the thrill of dominating and destroying another human being" (p. 158). Miller supports MacLean's notion of a fusion in the limbic areas that govern sex and aggression, but Miller believes these two drives become melded as a result not only of biology but of an abusive, hypersexualized upbringing as well.

Reid (2017b) recently reviewed various biological theories of sexual murder, beginning with the nineteenth century to the present. Her review included research on genetics, head injuries, gross structural/functional abnormalities, chromosomal anomalies, as well as other factors such as the effects of illness and exposure to toxins. The author also discussed various methodological problems with all of the theories and research findings and concluded that serial sexual homicide "is the result of a complex interplay of various organic and environmental developmental factors and that biology represents only one small part of its pathogenesis" (p. 59).

9.10 A Look to the Future

In many instances, one of the three theoretical models seems directly applicable to understanding a particular case of compulsive murder. For instance, Albert Fish, Peter Kürten, and Albert DeSalvo were all raised in terribly abusive social environments; Edmund Kemper and Edward Gein had disturbed relationships with their mothers; and Earl Nelson sustained a childhood head injury that caused brain damage. But for every case involving an abusive background, hatred of the mother, or some level of organicity, there are many other cases where these factors are totally absent. In fact, in many instances the compulsive murderer is raised in a family with other children, all with the same mother, and everyone (except the offender) turns out to be a reasonably well-adjusted citizen. Thus, the displaced-matricide theory now appears less applicable than it once did. Although disturbed (sexual) relationships with one's mother are never helpful in a child's upbringing (e.g. Schlesinger, 1999), many compulsive murderers have not had this experience, and many individuals who are abused in this way do not become sexual murderers.

Although social and psychological factors clearly play a role in compulsive murder, the biological component, as complicated as it might be, seems indispensable. In fact, the role of biology in most psychiatric and addictive disorders is paramount (Hedaya, 1996). Even general criminality has been demonstrated to have a strong biogenetic etiology (Raine, 1993; Mednick, Moffitt, and Stack, 1987), especially violent criminality (Volavka, 2002). There is a long list of well-known serial sexual murderers with a documented history of head trauma such as John Wayne Gacy (Amirante and Broderick, 2015), Henry Lee Lucas (Cox, 1991), and Albert Fish (Schechter, 1990). And Allely, Minnis, Thompson, Wilson, and Gillberg (2014) found over 20% of the serial and mass murderers they studied had suffered some type of head injury. Thus, a biological abnormality will surely be a necessary, but not a sufficient, part of any explanation of the compulsive murderer. Such an abnormality could arise from multiple factors (such as genetics, brain injury, hormones, and electrical and chemical difficulties), all of which might have an etiological role.

Within the next 50–75 years, as technology becomes more sophisticated, such an underlying neurobiological component will most likely be uncovered in the compulsive murderer. Ultimately, a biopsychosocial model, perhaps similar to an addiction model (Blanchard, 1995), that takes all three factors into account will be needed to explain compulsive murder, but it will have an indispensable neurobiological foundation (Rafter, 2000; Raine, 2014). The final theoretical model is likely to be as complex as the behavior of compulsive murderers themselves.

Because so many different things must go wrong in order for an individual to develop a compulsion to kill (multiple biological abnormalities and abusive social and psychological experiences), the incidence of compulsive, repetitive, sexually motivated murder should be low. In fact, the incidence of this type of offense is extremely low. The compulsive murderer has been present in different countries, in different cultures, and in different time periods. Compulsive murder has always been, and continues to be, a rare crime, with no evidence (contrary to popular myth) that it is increasing (Schlesinger, 2001a).

Prediction and Disposition 10

The ability of mental health professionals (MHPs) to make accurate predictions of future violence has generated an enormous amount of research, theory, and debate since the early 1970s. Initially, most researchers were pessimistic about the ability of MHPs to predict violence. They based their view on a number of studies such as the one conducted by Kozol, Boucher, and Garofalo (1972), who found that predictions of future dangerousness, even if arrived at by a team of mental health experts, were highly inaccurate. In fact, Ennis and Litwack (1974) argued that MHPs have neither a special ability nor specialized training or techniques for making violence predictions. These authors concluded that the accuracy of MHPs' predictions is not much better than that of laypeople.

Additional research, commonly known as the "Baxstrom" (Steadman and Cocozza, 1974) and the "Dixon" (Thornberry and Jacoby, 1979) studies, supported the earlier results. The investigators found that psychiatric patients who were confined for years because of a finding of dangerousness turned out not to be dangerous at all when they were eventually released. As a consequence of these and similar findings, Monahan (1981) concluded that MHPs were wrong twice as often as they were correct in their violence predictions and that, accordingly, significant changes in public policy needed to be made. However, further scrutiny uncovered a number of methodological weaknesses in what Monahan (1984) referred to as the "first generation" of research and thinking on this topic. Monahan stressed the need for a second generation of research, thought, and policy on violence prediction rather than just conducting additional studies to demonstrate the inaccuracy of MHPs in predicting future violence among mentally disordered individuals. He proposed the need to (1) study various methods of prediction, (2) use actuarial techniques that incorporate clinical information, (3) employ statistical tables on various situational factors (e.g., family, work, peer group environment), (4) study different populations of offenders, and (5) specify the time range of predictions.

Research and debate on the ability of MHPs to predict violence have continued (Menzies, Webster, McMain, Staley, and Scaglione, 1994; Monahan, 1996, 1997), with the current consensus being that some prognostic statements can, in fact, be made under some circumstances (Litwack and Schlesinger, 1987, 1999). Litwack and Schlesinger (1999) note that considerable strides have been made in research methodology, assessment of risk factors, development of actuarial risk assessment instruments, and guidelines for clinical assessment (Webster and Jackson, 1997). Although research findings and subsequent thinking have become more positive regarding the predictive ability of MHPs in comparison with the pessimistic view of the first generation of researchers, the criminal and civil justice systems have in fact never stopped relying on MHPs' violence predictions. Many statutes have even required that an MHP offer such a prediction. Borum (1996) notes:

> Despite a long-standing controversy about the ability of mental health professionals to predict violence, the courts continue to rely on them [MHPs] for advice on these issues [civil

commitment and parole recommendations] and in many cases have imposed on them a legal duty to take action when they know or should know that a patient poses a risk of serious danger to others [*Tarasoff v. Regents*, 1976]. (p. 954)

Research and thinking on dangerousness predictions continue to evolve. A recent controversy resurrects an old issue regarding the superiority of clinical vs. actuarial methods, a question initially framed by Meehl (1954) in a much different context. The debate centers on whether MHPs should use clinical judgments or statistically grounded instruments in offering their violence predictions. Quinsey, Harris, Rice, and Cormier (1999) have proposed the total replacement of clinical assessments of dangerousness with actuarial methods: "What we are advising is not the addition of actuarial methods to existing practice, but rather the complete replacement of existing practice [clinical judgments] with actuarial methods" (p. 171). These authors argue that psychometric instruments such as the "Violence Risk Appraisal Guide" (Quinsey et al., 1999) are far superior to judgments made by individual practitioners or groups of practitioners.

Although a number of researchers have taken the general position that actuarial assessments are superior to clinical assessments (Douglas, Cox, and Webster, 1999; Gottfredson, 1987), other researchers do not share this view. For example, Litwack (2001) investigated the evidence on which the purported superiority of actuarial assessments was based and found this position to be seriously flawed.

> It is frequently claimed, often as if it were hardly worth discussing, that actuarial assessments of dangerousness have proven to be superior to clinical assessments. However, the actual picture that emerges from the research is far more complex. In addition, apart from their relative merits vis-à-vis clinical assessments, far more is currently claimed regarding the utility of actuarial tools for assessing dangerousness than is merited by actual research findings. (p. 411)

In fact, Litwack concluded that not only is there little empirical support for the contention that actuarial assessments of dangerousness are superior to clinical assessments, but in some circumstances clinical assessments may actually be superior to actuarial assessments. As a practical matter, the author believes (and we strongly agree) that not only will clinical assessments of violent behavior continue, but it is "hard to imagine that the day will ever come when actuarial assessments of dangerousness can properly and completely substitute for clinical assessments" (p. 437).

The research, thinking, and debate regarding the best way to predict future violence has continued. No one is able to predict future violence (or future behavior) of an individual with a high degree of accuracy, and no one can ever guarantee an individual will or will not act out in a violent way. Accordingly, risk assessment—which is not and should never be considered a prophecy of future behavior—is an analysis of various factors in a case that can contribute to future acting out. To help in risk assessment, various risk assessment instruments have been developed, some that are very quantitative in nature (e.g., Miller, 2006) and others (e.g., Douglas, Hart, Webster, and Belfrage, 2013) that use a structured professional judgment approach. The HCR-20 (Douglas et al., 2013) encompasses static factors (behaviors in the subject's background that cannot change), as well as dynamic factors which can change (such as his response and compliance to treatment). An assessment of risk must take into account the nature, magnitude, probability, eminency, and frequency of violence. These factors, as well as response to psychotic symptoms, ability to mask or cover up symptoms, effectiveness of prior treatment, and openness with respect to discussing his history and various problems, are all important factors in predicting future violence. Predicting human behavior is exceptionally complex. There is no one method that can stand alone as being dispositive for predicting violence—all relevant factors must be taken into account. But in the final analysis, a clinical judgment by an experienced and informed mental health professional (MHP) has to be made.

10.1 Predicting Sexual Murder

In most violence-prediction research, the population studied has been mentally disordered offenders, insanity acquitees, and sex offenders. But is the research on mentally disordered offenders, or even the research on sex offenders (Barbaree and Marshall, 1988; Furby, Weinrott, and Blackshaw, 1989; Campbell, 1995; McGrath, 1991; Quinsey, Lalumiere, Rice, and Harris, 1995), applicable to other populations such as sexual murderers? Because perpetrators of sexual homicides are different from mentally disordered offenders, insanity acquitees, or sex offenders, the usefulness of the available research on violence prediction with such a very different group of subjects is questionable (Quinsey et al., 1999). Moreover, violence-prediction research has been based on individuals who have committed a violent act in the past (e.g., an assault or a sex offense) or who have made direct threats to do so. Risk assessment with the sex murderer is much more complex since this offender often has no overt mental disorder, usually does not make threats, and, in many cases, may not have any history of interpersonal violence. Hill, Rettenberger, and Haberman (2012) found that typical risk assessment instruments used in predicting risk with traditional sex offenders do not have predictive validity with sexual murderers. In addition, sexual murder is a very low base-rate crime, so comparatively few cases are available for checking the accuracy of predictions. Even when a potential offender is identified, perhaps by his expression of a fantasy or urge to commit a sexual homicide (e.g., Johnson and Becker, 1997), the murder itself may not occur for many years, perhaps even as many as 20 or 30 years in some cases (Revitch, 1965).

Individuals who have already committed a compulsive homicide have an extremely high risk for repetition. Over the years many authors have cited countless examples of such recidivism. For example, Guttmacher (1963) reported the case of a 40-year-old man who served 13 years in prison for killing and mutilating a prostitute. Shortly after his release, he was arrested again for attacking another prostitute in a similar manner. After serving a relatively brief term for this assault, he was paroled, only to then kill and behead another prostitute. Kozol, Cohen, and Garofalo (1966) reported the case of two young brothers who were sexually attacked and murdered by a man who had just been released from prison after having served a 10-year sentence for a similar sexual attack on a young boy. More recently, Ressler and Schachtman (1992) described the case of Arthur Shawcross, who killed 11 women, many of whom were prostitutes. These acts were carried out after the offender had served 14 years in prison for the sexual murder of an 8-year-old girl. Shawcross also admitted to killing a young boy, but for some reason the case was not prosecuted. In fact, it is rather rare for a sexual murderer to not have had prior contact with the criminal justice system in some way.

These types of repetitive sexual attacks and murders are by no means rare and have, over the years, served as a basis for many laws regulating the incarceration and discharge of potentially dangerous sexual offenders. As a consequence, many researchers (e.g., Douglas and Olshaker, 1995; Ressler and Schachtman, 1992; Revitch and Schlesinger, 1981, 1989) have concluded that the probability of an individual committing another compulsive murder after he has already committed one compulsive sexually motivated homicide is extremely high despite an absence of mental illness, good prison adjustment, high intelligence, denial of current sexually aggressive fantasies, and a display of good insight in psychotherapy. In fact, one could even add to this list of insignificant positive indicators "good scores" on various actuarial assessments purported to predict future violence (Quinsey et al., 1999). Because the type of violence in these cases is so malignant, it is not difficult to offer a prediction of future dangerousness in someone who has already acted out in this manner.

Potential sex murderers (those who have not yet acted out but who present serious concerns) constitute a much larger group of individuals for whom risk assessment is not only critical but even more complex. Not only is the offense a very low base-rate crime, but, as noted in Chapter 8, many studies indicate that the number of individuals who harbor sexually aggressive fantasies is much larger than the population of actual offenders. Therefore, in attempts to identify those who might commit such rare crimes, especially when there is no history of such behavior, the likelihood of false positives is understandably high. However, as Mulvey and Lidz (1995) note, concerns about high false positives are misplaced. These authors believe, and we strongly agree, that risk assessments should be reconceptualized as "clinical concerns" about a person's possible future violence, not necessarily as specific predictions that the person will act out. This view is consistent with that offered years earlier by Tanay (1975), who drew a distinction between a behavioral tendency and an exact prediction:

> The concept of prediction requires some elucidation and definition. The description of a behavioral tendency (propensity, proclivity) does not constitute a prophecy of an event. A tendency is a readiness to engage in specified behavior which is inferred from observational or historical data about the patient. ... The description of a tendency is frequently confused with prediction of the occurrence of a future event like homicide or suicide. (p. 23)

Although empirical validation of various red flags or ominous signs is highly desirable, this type of research is extremely difficult to carry out with the sex murderer and potential sex murderer, as noted in Chapter 1. But to say that we know so little about a sexual homicide that some type of prognostic statement cannot be offered to MHPs, the court, law enforcement, governmental agencies, and others who are involved with such potentially dangerous individuals is simply incorrect. In fact, the majority (6–3) of members of the U.S. Supreme Court reached a similar conclusion, in a somewhat different context, when they addressed the issue of dangerousness predictions in *Barefoot v. Estelle* (1983):

> There is no merit to petitioner's argument that psychiatrists [or MHPs], individually and as a group, are incompetent to predict with an acceptable degree of reliability that a particular criminal will commit other crimes in the future and so represent[s] a danger to the community. To accept such an argument would call into question other contexts in which predictions of future behavior are constantly made. ... The suggestion that no [MHP's] testimony may be presented with respect to a defendant's future dangerousness is somewhat like asking us to disinvent the wheel. ... If it is not impossible for even a lay person sensibly to arrive at that conclusion, it makes little sense, if any, to submit that [MHPs], out of the entire universe

of persons who might have an opinion on the issue, would know so little about this subject that they should not be permitted to testify. (pp. 14–16)

The prediction of a sexual homicide is based on two general considerations: (1) for those offenders who have already committed a murder, the offense must be placed along the motivational spectrum, as outlined in Chapter 3; and (2) for those individuals who have not committed a homicide, the presence, in considerable combination, of ominous signs that have been found in the backgrounds of individuals who have already committed a sexual homicide needs to be identified and evaluated.

10.1.1 Prediction Based on the Motivational Spectrum

The motivational spectrum as outlined in Chapter 3 serves as a device not only for classifying crime (including homicide) but also for predicting future violence on the basis of an analysis of the antisocial act already committed. The motivational stimuli are spectrally distributed, with purely exogenous (or sociogenic) stimuli on one end of the scale and purely endogenous (or psychogenic) stimuli on the extreme opposite end. Thus, the offenses are divided into (1) environmental or social, (2) situational, (3) impulsive, (4) catathymic, and (5) compulsive. The external sociogenic factors play less and less of a role as one approaches the other end of the spectrum occupied by the compulsive offenses, which are almost entirely internally driven. Offenses that result from paranoid, organic, or toxic states form a group of their own apart from the motivational spectrum. If an individual commits a homicide as a direct result of one of these psychiatric conditions, such as in response to command hallucinations or delusions, the likelihood of recommitting the offense is reduced if the offender is relieved of these symptoms.

Situational murders constitute the majority of all homicides and have the best chances of not being repeated. Wolfgang (1958) found that murders stemming from domestic disputes (which are basically situational) are unlikely to occur again. Halleck (1978) further noted that in situationally stimulated homicides the offender is no longer a threat the moment the murder has taken place. Tanay (1975) also echoed this view: "The overwhelming majority of homicide[s] … are of the interpersonal variety, where the dissolution of the conflict-ridden relationship terminates the [future] homicidal risk" (p. 17).

The fate of the environmentally (or socially) stimulated offender depends largely on his opportunities, associations, level of maturity and value system, and particularly the setting he returns to following the crime or after a period of incarceration. A person who, for example, commits a cult or contract murder (or what Miller and Looney (1974) referred to as an act that was socially and interpersonally validated) will behave similarly if the same social pressures or influences affect him in the same way they did previously.

The impulsive offender's lifestyle is characterized by unpredictability, spontaneity, and multiple antisocial actions. In most cases, he lacks the capacity to modulate emotional stimulation and acts out accordingly. Thus, the impulsive offender who commits a murder may continue in various criminal activities, but these acts will not necessarily be of a homicidal nature.

Individuals who have already committed a sexual murder, either catathymic or compulsive, have a much higher potential for repetition than the environmentally, situationally, or impulsively stimulated offender because a sexual murder is not a reaction to circumstances but stems from internal psychogenic sources. Most catathymic homicides are one-time incidents. However, in several cases the catathymic offender after years of incarceration committed another catathymic murder when similar unresolved conflicts were again ignited. Therefore, if the underlying (sexual) conflicts that fueled a catathymic homicide are not resolved, possibly by the murder itself or through some type of intervention, the likelihood for repetition is high.

The type of offender who clearly has the worst prognosis is the individual who has already committed a compulsive sexually motivated murder. These individuals do not kill in response to hallucinations or because of social influence, circumstantial pressure, or even the triggering of unresolved sexual conflicts that overwhelm their psychic homeostasis. Compulsive murderers have a need to kill that drives them to seek out victims. Consequently, they are the most dangerous and present the highest risk for repetition.

10.1.2 Prediction Based on Ominous Signs

Experience with sexual murderers, particularly compulsive murderers, reveals some common characteristics in their backgrounds and prehomicidal behaviors. Therefore, the presence of such signs should serve as a red flag or should raise what Mulvey and Lidz (1995) refer to as "clinical concerns" about the likelihood that such individuals will commit a sexually motivated compulsive murder in the future. Schlesinger (2001b) has described ten such ominous signs to be used as a guideline for practitioners confronting potential sex murderers. Although not yet empirically grounded, these signs can provide a direction for research with this relatively small criminal population. In fact, Douglas et al. (1999) have pointed out the heuristic benefit of this type of clinical finding; they call for a "collaboration among researchers and clinicians [where it is hoped their partnership will] benefit some patients, convicted persons, and even young children inclined towards early aggression and violence" (p. 149).

The usual signs and behaviors that the violence-prediction research has focused on—mental disorder, threats, prior violence—are not applicable to the potential compulsive sex murderer. Compulsive murderers rarely have a major psychiatric disorder like an overt psychosis (Meloy, 2000; Revitch, 1965; Revitch and Schlesinger, 1981, 1989; Schlesinger, 2000a). In fact, Meloy (2000) notes that "with few exceptions … most sexual homicide perpetrators are not psychotic and do not have a diagnosable psychotic disorder if evaluated" (p. 7). In addition, as Rappeport (1967) has pointed out, most psychotics, contrary to popular belief, are not particularly prone to commit homicide and are rarely assaultive.

Unlike psychiatric patients who are involuntarily committed because they have made a threat to commit violence, compulsive murderers rarely threaten to kill. Unfortunately, the important relationship between threats to kill and carrying out such warnings has rarely been studied except for some early work by MacDonald (1963, 1967, 1968). In one of the few studies of its kind, MacDonald (1967) found that out of 100 patients admitted to a psychiatric hospital because of homicidal threats, four committed suicide, and only three committed homicide in a 5- to 6-year follow-up. Thus, there seems to be a connection between homicidal threats and suicide as well as homicide, a finding substantiated by Rhine and Mayerson (1973). In any case, relatively rarely does an individual who makes a homicidal threat carry out the act. In cases of compulsive murder, the problem is compounded since these offenders keep their fantasies private and typically do not directly notify others of their inner thoughts.

Moreover, many compulsive murderers have a history neither of interpersonal violence nor of the usual sex crimes and sexual offenses. If a community is terrorized by a series of sex murders or sex assaults, the police often target known sex offenders—most who are child molesters—who have been recently released. However, for many years researchers (Brancale, Ellis, and Doorbar, 1952; Brancale, McNeil, and Vuocolo, 1965; Guttmacher, 1963) have found that most sex offenders are passive, inadequate individuals who may repeat their specific crime but rarely commit a sexual murder. In fact, Revitch (1965) found that only 3 out of 43 (6%) violent sex offenders and sex murderers had a previous history of sexual crimes. Other than fetishism (which is generally not a crime) and voyeurism (which can be a crime but is often considered a misdemeanor), most of the sex murderers described in this book did not have a history of traditional sex offenses. In some cases individuals do commit sex crimes and escalate their acting out until it culminates in sexual murder. But these cases are not typical; most rapists, for example, do not go on to kill their victims (Groth, 1979; Podolsky, 1966; Ressler, Burgess, and Douglas, 1983).

The ten ominous signs that Schlesinger (2001b) described are listed in order of increasing prognostic significance (see Table 10.1). Early in the list are disturbed childhood experiences of abuse and inappropriate maternal (sexual) conduct. Childhood sexual abuse, which is quite prevalent in nonclinical, psychiatric, and other criminal populations, has a little discriminate capacity and therefore accrues little weight. As the list of behaviors advances from maternal sexual conduct to pathological lying to animal cruelty, more serious forms of acting out are involved. These escalating forms of disturbed behavior are typically found in the histories of compulsive murderers, and they accrue more significance accordingly. Firesetting, sexual burglary, unprovoked attacks on women, and ritualistic behavior are increasingly more ominous and therefore should be assigned the most prognostic weight.

In making a prediction, as in arriving at a diagnosis, specific signs, symptoms, behaviors, and test results are usually not sufficient. In the final analysis, clinical judgment must be exercised. As Douglas et al. (2013) have noted, the risk of future violence depends on numerous factors including types of supervision, treatment, motivation to live a noncriminal life and whether the individual will experience adverse life events (Otto, 2000). Malamuth (1986) found predictions of future sexual violence should be based on a dynamic interaction of various indicators, rather than on the static summation of them. Malamuth also argued that the assessments should be placed on a continuum of degrees of inclination to act aggressively. In fact, the statistical cookbook-like approach (Borum, 1996) may

Table 10.1 Ominous Signs (When Seen in Combination) Indicate Risk for a Potential Sex Murderer

- Childhood abuse
- Inappropriate maternal (sexual) conduct
- Pathological lying and manipulation
- Sadistic fantasy with a compulsion to act
- Animal cruelty, particularly toward cats
- Need to control and dominate others
- Repetitive firesetting
- Voyeurism, fetishism, and sexual burglary
- Unprovoked attacks on females, associated with generalized misogynous emotions
- Evidence of ritualistic (signature) behavior

Source: From Schlesinger, L.B., *Journal of Threat Assessment, 1*, 2001, p. 50. With permission.

miss the essence of the subject (Grubin, 1997). Psychometric measures used to help predict future sex crimes—standardized with traditional (nonhomicidal) sex offenders (Witt, Del Russo, Oppenheim, and Ferguson, 1996)—may be of value, particularly when used in conjunction with the ten ominous signs. However, the clinician needs to remain aware that traditional sex offenders are very different from sexual murderers. Moreover, Litwack and Schlesinger (1999) argue:

> The distinction between actuarial [cookbook] and clinical assessments is blurring to the point where there is often no meaningful distinction between the two. For example, good clinical assessment routinely takes into account such actuarial predictors as a history of violence; conversely, the most powerful actuarial predictor in recent studies—the PCL-R [Hare, 1991] score—is, in significant part, a clinical variable. (p. 188)

While the ten ominous signs described in detail in the following sections have not been empirically validated as a group, it is hard to believe that an individual who has engaged in this type of conduct is headed for a good adjustment in later life. Perhaps the person who commits sexual burglaries, sets fires, kills cats, attacks females in an unprovoked manner, and displays some ritualistic behavior may not commit a sexually motivated murder. However, these behaviors in and of themselves (notwithstanding the lack of empirical predictive validity) certainly should raise a major red flag and require some form of intervention. We hope that future efforts will be aimed at validating and weighing the significance of the ten ominous signs. In the meantime, however, clinical judgments and clinical concerns should be expressed without fear of making some false-positive predictions, which are to be expected under the circumstances. With this group of offenders, a false-negative prediction can be particularly devastating and should not be rationalized on the basis of lack of statistical verification.

10.1.2.1 Childhood Abuse

The prevalence of childhood abuse in the general (i.e., nonpsychiatric and noncriminal) male population is much higher than commonly believed. Lisak, Hopper, and Song (1996) surveyed a nonclinical population of approximately 600 college men to determine the incidence of abuse in the male population. They phrased questionnaires carefully to eliminate ambiguity, to ensure anonymity, and to increase the likelihood of accuracy in responses. The researchers found that 18% of their sample reported sexual abuse (involving direct contact) by age 16; when noncontact sexual abuse was included, the figure rose to 28%. Moreover, 34% of these men also reported a history of nonsexual physical abuse. The onset of sexual abuse was at about 10 to 15 years; physical abuse began earlier, at about 7 years. Also, 36% of those who were sexually abused reported the use of force, intimidation, or threats in conjunction with the abuse. Most of the men who were sexually abused were victimized by other men (61%), but 28% were abused by women. The majority of the sexual abuse (79%) was extrafamilial, while most of the physical abuse (79%) came from a family member.

Although the prevalence of abuse among men in general is rather high, the prevalence of abuse among sexual murderers is even higher. In fact, Ressler et al. (1988) found that every one of the 36 sexual murderers they studied had a history of some type of severe abuse or neglect. It is seen that 43% of their subjects had been victims of sexual abuse, and 73% had been party to sexually stressful events such as witnessing sexual violence or sexual activity of a parent or receiving harsh punishment for engaging in sexual activities such as masturbation. In fact, Ressler, Burgess, Hartman, and Douglas (1986) noted that sex murderers who had a history of sexual abuse had more serious sexual deviations such as zoophilia, fantasized about rape at a younger age, and often mutilated their victims in contrast with sex murderers who did not have such a history. Myers and Blashfield (1997) noted similar findings: 93% of their sample of 14 juvenile sexual murderers had chaotic families, 69% reported having experienced physical abuse, 62% emotional abuse, and 15% sexual abuse. In a study by Dietz, Hazelwood, and Warren (1990) of 30 sexually sadistic offenders—22 of whom had committed at least one murder—about 20% self-reported a history of physical abuse, and about 50% self-reported sexual abuse. And Prentky, Knight, Sims-Knight, and Straus (1989) found that 90% of offenders who used extreme sexual aggression in their criminal acts had backgrounds of abuse and came from families where sexual deviations were common.

Some studies, however, have uncovered somewhat contradictory results. For example, Gratzer and Bradford (1995) and Meloy (1997) did not find physical or sexual abuse to be that frequent in their sample of sadistic murderers. However, it is hard to understand why the prevalence of abuse among a sample of compulsive murderers would be lower than that of the general population. This finding raises the important issue of the truthfulness of self-reported incidences of abuse, especially among a population of sadistic murderers who, as noted consistently throughout the literature, are notorious liars. In some instances, abuse can be verified and documented, but in most cases researchers must rely solely on the offender's self-report. Therefore, the low incidence of abuse reported by some subjects may not reflect the absence of abuse but may instead reflect a lack of truthfulness, especially in those subjects who were particularly sadistic in their criminal conduct. The markedly sadistic compulsive murderer often likes to appear in control and dominant and may not want to be seen as weak, submissive, or victimized. Notwithstanding the results of these few studies, we generally agree with Myers (2002) who found that "the family background of the sexual homicide perpetrator is usually marred by irresponsible, abusive parenting, and an unstable, impoverished childhood" (p. 28).

Being abused has consistently been found to be unhelpful in a person's development. Recent research by Widom and Massey (2015) has found that being a victim of childhood sexual abuse and its relationship to future sex offending is more complex than previously thought. Although every abused individual may not experience major deleterious effects, researchers found many abuse victims to have significant problems in contrast to people who have not been abused: lower levels of empathy (Miller and Eisenberg, 1988), increased aggressive acting out (Vanderkolk, 1989), more suicide attempts (Cavaiola and Schiff, 1988), more antisocial personalities (Luntz and Widom, 1994), and more general criminality (Widom, 1989a, 1989b). James, Proulx, and Lussier (2018) reviewed a cross-cultural sample of sexual murderers and found a background of childhood victimization (physical, psychological, sexual) occurred anywhere from 32% to 67%. There is a long list of compulsive murderers who have experienced various forms of childhood abuse. For instance, Albert DeSalvo was subjected to cruel punishment by his violent father, who had sexual relations with prostitutes in front of family members and sold his children to work as farm laborers (Rae, 1967). The notorious Albert Fish was raised in an orphanage where he was regularly subjected to severe beatings, often while naked, in front of other children (Schechter, 1990). Henry Lee Lucas reported a brutal upbringing; he said he was "treated like what I call the dog of the family. I was beaten. I was made to do things that no human bein' would want to do" (quoted in Schechter and Everitt, 1996, p. 294). In cases such as those of Ted Bundy and Jeffrey Dahmer, a history of sexual abuse was strongly suspected but was difficult to document and even more difficult to corroborate (Fox and Levin, 1994).

10.1.2.2 Inappropriate Maternal (Sexual) Conduct

The strange relationship between some sexual murderers and their mothers was first pointed out by Krafft-Ebing (1886). He described the case of Vincenz Verzeni who, after killing a woman, hid part of the victim's body in a haystack "for fear his mother would suspect him" (p. 66). Revitch (1965) noted that a disturbed sexualized relationship an offender has with his mother contributes to his crimes. This author argued that the future offender develops ambivalent feelings involving both a hostile and sexualized relationship with his mother that is transferred to other women.

> The common denominator behind all enumerated factors leading to transfer of hostility from mother to womanhood is believed to be the struggle with an attempt at rejection of repressed incestuous wishes. These wishes are stimulated by maternal over-protection, seductiveness, and sexual promiscuity. This may be coupled with either father's brutality, weakness, or unavailability. Outright maternal rejection may create a need to possess her. (p. 643)

Meloy (2000) finds that an offender's rage against his mother is a "product of a lack of differentiation from the mother when the perpetrator was a boy. Many social factors could contribute to this, including aggression, dominance, control, manipulation, or sexualization by the mother" (p. 14). Liebert (1985) believes that aggressive aspects of the early mother–son relationship are internalized and then projected onto a female victim.

Brittain (1970) notes that the sadistic murderer often harbors "a deep hatred for [his mother], not superficially obvious and not always acknowledged even to himself ... [he] often tells of having, as a child, seen his mother undressed" (p. 202). Brittain described these men as having "a strong ambivalent relationship to [their] mother[s], of loving her and hating her. He is ... emotionally closely bound to her, bringing her gifts to a degree beyond the ordinary. He is a 'mother's boy' even when adult" (p. 202).

The offender's mother may be rejecting, punitive and hated, or she may be overprotective, infantalizing, and seductive. Brittain (1970) provides insight into the personalities of some mothers of offenders; he found them to be

> pleasant, very motherly, kindly persons, distressed by the murder the son had committed but remaining devoted to him. Later, it is sometimes found that when they come to visit [their sons], they bring books or magazines, and when these are examined they are found to deal with matters of a sadistic, criminal or pornographic nature. (p. 202)

Revitch and Schlesinger (1989) emphasized the image and behavior of the mother in the psychosexual development of adolescent males. Adolescent boys more than adolescent girls need to have a nonsexual view of their mothers, and the notion that the mother might be sexually promiscuous can be destabilizing for such youngsters. "For some reason, possibly cultural, a boy's perception of his mother's infidelity and sexual looseness is far more traumatic than a girl's perception of the same behavior in the father" (p. 108).

In some cases incestuous feelings are markedly overt and are not displaced; here, the mother may become the victim. For example, Schlesinger (1999) reported the case of a

16-year-old who committed a sexual matricide including vaginal and anal necrophilia following about 8 years of mother–son incest. Edmund Kemper (Strentz and Hassel, 1970) also had a disturbed relationship with his mother, who treated him with cruelty accompanied by sexual innuendos. Kemper went on to kill six women, some of whom he decapitated and cannibalized. He finally killed his mother, cut out her larynx, and threw it in the garbage disposal. Following the matricide, Kemper called the police and turned himself in. Bobby Joe Long (Hunter, 2017) slept in his mother's bed until he was a teenager and resented her numerous boyfriends. He subsequently tortured and killed ten women in fairly rapid sequence. In many other cases (e.g., Scherl and Mack, 1966; Wertham, 1941), adolescents became so enraged at their mothers' sexual indiscretions that matricide resulted.

In some young men anger toward their mothers is displaced and becomes an obvious cause for a subsequent sexual attack or murder. For instance, Revitch (1980) reported the case of an 11-year-old boy who made multiple attempts to choke little girls. Under the influence of sodium amytal, he revealed witnessing his mother having sex with various men. This boy was sexually preoccupied and made disparaging remarks about his mother's conduct. "Choking girls, he said, made him feel glad" (p. 9). Revitch (1980) described another case of a 14-year-old who beat, choked, and stabbed a 10-year-old girl. He expressed dislike for all girls and had a fantasy of his mother's sexual purity and lack of sexual relations, even with his father.

Johnson and Becker (1997) reported the following case: A youngster

> recalled his mother being very sexually provocative throughout his youth, exposing herself to him or watching him undress and making erotic comments. His parents once engaged in sexual intercourse in front of him, and he recalled his mother moaning in what he felt was a haunting and deathlike manner. (p. 339)

At age 14, this youngster began to fantasize about having sexual relations with his mother; the fantasy involved listening to her moan, killing her, and then engaging in necrophilia. He masturbated about eight times a day, using his mother's underwear as a fantasy aid. At age 17, he killed a woman by strangulation and had sex with the corpse for 3 days following her death. Lauerman (2001) reports an interesting case of a 36-year-old male with Klinefelter's syndrome who blamed his mother for his physically poor sexual development, including undescended testicles. He had long-standing urges to damage female genitals and eventually committed a sexual homicide by strangulation.

10.1.2.3 Pathological Lying and Manipulation

Lying is a ubiquitous phenomenon. In Ford's (1996) comprehensive review of multiple studies of lying and deceit, he found that about 90% of the general population admitted to frequent lying, especially about their true feelings, income, accomplishments, sex life, and age; lying was also prevalent in dating relationships, the workplace, advertisements, politics, and even science and the practice of medicine under some circumstances. Therefore, it is not surprising that criminals also lie and do so even more frequently than the general population. In fact, lying and manipulation are common characteristics of individuals with antisocial and conduct disorders. Here, the lying is frequently used as a means of escaping responsibility for wrongdoing.

For the potential sex murderer, lying serves a different function. The compulsive murderer lies not only as the average person or typical criminal does but also specifically to achieve a sense of control, domination, and mastery over others (Douglas and Olshaker, 1995). Sexual murderers frequently lie and manipulate when they do not have to, and sometimes the desire to put something over on someone is so strong that they manipulate even when it is to their ultimate disadvantage. Bursten (1972) found that many individuals have a "manipulative personality" involving a fragile narcissism along with contempt for people. Such a person tries to "influence others by employing a deception of some sort, and [has] a feeling of exhilaration at having put something over on the other person if the deception is successful" (p. 319). Bursten believes that these individuals are "driven to manipulate as a lifestyle" (p. 319) and argues that

> it is the manipulation itself which is the primary goal of the manipulative personality, and the fact that a manipulation may not work, or may lead to punishment may have no more effect on his need to manipulate than the inconvenience of promptness may have on the needs of the obsessive compulsive personality. (p. 318)

Blatant and persistent pathological lying and manipulation by compulsive murderers have been described by Krafft-Ebing (1886) as well as by Brittain (1970). Krafft-Ebing noted that offenders lied when they were caught, tried to cast suspicion on others, and had a long history of lying and manipulation. Brittain found that many of his subjects were convinced that they could "escape detection by being more clever than the police" (p. 199). Meloy (2000) also notes that offenders who have a narcissistic or psychopathic personality—primarily those who plan their murders in detail—are most prone to deceptiveness and manipulation.

Researchers have not focused on lying and manipulation directly among sexual murderers, probably because lying and manipulation in various sex murder cases are secondary to these offenders' more striking behaviors such as manifestations of sadistic fantasy and intricate MOs. However, Ressler et al. (1988) found that 75% of their subjects self-reported lying constantly as adolescents and 68% as adults. Myers and his associates (1998) also found that almost all their juvenile sexual murderers had a diagnosis of conduct disorder, which presumably would involve various forms of repetitive lying and deceptiveness, although this conclusion was not explicitly stated. Recent research by James, Lussier, and Proulx (2018) compared serial and nonserial sexual murderers on a number of background characteristics and found 40% of serial offenders, compared to 17.8% of nonserial offenders, evidenced chronic lying in their histories.

Lying, manipulation, and deception begin in childhood and develop in adolescence when the future compulsive murderer hones his technique. As an adult, he lies and manipulates with ease and uses his skill to obtain victims. Many compulsive murderers have engaged in deceit and manipulation in order to abduct victims, as well as to redirect the criminal investigation. Harvey Glatman (Nash, 1973), for example, placed ads in newspapers for female models who allowed him to tie them up under the pretext of being photographed for detective magazines. Once Glatman had the women bound, he overpowered and killed them. Albert Fish (Schechter, 1990) cleverly abducted a 12-year-old girl by telling the child's parents he was taking her to a birthday party organized by his sister. And Ted Bundy (Rule, 1988) placed a fake cast on his arm so that potential victims would believe he was disabled and not a threat. Even when apprehended, these offenders typically continue to lie to attorneys, experts, judges, and police, even long after their conviction and in some cases right up to their execution. The extremely devious Trevor Hardy filed his teeth so authorities could not match bite marks found on a victim's body. He was so manipulative that he was released from custody several times, only to commit more offenses (Wilson, Tolputt, Howe, and Kemp, 2010). Their need to lie, manipulate, and con others seems almost insatiable. As one offender's father said, "Don't believe anything he tells you. Don't even believe when he tells you what he had for lunch. He is not capable of telling the truth. He lies about absolutely everything."

10.1.2.4 Sadistic Fantasy with a Compulsion to Act

The importance of sadistic fantasy as an indication of a potential sex murderer cannot be overstated. Individuals who commit compulsive homicides do not develop sadistic fantasies weeks or even months prior to acting out; instead, the fantasies begin in childhood, and the offenders remain deeply immersed in these inner thoughts for most of their lives. Fantasies typically involve themes of control, domination, revenge, and sexually sadistic aggression. The fantasies of those who plan their crimes with some level of sophistication are usually detailed and intricate. The compulsive murderer who commits unplanned crimes also harbors fantasies, but these are much less differentiated and more global. Myers, Husted, Safarik, and O'Toole (2006) concluded that the main motivating force in serial sexual homicide is "pursuit of sadistic pleasure" (p. 900).

Ressler et al. (1988) found that sexual murderers' sadistic fantasies "begin in childhood, [and] develop and progress until … these men are motivated to murder by way of their thinking" (p. 34). In some cases, "what begins in fantasy may end as part of a homicidal ritual" (Ressler and Shachtman, 1992, p. 99). Ressler and Shachtman (1992) cite the case of a man who, as a child, pulled the heads off Barbie dolls; as an adult, he decapitated his female victims. Another individual chased a friend with a hatchet during childhood; as an adult he used a hatchet to murder a woman.

Johnson and Becker (1997) described the homicidal fantasies of nine adolescents who expressed the desire to commit sadistic murders. One subject admitted to fantasizing about killing humans and had recurrent thoughts of rape involving strangulation, necrophilia, and mutilation. He also fantasized about keeping sexual organs and skulls. Another subject fantasized about killing many people, disemboweling them, playing with the viscera, and eating part of the corpses. One young man reported fantasies of tarring and feathering people and of tying victims to trees and cutting and peeling off their skin with a knife while they were still alive. Still others fantasized two to three times a day about killing humans by shooting them; by cutting off their fingers, toes, and limbs while alive; or by committing mass murder.

How, if one's thoughts are private, can we know that an individual, especially an adolescent, is having sexually violent fantasies? Frequently, adolescents reveal their fantasy life through their drawings and writings, as well as their interest in weapons, war criminals, Nazi atrocities, or hard-core pornography. Brittain (1970) noticed an interest in sadistic pornography in his cases. He found his subjects used fantasy aids such as military or soldier-of-fortune magazines portraying "scantily clad young females in danger or distress; words such as sin, lust, sex, nude, death, virile, vice, satan, devil, etc. The sadistic man may have made additions to the pictures, for example, manacles may be drawn on the wrists" (p. 203).

In addition to an interest in hard-core pornography, war, captivity, prisons, and dungeons, the potential compulsive murderer may have a particular interest in detective magazines. Detective magazines are filled with descriptions and pictures of actual sexual homicides and sexually motivated crimes. Detective magazines frequently have advertisements focused on their readership. For instance, there are ads on how to become a locksmith (with the ability to order locksmith tools and picks), as well as offering courses on criminal investigative methods. Dietz, Harry, and Hazelwood (1986) found that detective magazines serve as a fantasy aid for compulsive murderers. In addition, detective magazines are, in some sense, how-to manuals for committing a sexual homicide. The magazine articles provide details of criminal investigations and mistakes the offenders made that resulted in their apprehension. Sometimes the stories provide an idea for the fledgling compulsive murderer, such as taking photographs of the crime scene. Detective magazines report not only recent crimes but also notorious crimes from the past, especially those with intricate and clever MOs. One young offender's mother commented during an evaluation, precipitated by the adolescent's unprovoked attacks on female classmates, that her son collected detective magazines. "I'm glad he is not into pornography; maybe he wants to go into law enforcement because he reads detective magazines all the time." This mother reflected the typical uninformed view of many who do not recognize the significance of detective magazines as an indication of emerging criminal fantasies. Detective magazines have now either ceased publication or have a broader scope of the types of crimes they cover. With the internet, individuals can now find much of this material online.

The number of individuals who have sadistic fantasies is much larger than the small subgroup of those who act the fantasies out. Nevertheless, any indication of the presence of such disturbed fantasies should still be considered a strong red flag. Some individuals have entertained sadistic fantasies for over 30 years before eventually acting on them, as reported by Revitch (1957, 1965). Accordingly, Johnson and Becker (1997) advise that "adolescents who demonstrate sexually sadistic fantasies, especially of a violent nature that end in killing, should be 'red flagged,' followed closely, and offered treatment to help extinguish or combat the deviant fantasy before it becomes a reality" (p. 346).

10.1.2.5 Animal Cruelty, Particularly toward Cats

MacDonald (1963) was the first to observe the relationship of childhood enuresis, firesetting, and animal cruelty to sadistic behavior as an adult. The first empirical study of the triad, which was carried out by Hellman and Blackman (1966), seemed to lend support to MacDonald's clinical observations. Additional research into the triad has generated a variety of findings, depending on the subject populations (Felthous and Bernard, 1979; Justice, Justice, and Kraft, 1974; Wax and Haddox, 1974a, 1974b). Persistent enuresis by itself is not very significant since it is found in those with a wide range of psychiatric conditions having little to do with violence. But animal cruelty—seen alone or in combination with firesetting—is a significant indicator of major problems brewing.

Adults who act in a sadistic manner toward humans almost always have a history of having committed sadistic acts toward animals. Krafft-Ebing (1886) noted that a number of his subjects who committed sexual murders as adults displayed cruelty toward animals as children. For example, Vincenz Verzeni "noticed, when he was 12 years old, that he experienced a peculiar feeling of pleasure while wringing the necks of chickens. After this, he had often killed great numbers of them" (p. 67). Another of Krafft-Ebing's cases, Sergeant Bertrand (a necrophiliac who mutilated bodies subsequent to having sex with them) was also cruel to animals as a child: "He would cut open the abdomen [of animals], tear out the entrails, and masturbate during the act" (p. 69).

The empirical research on the relationship of animal cruelty in general, and cruelty to cats in particular, is scant and suffers from methodological problems such as small sample size and reliance on self-report. Among Johnson and Becker's (1997) subjects, 44% reported severe animal cruelty. One child shot, drowned, stabbed, or set on fire various animals, sometimes injuring or killing ten animals a day. Another youngster felt sexual arousal after dissecting animals once he killed them; he kept many of their skulls as trophies in his bedroom. Another killed dogs by snapping their necks while they were alive; still another killed snakes and rabbits and searched for road kill, as he enjoyed looking at the dead animals' organs or cutting them open. Myers, Burgess, and Nelson (1998) found that 4 out of 14 (28%) of their group of adolescents who committed a sexual murder had a history of animal cruelty. Wright and Hensley (2003) reported five cases of sexual murderers who killed cats as children and then humans as adults. Gleyzer, Felthous, and Holzer (2002) found a relationship between childhood animal cruelty and later adult antisocial conduct (in a sample of 48 subjects), but animal cruelty was not related to psychosis, mental retardation, or alcohol abuse.

A number of compulsive murderers not only killed animals but tortured them as well. For example, Peter Kürten (Wilson and Pitman, 1962) became friendly with a sadistic dog catcher who tortured dogs. During Kürten's adolescence, he had sex with animals while stabbing them. Ressler and Shachtman (1992) reported the case of a compulsive murderer who, as a child, cut a dog's stomach open to see how far it could run before dying. Revitch and Schlesinger (1989) also reported the case of a sadistic compulsive murderer who, from an early age, tortured animals. He cut off cows' udders, inserted lit firecrackers into horses' rectums, and enjoyed watching these animals in pain. Brittain (1970) also observed extreme animal cruelty in the childhood backgrounds of sadistic murderers. "Such cruelty is particularly significant when it is related to cats, dogs, birds, and farm animals" (p. 202). Felthous and Keller (1987) advise those who treat or observe children "to be alert to the particularly ominous significance of this behavior [animal cruelty] in childhood and the advisability of concerned, helpful intervention" (p. 716).

Revitch and Schlesinger (1981, 1989), Schlesinger and Revitch (1997b), and Davis and Schlesinger (2016) noted that cruelty to cats, in particular, was in the backgrounds of individuals who committed compulsive homicides. Perhaps this is because cats are a female symbol more than other animals such as dogs, and they arouse anger in the potential sex murderer. Lockwood (2005) noted that "cats were associated with femininity, fertility, and sensuality in ancient religions. … Many cultures have equated promiscuous sexuality with cats" (pp. 17–18). Tapia (1971) found that out of 18 subjects with a history of violence, only one had not hurt a cat. Felthous (1980) concluded from his research on animal cruelty that

> cats more than dogs seem to induce a child's sadistic projections and cruel behavior. A number of subjects in this study who had tortured cats admitted an intense dislike of this animal, in particular, but disclosed no insight into the animosity. (p. 175)

Revitch (1978) reported the case of an adolescent who set cats on fire and experienced a euphoric feeling while watching them burn. He compared cats to women, observing similarities in their looks and behavior. Ressler and Shachtman (1992) described two serial murderers who had tortured cats when they were children. One individual "attached cherry bombs to cats' legs and made many cats in his neighborhood three-legged" (p. 96).

Albert DeSalvo, the Boston Strangler, tortured cats during his childhood, and described his attitude on this topic:

> I don't like cats. ... I used to shoot cats with a bow and arrow, put it right through their belly, and sometimes they ran with the arrow right through them, yowling, and I don't recall being too upset by that. ... Sometimes when I would see them, before the shoot, I'd get such a feeling of anger that I think I could tear those cats apart with my bare hands. I don't understand this, but just that I hated them and they had done nothing to me. (quoted in Rae, 1967, p. 61)

Olsen (2002) reported the case of Keith Jesperson who claimed responsibility for killing over 100 women; he had a history of killing numerous cats as a child.

10.1.2.6 Need to Control and Dominate Others

The need to control others is a major aspect of compulsive murderers' gratification; in fact, it is at the core of their motivational dynamics. Krafft-Ebing (1886) and MacCulloch, Snowden, Wood, and Mills (1983) note the desire for control as the primary driving force in compulsive murder and the primary element of sadism. Weinberg and Levi (1983) also believe that obtaining total control is critical to the sexually sadistic killer. And Langevin (1991) concluded that the offender's "ultimate control" over the victim provides the most motivation.

According to Brittain (1970), sadistic murderers'

> desire to have power over others is an essential part of their abnormality and if the victim resists they become more determined and brutal. If the subjugation of the victim to their power is more important to them than the infliction of pain, this may help us to understand why they do not feel cruel, for they may be unaware that cruelty is not their primary objective but only the means whereby they achieve their end. (p. 204)

Johnson and Becker (1997) found that many of their adolescents expressed the need for total control over other people.

> It's the killer's need to have ultimate control over his victim that causes the sexual excitement. He probably does this because of his own poor feelings of self worth and inadequacies. Complete control is the only way to overcome this inadequacy ... the actual death itself could be anti-climactic. (p. 345)

The need to control others often begins in childhood and manifests itself in a variety of ways. For example, the future offender may attempt to directly control other children through acts of play that get out of hand, or he may intimidate other children by threats of direct violence. Ressler et al. (1988) found that over half their 36 sexual murderers were cruel to their peers as children and adolescents. The future sexual murderers were "filled with troublesome, joyless thoughts of dominance over others. These thoughts [were] expressed in a wide range of actions towards others ... abusive[ness] ... destructive play patterns, disregard for others, firesetting, stealing, and destroying property" (p. 74). Myers et al. (1998) found that 92% of their group of juvenile sexual murderers had histories of fighting, including the use of weapons to intimidate other adolescents.

A long tally of compulsive murderers intimidated, controlled, or held captive their victims. Sometimes this behavior began early. As an adolescent, Jerome Brudos (Rule, 1983) abducted girls at knife point, forced them to undress, photographed them, and kept them for hours in the family barn. As an adult, Brudos abducted and then killed several women. Ressler and Shachtman (1992) report the case of John Crutchley who committed sexual murders as an adult. As an adolescent, he "liked to control people and often made them do his bidding" (p. 172). Gary Heidnick (Englade, 1988) also gained total control over his victims. After abducting them, he kept them captive in his basement, which was converted into a torture chamber. In this case the control, captivity, and total domination seemed just as arousing as the (eventual) sadistic murders. Jeffrey Dahmer tried to render his victims helpless by injecting acid into their brains so that he could control them and get them to do whatever he wanted (Jentzen, Palermo, Johnson, Ho, Stormo, and Teggatz, 1994). Serial sexual murderer Dennis Rader called himself the BTK Killer—bind, torture, kill—illustrating how motivating control of his victims was for him (Ramsland, 2016).

10.1.2.7 Repetitive Firesetting

Notwithstanding controversy, pyromania continues to be a stand-alone diagnosis in the *DSM-5* (2013) with criteria including emotional arousal, fascination, and relief watching fire. Several early authors such as Stekel (1924) and Lewis and Yarnell (1951) described cases of repetitive firesetting with overt sexual dynamics involving a display of genitality such as expressed feelings of sexual arousal or masturbation when observing the flames. Although some contemporary cases are of this nature, most repetitive firesetting involves less obvious or covert sexual dynamics. In fact, many times the underlying sexual aspects of an arson are completely missed (Banay, 1969; Schlesinger and Revitch, 1997b) simply because there are no overt or obvious manifestations of sexuality. Perhaps one reason some researchers (e.g., Geller, Erlen, and Pinkus, 1986) have found relatively few individuals with classic pyromania is that in many cases of repetitive firesetting the sexual aspect is not obvious. The sexual motivation in many cases of arson may be more frequent than thought because the sexual element may not be able to be elicited in one or two interviews but may emerge only after prolonged therapeutic involvement. Mavromatis (2000) finds revenge and retaliation to be the most commonly expressed motives of children who set fires. However, on closer inspection, these motives often prove to be an outgrowth of a more basic need for control which itself can be eroticized. The sense of mastery and dominance gained through firesetting can be powerful as an adolescent can destroy property, burn large buildings, or kill others by simply lighting a match.

Brittain (1970) also noted a history of firesetting in his group of sadistic murderers. Ressler et al. (1988) found that 56% of their subjects set fires as children, 52% during their adolescence, and 28% in adulthood. In Myers et al.'s (1998) study of adolescent sexual murderers, 36% had a history of firesetting. One of their subjects set a van on fire, attempted to burn down his mother's home on three occasions, and set his aunt's bed on fire because he "wanted to see someone burn" (p. 343). Burton, McNeil, and Binder (2012) updated the research and thinking on firesetting, arson, and pyromania and found firesetting for sexual purposes to be rare. Grant and Kim (2007), however, found their sample of pyromanics all experienced a "rush" when watching fires but denied sexual arousal—not a surprising self-report finding. James et al. (2018b) found firesetting to have occurred in the backgrounds of serial sexual murderers 10% of the time and 6.7% in nonserial sexual murderers.

As an adolescent, Peter Kürten (Wilson and Pitman, 1962) committed many acts of arson before he began to kill women. In fact, he entertained fantasies of annihilating entire communities by fire and dynamite. Thomas Piper (Schechter and Everitt, 1996) set numerous fires prior to raping and bludgeoning four victims, including a 5-year-old girl. More recently, David "Son of Sam" Berkowitz set 1,488 fires, which he meticulously documented in his diary, before going on to kill six women in New York City. Ressler and Schachtman (1992) concluded that Berkowitz's firesetting—as well as his torture of animals—was an outgrowth of his "control fantasies involving power over living things. ... These fires were all a prelude to his moving into the arena in which he could exercise the ultimate control, homicide" (p. 80).

10.1.2.8 Voyeurism, Fetishism, and Sexual Burglary

Voyeurism and fetishism are important paraphilias that need to be considered in the risk assessment of compulsive murder. Brittain (1970) noted a history of voyeurism and fetishism in the backgrounds of his subjects, but he was unaware of the significant association between these acts and subsequent acts of sexual violence and homicide. Ressler et al. (1988) also found that sexual murderers have frequently engaged in voyeurism and fetishism since childhood, perhaps even beginning at a somewhat earlier age than that of those who developed these paraphilias but did not subsequently commit an act of sexual aggression (Abel, Osborn, and Twigg, 1993). In Ressler and his colleagues' sample of sexual murderers, 71% engaged in voyeurism and 72% in fetishism; Prentky, Burgess, Rokus, Lee, Hartman, Ressler, and Douglas (1989) noted similar findings. Langevin (2003) found both voyeurism and fetishism in his sample of 33 sexual murderers. Habermann and Briken (2007) found voyeurism to be more common in his sample of serial sexual murderers than the nonserial cases.

In some cases, voyeurism and fetishism are connected directly to acts of burglary and subsequent murder. For example, an individual who has a fetish for female underwear often begins by stealing from clotheslines. When the fetishistic object is no longer easily available, the subject may commit a burglary in order to obtain it. Similarly, voyeurs sometimes escalate their behavior from peeping in windows to entering the dwelling in order to look through rooms and drawers. Although most burglaries are committed for material gain, this subgroup of sexually motivated burglaries is symbolic, often ego-dystonic, and sometimes outright bizarre. The connection between fetishism, voyeurism, burglary, and subsequent assault arises because, according to the UCR (2018), about half of all burglaries are committed in the evening, when the occupants are likely be home.

In fetish burglaries, the sexual dynamics are overt and obvious since the offender is typically stealing female underwear, shoes, scarfs, or hairbrushes. Ressler and Schachtman (1992) note that fetish burglars "take these [items] for auto erotic purposes" (p. 8). The most typical fetish burglar with obvious sexual dynamics is William Heirens, described in Chapter 7. Heirens developed a fetish for female underwear at 9 years of age and began to steal and collect it when he was slightly older. Prior to killing two women and a 6-year-old child whom he dismembered, Heirens committed hundreds of burglaries. "He had sexual excitement or an erection at the sight of an open window at the place to be burglarized. Going through the window he had an emission" (Kennedy, Hoffman, and Haines, 1947, p. 117). In fact, Heirens was apprehended not for committing a murder but for an attempted burglary. David Russell Williams had 82 documented cases of fetish burglary before committing multiple sexual homicides (Brankley, Goodwill, and Reale, 2014).

Krafft-Ebing (1886) noted a relationship between fetishism and various crimes, all of which he considered rather "peculiar." He found that many fetishists have an impulse to "injure the fetish—which represents an element of sadism toward the woman wearing the fetish" (p. 183). He described the case of a man with a long-standing fetish for female underwear, who was eventually executed for murder.

In some cases, the offender may rip and destroy the female clothing, and on other occasions he may soil the premises through defecation, urination, or ejaculation. Heirens defecated and urinated in some of the rooms that he burglarized. Sargent (1979) contends that burglars who soil the premises of the homes they enter are expressing repressed rage directed at the occupants, who may symbolize the burglars' parents.

In voyeuristic burglary, the sexual motivation is less overt since these burglars are stimulated by a generalized urge to look and inspect rather than to steal; their fantasy is about seeing a naked woman. Thus, the sexual dynamics in these cases are not as obvious as in fetish burglary and often missed. Frequently, voyeuristic burglars steal something of minimal value to help them rationalize their conduct, which they do not understand. One voyeuristic burglar stated, "I'd feel stupid if I broke in and didn't take nothing." Yalom (1960) noted the relationship between voyeurism and aggression. He reported eight cases of voyeurs who progressed to rape, assault, and firesetting. Three of these cases involved burglary with severe violence. Fenichel (1945) also found a connection between voyeurism and violence. "Very often sadistic impulses are tied up with scoptophilia: the individual wants to see something to destroy it … often, looking itself is unconsciously thought of as a substitute for destroying" (p. 71). Schlesinger and Revitch (1999) reported the case of a 17-year-old who was arrested for masturbating while looking through the window of a woman whom he followed home. Seven years later, while on parole after serving a sentence for committing various other voyeuristic acts, he broke into an apartment and hit a sleeping woman on the head with a pipe.

Both voyeurism and fetishism begin in late childhood, but the burglaries usually do not begin until adolescence. Because the sexual aspects in voyeuristic burglary are often not recognized by law enforcement or forensic examiners such offenders are infrequently referred for evaluation unless the voyeurism is independently noted to be distinct. Unfortunately, cases of sexually motivated voyeuristic burglary are often incorrectly viewed as an unsuccessful attempt at burglary for gain (Schlesinger, 2000b). Table 10.2 lists the differentiating characteristics of fetish and voyeuristic burglaries.

Despite the seriousness of the connection between voyeurism and fetishism to burglary, Revitch (1997) pointed out the absence of research in this area. In one of the first empirical studies of burglary and its relationship to sexual murder, Schlesinger and Revitch (1999) found that 42% of a total of 52 sexual murderers had a history of burglary; of those who burglarized, 32% committed predominantly fetish burglaries, while 68% committed

Table 10.2 Differentiating Characteristics of Fetish and Voyeuristic Burglaries

Type of Burglary	Sexual Dynamics	Behaviors
Fetish	Overt: stimulated by sexual attraction to nonliving objects	Fetishism (begins in the late childhood). Burglary to get fetish objects (begins in adolescence). Steals objects, commonly female underwear, shoes, hairbrushes; sometimes soils premises.
Voyeuristic	Covert: stimulated by the urge to look	Voyeurism (begins in late childhood). Burglary with the urge to look and inspect premises (begins in adolescence). Steals objects of minimal value; stealing is rationalized.

Source: From Schlesinger, L.B., *Serial Offenders: Current Thought, Recent Findings*, CRC Press, Boca Raton, FL, 2000, p. 9. With permission.

predominantly voyeuristic burglaries. Interestingly, among the victims who were killed in their residences, 77% were killed by an individual who had a history of burglary. In a replication study, Schlesinger, Pinizzotto, and Pakhomon (2004) found 61% of sexual murderers had a history of burglary. These findings not only have clinical interest but significant investigative implications as well. In more recent research on sexual burglaries, Pedneault, Beauregard, Harris, and Knight (2015) found sexual burglars to have acted based on situational factors, very different from the method of nonsexual burglars. Pedneault, Harris, and Knight (2012) proposed a typology of sexual burglaries: fetish noncontact, versatile contact, and sexually oriented.

The combination of fetishism, voyeurism, and burglary occurs in the case histories of numerous compulsive murderers. Frequently, an author lists burglaries in an offender's background information without realizing the significance of this behavior and its connection to sexual murder. Table 10.3 lists 14 fairly notorious compulsive murderers who had a history of fetish or voyeuristic burglary. In fact, 30% of them were apprehended not for committing a murder but for committing a burglary.

Therefore, adolescent burglaries—particularly those committed solo and under bizarre circumstances, where the material gain is minimal or rationalized—often have a strong underlying sexual basis with ominous significance. This finding was also noted by Langevin (2003). In some cases, voyeurism in adolescence is preceded by an obsessive interest in pornography, which is, in essence, "voyeurism lite." Ted Bundy, who was alleged to have killed 40 women, claimed his problem began with pornography. Rather than being another example of Bundy's lying—which had been assumed when he made this comment just prior to his execution—his claim provides useful information regarding the genesis of his acting out. In this case, Bundy's obsessive interest in pornography escalated, and he went on to commit acts of voyeurism, which then led to burglary, sexual assault, and finally sexual homicide.

10.1.2.9 Unprovoked Attacks on Females, Associated with Generalized Misogynous Emotions

Unprovoked aggression against females, even if relatively minor, often precedes a compulsive homicide by weeks, months, or sometimes many years. Usually these attacks do not involve an overt manifestation of genitality, such as erection, penetration, or ejaculation, but rather the victims are battered, choked, pushed, or knifed (Revitch, 1980). At times, offenders may rip the women's clothes, expressing some level of sexual arousal, or they may unnecessarily attack a woman during a mugging or robbery, displaying much more force than is necessary to accomplish what would seem to be the primary crime. This type of behavior was noted in Case 9.4, where the offender, during a mugging, threw the victim to the ground, kicked her, and threatened to kill her. Several years later, he committed sexual assaults and finally a sexual murder. Such unprovoked attacks, even if they seem minor, are often an important indication of an underlying fantasy with a developing compulsion to act. In some cases, however, the offender has a history of rape beginning in adolescence (Ressler et al., 1983) or violent sexual assaults that escalate to sexual murder (Healey, Beauregard, and Beech, 2016). The latter is illustrated by the case of Altemio Sanchez (Beebe and Becker, 2009), who committed approximately 15 rapes that escalated to four sexual murders.

Krafft-Ebing (1886) described a number of compulsive murderers who had previously engaged in unprovoked attacks on women. For example, he described the case of a

Table 10.3   Notorious Sexual Murderers Who Committed Burglaries

Offender	Type of Burglary[a]	Number Murdered and Location of Murders[b]
Jerome Brudos	Fetish burglary began at age 16; shoe and foot fetish.	Murdered four women in his home and outside of home.
Ted Bundy	Voyeurism in adolescence led to voyeuristic burglary and "cat" burglary.	Murdered 30 to 40 women in and outside their residences.
Richard Trenton Chase	Committed fetish burglary and soiled premises.	Murdered ten women in their homes; engaged in vampirism.
Nathaniel Code	Numerous undescribed "cat" burglaries; ejaculated on premises.	Murdered eight victims in their homes.
Albert DeSalvo	Voyeurism began in adolescence; voyeuristic burglaries began during military service; ejaculated on premises.	Murdered 13 women in their homes.
Robert Hansen	Undescribed burglaries began in early twenties.	Murdered four prostitutes outside and inside their residences.
William Heirens[c]	Fetish burglary began at age 13; soiled premises by defecation and urination.	Murdered two women in their homes; dismembered a child.
Cleophus Prince[c]	Found guilty of 21 undescribed daytime "cat" burglaries.	Murdered six women in their homes.
Richard Ramirez	Voyeurism since childhood; numerous voyeuristic burglaries.	Murdered 13 women and men, mostly in their homes.
Monte Rissell	Numerous undescribed burglaries began at age 12.	Murdered five women, prostitutes, and others outside their homes.
Danny Rolling	Voyeurism, voyeuristic burglaries, and regular burglaries.	Murdered five women plus three men and a child in their homes.
George Russell[c]	Numerous undescribed burglaries began in early adolescence.	Murdered three women, two in their homes, one outside.
Arthur Shawcross	Numerous undescribed burglaries.	Murdered 11 women, two in their homes.
Timothy Spencer[c]	Numerous undescribed burglaries began at age 14; considered a "cat burglar extraordinaire."	Murdered four women in their homes.

[a] In various reports of these cases, the details of the burglaries were not always provided.

[b] The number of victims is usually the number the offender was legally charged with; in many cases, this number is less than the actual number of murders committed.

[c] Apprehended while committing a burglary; subsequently charged with murder.

Source: From Schlesinger, L.B. and Revitch, E., *Journal of the American Academy of Psychiatry and Law, 27,* 1999, p. 230. With permission.

20-year-old man who attacked and stabbed girls in the genitals in broad daylight. Revitch (1980) reported the case of a 19-year-old compulsive murderer who had broken into women's homes since age 12 with the intent of hitting the sleeping women with a brick. The offender described a feeling of relief during the assaults. Revitch also reported the case of a 23-year-old who killed and mutilated a 15-year-old girl. The victim's skull was crushed, her right breast showed some indication of biting, her left eye was destroyed, and her jaw was fractured. Several years earlier, in adolescence, the offender had been placed on probation for attacking a girl, throwing her to the ground, and then exposing himself to her.

Revitch and Schlesinger (1989) detailed the case of an 11-year-old who was evaluated because of unprovoked choking of little girls on the school playground and school bus. He had also set several cars on fire. In addition, this child uttered profanities directed primarily against girls. His family background was sordid: an absent father and a promiscuous and rejecting mother with whom the subject may have engaged in some type of sexual activity. He said that he enjoyed choking girls, as it made him "feel happy." The young offender also said that he enjoyed hurting others and wanted to kill females, which he eventually did. Another offender (Revitch and Schlesinger, 1989) was seen at ages 16, 17, 21, and 24 for increasing unprovoked violence against females. He hit one woman on the head with a stick because "I was mad at the whole female race. I was mad at all females and did not care which one I hit." He fantasized killing women and keeping them as slaves. Eventually, he broke into a house and killed a sleeping woman by hitting her on the head with a pipe. Johnson and Becker (1997) briefly referred to one of their subjects who had a 5-year history of unprovoked attacks on women involving cutting and had as well attempted to kill his foster mother with a butcher knife.

Ressler et al. (1988) did not look specifically at the variable of unprovoked attacks in their subjects' histories. Nevertheless, they did note that between 50% and 65% of their sample, as children and adolescents, were cruel to age-mates and were also assaultive toward adults. Unfortunately, the nature of the cruelty and the sex of the victims were not listed. Similarly, Myers et al. (1998) and Myers (2002) recorded the prevalence (close to 90%) of violence in their juvenile, sexual homicide subjects, but the researchers did not report if any of the aggression involved unprovoked attacks on females. James and Proulx (2014) found that nonserial sexual murderers, more than serial murderers, are easily angered and likely have a history of explosive interpersonal violence. Once an adolescent strikes out against a female—particularly if the attack is unprovoked and especially if it is associated with expressions of contempt, hatred, or dislike for women—an ominous signal has been sent. Here, the individual has already begun to behave in a directly violent interpersonal manner, beyond just fantasizing.

10.1.2.10 Evidence of Ritualistic (Signature) Behavior
Some compulsive murderers exhibit repetitive ritualistic behavior at the crime scene that goes beyond what is necessary to carry out a homicide. In such cases, the offender injects part of his personality into the criminal act itself, which is an outgrowth of his fantasies that have been developing in him for years.

> An offender's fantasies often give birth to violent crime. As the offender broods and daydreams, he develops a need to express these violent fantasies. When he finally acts out, some aspect of the crime will demonstrate a unique, personal expression or ritual based on these fantasies. Committing the crime does not satisfy the offender's needs. This insufficiency compels him to go beyond the scope of perpetration and perform his ritual. (Douglas, Burgess, Burgess, and Ressler, 1992, p. 261)

There has been some confusion regarding the difference between the terms "ritual" and "signature" since various authors have used these terms interchangeably. As noted in Chapter 8, we believe signature (unique behavior) is a subset of ritual (repetitive behavior beyond what is necessary to kill the victim). Schlesinger et al. (2010) emphasized the complexity and variation of crime scene behavior of sexual murderers.

Keppel (1995, 1997) refers to "signature behavior" as an offender's "calling card"; through this behavior the murderer leaves his own psychological imprint at the crime scene. According to Douglas et al. (1992), examples of signature behavior include mutilating or carving the body, overkill, leaving messages, positioning the body, engaging in postmortem activity, or making the victim respond verbally in a specified manner. In some cases, the "signature" (or ritual) is exactly the same in different crimes; in other cases, it develops and becomes more elaborate or it appears superficially different, but the underlying theme remains constant. At times, an offender may not be able to carry out the specific ritualistic behavior for a variety of reasons: the unanticipated appearance of a third party or an unexpected victim reaction requiring the offender to leave the crime scene quickly.

Krafft-Ebing (1886) described ritualistic behavior in several of his subjects, including one offender who was compelled "to pull the hairpins out of the hair of my victims" (p. 67), another to press the hands of victims together, and yet another to fill the mouths of his victims with dirt. Revitch and Schlesinger (1989) reported the case of a 14-year-old who forced two female classmates to undress; he then stuffed their mouths with tissue paper and let them go. A week earlier, he had broken into a neighbor's house, had ripped clothing belonging to the female occupant, and had thrown paper, coffee, and sugar throughout the residence. Four years later, at age 18, he drove a 15-year-old girl to an isolated spot where he tore off her clothes and strangled her with a plastic belt. After she was dead, he stuffed her mouth with tissue paper and dragged her body into some bushes. In this case, the ritualistic behavior associated with the homicide was apparent 4 years earlier.

Ritualistic behavior stems from the offender's fantasies, which have been developing for years.

> Most serial killers have been living with their fantasies for years before they finally bubble to the surface and are translated into behavior. When the killer finally acts out, some characteristic of the murder will reflect the unique aspect played over and over in his fantasies. (Keppel, 2000, p. 125)

And because some of these behaviors, or combination of behaviors, have been distinctive, or unique, the behaviors have been used to link a series of crimes to the same individual (Hazelwood and Warren, 2003). Any type of odd, unnecessary, unusual, or somewhat bizarre behavior associated with interpersonal control—with or without violence—must be thoroughly evaluated with a recognition that a ritualistic element may be emerging. If a ritualistic behavior is found in an adolescent, the development of dangerous fantasies and the beginning of some form of serious acting out—even if not initially aggressive— should be strongly suspected. Such activity by an adolescent should not be rationalized as an expression of eccentricity or an outgrowth of psychosis; it is difficult to imagine a more ominous indication of a budding compulsive offender.

10.1.3 Immediate Triggers for a Compulsive Murder

The time period from the emergence of various ominous signs to an eventual homicide is likely to be many years. Therefore, the question arises as to what might trigger an individual who has engaged in violent fantasy and nonlethal forms of aggression to actually commit murder. Various factors that reduce controls and inhibitions, especially in predisposed individuals, are important immediate triggers for a compulsive homicide. Depression, frustration, or anything else that can weaken inhibitory controls, including alcohol and drugs, can potentially precipitate a murder by an individual who is struggling with a compulsion to act.

Revitch (1980) noted that "some of the attacks by predisposed individuals may be unleashed by a suggestive stimulus" (p. 8). He cited a number of cases where an individual committed his first sexual homicide after watching a TV show or reading press reports about similar crimes. Malamuth (1986) and Wertham (1968) referred to the disinhibiting influence of the media, particularly television and movies. In fact, Wertham (1968) argued that media violence could facilitate "a transition from daydreams into actions" in susceptible individuals (p. 199). Pennell and Browne (1999) reported on the relationship between film violence and subsequent aggressive acting out in predisposed viewers. Meloy and Mohandie (2001) also studied the connection between "screen violence" and homicide committed by vulnerable adolescents. These authors described seven cases where the offenders viewed violent movies prior to the commission of a homicide and concluded that media violence can increase the risk of violent criminality, especially among the predisposed. However, Meloy and Mohandie, caution that "screen violence alone should never be used to predict risk, but it is one of a number of static (historical and dispositional) and dynamic (clinical and situational) variables that contribute to violent behavior" (p. 1117).

Several researchers (Brittain, 1970; Douglas and Olshaker, 1995; Ressler and Schachtman, 1992) have found that a compulsive murder may be triggered by a severe loss such as rejection in a relationship or discharge from a job. For example, in Case 8.1 an army drill sergeant committed the first of his six compulsive murders following a dishonorable discharge because of exploitation of subordinates. In Case 9.10 the offender had harbored violent fantasies and was preoccupied with the future victim but acted out only after having been fired from his job at a gas station. A failed relationship was a trigger in Cases 8.4 and 9.9.

Various other traits, characteristics, and behaviors have been associated with individuals who committed compulsive sexually motivated murders. For example, difficulty with authority (Douglas and Olshaker, 1995), persistent enuresis into adolescence (Ressler et al., 1988), absence of conscience (Hazelwood and Douglas, 1980), and social isolation (Grubin, 1994) have all been regularly noted in the histories of sex murderers. However, these signs do not differentiate a potential compulsive murderer from individuals who might engage in other types of criminal violence, including nonsexually motivated homicide or even various forms of noncriminal behavior. Antisocial personality disorder, for example, is found in individuals who commit various crimes involving violence, but it is not determinative or dispositive in predicting a homicide (Revitch and Schlesinger, 1981). Accordingly, we believe that the ten signs discussed, especially when seen in considerable combination, are more effective than these other characteristics in pointing out a predisposed individual who might eventually commit a compulsive homicide.

10.2 Disposition and Intervention

What should be done with a potential sex murderer once some type of negative prognostic judgment is reached? Most mental health professionals (MHPs) would agree that a person who has exhibited a considerable number of the ominous signs outlined above needs some type of intervention, treatment, or restraint. These behavioral indicators, at least from a common-sense perspective, do not point to a healthy future adjustment. Typically, when a child or adolescent exhibits such conduct (e.g., killing cats, firesetting, unprovoked assaults), he is often hospitalized, usually out of desperation or lack of a more acceptable immediate alternative. Such hospitalizations, however, are usually brief and often unproductive. In fact, when the treatment staff is confronted with such an individual, they are often not sure what (symptoms) they are treating, as there is no overt psychosis and often no behavioral display while on the unit. If the youngster presents with a psychosis (which is rare) or, more often, anxiety, depression, or attentional difficulties, these symptoms are treated with medication, the patient is discharged, and outpatient psychotherapy is recommended as follow-up.

But the psychotherapeutic treatment of the sex murderer or potential sex murderer has been hardly studied. Despite a voluminous literature on various therapeutic approaches with traditional sex offenders (e.g., rapists, pedophiles, exhibitionists), no one has empirically studied the effectiveness of any type of treatment modality with the sex murderer, who is different from the sex offender or individuals who engage in various other forms of sexual violence (Kafka, 1995). And even with the usual sex offender, the effectiveness of the therapeutic intervention is debatable. For example, Grossman, Martis, and Fichtner (1999) found that many studies of the effectiveness of treating sex offenders were flawed; however, the various treatment approaches did seem to decrease future offending to some extent. Treatments created specifically for traditional sex offenders—such as behavioral interventions to moderate deviant sexual arousal, programs to increase empathy, methods to enhance the capacity for intimacy, modification of cognitive distortions, and relapse prevention (see Table 10.4)—all seem to have some positive impact depending on the

Table 10.4 Treatment Modalities with Traditional Sex Offenders

Type of Intervention	Purpose
Individual and group therapy	Provide insight into personal and interpersonal psychodynamics and conflicts.
Aversion therapy and covert sensitization	Pair deviant sexual fantasies with negative reinforcement.
Imaginal desensitization	Utilize the technique of relaxation to help subject tolerate the feelings associated with deviant fantasies without acting out.
Masturbatory reconditioning	Eliminate deviant sexual arousal by pairing the effects of orgasm with nondeviant fantasies.
Cognitive restructuring	Change distorted beliefs that the subject may use to rationalize deviant behavior.
Social skills training	Help the subject develop various social skills to enhance interpersonal relationships.
Victim empathy training	Help the subject understand the impact of their behavior on victims.
Relapse prevention	Help the subject maintain progress and avoid triggers that can lead to reoffense.
Surgical intervention (neurosurgery and castration)	Removal of brain centers connected with sexual arousal; orchiectomy.
Psychopharmacology	Help offenders with co-morbid psychosis or mood disorder.
Antiandrogen medications	Reduce the serum levels of testosterone.
New hormonal therapies and serotonergic agents	Decrease testosterone levels.

Source: Adapted from Grossman, L.S., Martis, B., and Fichtner, C.G., *Psychiatric Services, 50*, 1999, pp. 349–361.

individual's motivation, level of deviancy, and level of accompanying antisocial thinking. Unfortunately, sex murderers often have the characteristics—high levels of deviancy, sadism, and antisocial thinking—that are poor prognostic indicators.

Hanson and Bussiére (1998) analyzed 61 follow-up studies of sexual offenders who were discharged from treatment programs and found a 13.4% (n = 23,393) recidivism rate, which is rather low. Because these researchers studied the crime rather than categorizing the specifics of the offense, their study did not always differentiate the true compulsive offender (with a poor prognosis) from the situational sex offender (with a much better prognosis). As noted in Chapter 3, the crime tells us little about the motivational dynamics of the offender, which is directly connected to prognostication in terms of repetitiveness. Interestingly, Hanson and Bussiére also found that offenders with increased sexual deviancy and antisocial behavior—which sex murderers have an abundance of—were more difficult to treat. This finding is consistent with Lowenstein's (1992) contention that the traditional sex offender's prognosis seems to be poor when psychopathy and sexual sadism are involved. However, Lowenstein also reported some treatment success with adolescent males in a therapeutic community program.

There has been some recent experience with the psychotherapeutic treatment of sexual murderers in secure settings (Perkins and Carter, 2018), as well as in the community (Darjee and Baron, 2018). But a close examination of these treatment experiences and discussion of the topic is really a restatement of the problem—that offenders and potential offenders need some type of treatment in order to protect others. Maniglio (2010) notes that "provision of services designed to prevent the progression from fantasy to actual killing may decrease the incidents and prevalence of sexual homicide in our society" (p. 301). There is no disagreement here, but exactly how is the prevention of the progression from fantasy to murder actually accomplished? There has been some experience with pharmacotherapy with sexual murderers, including antihormonal intervention, which seems to hold promise (Bradford, 2000; Briken, Hill, and Berner, 2003). But as Darjee and Baron (2018) state "serial sexual killers, sadistic killers for whom there is uncertainty over whether sadistic fantasy is ongoing, and highly psychopathic sexual killers, should probably never be released unless there is overwhelming and compelling evidence of amelioration in risk" (p. 398), which would seem to be extremely hard to demonstrate.

But as a practical matter, some sexual murderers will be released and the potential sex murderer is already in the community. Schlesinger and Revitch (1990) have argued that an essential ingredient in the treatment of the sex murderer and potential sex murderer is patient rapport. The clinician must be able to establish a connection with the patient, notwithstanding revulsion toward the offender's conduct or fantasies. Meaningful therapeutic work is difficult to achieve if the patient detects uneasiness, anxiety, or disgust in his therapist. The various techniques used with traditional sex offenders may be helpful with some sex murderers; however, in addition to methods or techniques, the treatment provider must demonstrate interest in the patient and, at the least, should have some experience with sexually aggressive individuals.

Sex murderers are most available for treatment while they are incarcerated. However, the history of penology reflects changing views on how to handle incarcerated offenders (Lyle, 1973; Morris and Rothman, 1995); most of these views historically do not include the provision of treatment. During the 19th century, many criminologists had progressive ideas regarding punishment and its applicability to individual offenders, but these ideas still did not involve psychological treatment (Friedman, 1993). In the latter half of the 20th century, psychological treatment or "rehabilitation"—that included some forms of psychological treatment of incarcerated offenders—was instituted but was found to be largely ineffective (Martinson, 1974). Beginning in the early 1950s with the establishment of various sexual-psychopath laws, sex offenders were provided with specialized treatment programs and, in some states, specialized institutions. But sexual murderers were not—and as a general rule still are not—handled any differently than other murderers, and relegated to the general prison population.

Most sex murderers will eventually be released from prison, except perhaps for those whose offenses were particularly heinous, repetitive, or against children. And potential sex murderers will not be institutionalized (for long) prior to committing a crime. Therefore outpatient treatment of these offenders and potential offenders emerges out of necessity (Clarke and Carter, 2000). However, many problems are associated with the outpatient treatment of this population. In particular, many therapists refuse to treat violent or potentially violent individuals, especially on an outpatient basis, because of liability concerns stemming in part from cases such as *Tarasoff v. Regents* (1976). Here, the court declared that psychotherapists have a duty to warn potential victims of their patients' threats, and failure to protect third parties leaves the therapist vulnerable to liability and malpractice claims. As a result, "legal standards that were developed to protect citizens, in actuality may result in less protection, because patients are again being shunned by practitioners due to the fear of legal entanglements" (Schlesinger and Revitch, 1990, p. 177). In some cases, treatment of the most dangerous patient is left to staff members with the least training and experience, as the most qualified and senior staff are in a position to refuse such patients. This problem only compounds itself; when therapists decline such cases, they also forego an opportunity to gain experience in treating this population of offenders.

10.3 Comment

For many years, there has often been a disconnect between behavioral science research and clinical practice. For example, during the past 50 years, researchers have debated the ability of MHPs to predict violence, while at the same time—in actual practice—clinicians have routinely been offering predictions and are often required to do so by law (Borum, 1996). This same disconnect has also existed in the area of psychotherapy research and psychotherapy practice, as noted in Chapter 7. Over the same time period, statistical studies have repetitively demonstrated (e.g., Morris, Turner, and Szykula, 1988) that psychotherapy is basically not very effective. But notwithstanding numerous validation studies that demonstrated how those on waiting lists (who did not receive psychotherapy) improved at the same rate as those in psychotherapy (Strupp, 1973), clinicians continued to practice, patients improved, and laws were passed to reimburse individuals for treatment. In fact, the pool of potential therapists (limited initially to psychiatrists) increased to include psychologists, social workers, and counselors, all obtaining insurance reimbursement for treatment that patients found effective but which researchers could not empirically validate.

With some distance, we now realize that the psychotherapy research was misleading because the wrong questions were being asked. General questions such as "Does psychotherapy work?" should probably have been replaced by more specific questions such as, "What type of therapies work best, with what types of patients, under what types of conditions?" The same issue applies to the problem of violence prediction. "Can we predict violence?" is the wrong question. The more appropriate one is "What types of predictions can we make, with what types of individuals, under what types of circumstances?" When these sorts of questions are asked, a prognostic statement can and should be offered.

A purely legal approach to the compulsive, repetitive, sexual murderer, or potential murderer will not only fail to prevent recidivism, but it will also fail to protect society or help the offender. Confinement is not always the most satisfactory (or possible) solution for prevention and public safety or for rehabilitation, treatment, and intervention. This is not to negate the importance of retribution, but the law rigidly applied often deals not with the offender but with the legal definition of the crime, which emphasizes the degree of intent. Thus, an individual who commits a crime with a high level of intent will, according to sentencing guidelines, very likely be incarcerated regardless of his personality structure, motivational dynamics, or dangerousness. On the other hand, a relatively minor assault might (legally) call for a shorter period of incarceration even if the offender was toying with strong gynocidal fantasies and a pressure to act. Such a person is potentially more dangerous than an individual who may have committed, for example, a homicide with a strong situational (and noncompulsive) element. Thus, the disposition of offenders—especially homicidal offenders—based solely on the crime rather than on prognostic possibilities actually creates a dangerous situation for the public.

Specialized forensic centers are desperately needed to provide evaluation and treatment of pathological murderers, sex murderers, and potential sex murderers. These programs should not be bogged down by bureaucratic and legalistic restrictions; instead, they should focus on research, study, and teaching (Arrigo and Purcell, 2001). Such settings should be connected to medical schools and graduate schools in psychology and criminology. This model would provide an excellent opportunity for practitioners to gain clinical experience with this population of offenders as well as to engage in research and provide training. In the long run, this would protect society from a subgroup of dangerous individuals whom we desperately need to study further.

Such an approach to the evaluation, treatment, and prevention of pathological murder would be well worth the effort. The serious scientific study of sex murder has been neglected. Our government devotes vast resources to the apprehension, legal disposition, incarceration, and punishment of such offenders. However, it expends little effort on prevention, treatment, or the scientific study of the problem. Friends and relatives of the victims demand retribution, which serves a restorative psychological function as well as one of justice. But there is no reason why the punishment of sex murderers cannot also involve a concerted effort to learn more about them.

References

Abel, E.L. (1977). The relationship between cannabis and violence: A review. *Psychological Bulletin, 84*, 193–211.

Abel, G.G., & Blanchard, E.E. (1974). The role of fantasy in the treatment of sexual deviation. *Archives of General Psychiatry, 30*, 467–475.

Abel, G.G., Osborn, C.A., & Twigg, D.A. (1993). Preventing sexual aggression in adulthood through intervention in adolescence. In H.E. Barbaree, W.L. Marshall, & S.M. Hudson (Eds.), *The juvenile offender* (pp. 104–117). New York: Guilford Press.

Abelson, R.P. (1997). On the surprising longevity of flogged horses: Why there is a case for the significance test. *Psychological Science, 8*, 12–15.

Ainsworth, P.B. (2001). *Offender profiling and crime analysis.* Devon: William Publishing.

Allely, C., Minnis, H., Thompson, L., Wilson, P., & Gillberg, C. (2014). Neurodevelopmental and prosocial risk factors in serial killers and mass murderers. *Aggression and Violent Behavior, 19*, 288–301.

Alvarado, N. (1994). Empirical validity of the Thermatic Apperception Test. *Journal of Personality Assessment, 63*, 57–79.

American Psychiatric Association. (1952). *Diagnostic and statistical manual of mental disorders.* Washington, DC: Author.

American Psychiatric Association. (1968). *Diagnostic and statistical manual of mental disorders* (2nd ed.). Washington, DC: Author.

American Psychiatric Association. (1980). *Diagnostic and statistical manual of mental disorders* (3rd ed.). Washington, DC: Author.

American Psychiatric Association. (1987). *Diagnostic and statistical manual of mental disorders* (3rd ed., rev.). Washington, DC: Author.

American Psychiatric Association. (1994). *Diagnostic and statistical manual of mental disorders* (4th ed.). Washington, DC: Author.

American Psychiatric Association. (2000). *Diagnostic and statistical manual of mental disorders* (4th ed., text rev.). Washington, DC: Author.

American Psychiatric Association. (2013). *Diagnostic and statistical manual of mental disorders.* (5th ed.). Washington, DC: Author.

Amirante, S.L., & Broderick, D. (2015). *John Wayne Gacy: Defending a monster.* New York: Skyhorse Publishing.

Ansevics, N.L., & Doweiko, N.E. (1991). Serial murderers: Early proposed development model and typology. *Psychotherapy and Private Practice, 9*, 107–122.

Arendt, H. (1966). *Eichmann in Jerusalem: A report on the banality of evil.* New York: Viking Press.

Arieti, A., & Schreiber, R.F. (1981). Multiple murder of a schizophrenic patient: A dynamic interpretation. *Journal of the American Academy of Psychoanalysis, 9*, 501–524.

Arlow, J.A. (1978). Pyromania and the primal scene: A psychoanalytic comment on the work of Yukio Mishima. *Psychoanalytic Quarterly, 47*, 24–51.

Aronow, E. (1994). *Rorschach technique: The perpetual basis, content interpretation and application.* New York: Allyn & Bacon.

Arrigo, B.A., & Purcell, C.E. (2001). Explaining paraphilias and lust murder: Toward an integrative model. *International Journal of Offender Therapy and Comparative Criminology, 45*, 6–31.

Askill, J., & Sharpe, M. (1993). *Angel of death: Killer nurse Beverly Allitt.* London: Michael O'Mara Books.

Attick, R.D. (1970). *Victorian studies in scarlet.* New York: Norton.

Auerhahn, K., & Parker, R.N. (1999). Drugs, alcohol, and homicide. In M.D. Smith & M.A. Zahn (Eds.), *Studying and preventing homicide* (pp. 97–114). Thousand Oaks, CA: Sage.

Bachet, M. (1951). The concept of encephalosis criminogenes. *American Journal of Orthopsychiatry, 21,* 794–799.

Balmer, D. (2017). *Living with a serial killer.* London: Ebury Press.

Banay, R.S. (1969). Unconscious sexual motivation in crime. *Medical Aspects of Human Sexuality, 3,* 91–102.

Bandura, A. (1986). *Social foundation of thought and action: A social cognitive theory.* Englewood Cliffs, NJ: Prentice Hall.

Barbaree, H.E., & Marshall, W.L. (1988). Deviant sexual arousal, offense history, and demographic variables as predictors of re-offense among child molesters. *Behavioral Sciences and the Law, 6,* 267–280.

Barbaree, H.E., & Marshall, W.L. (1989). Erectile responses among heterosexual child molesters, father-daughter incest offenders, and matched nonoffenders: Five distinct age preference profiles. *Canadian Journal of the Behavioral Sciences, 21,* 70–82.

Barefoot v. Estelle. 103 S. Ct. 3383 (1983).

Barrett, A. (1990). *Caligula: The corruption of power.* New Haven, CT: Yale University Press.

Bartholomew, A.A., Milte, K.L., & Galabally, F. (1975). Sexual murder: Psychopathology and psychiatric jurisprudential considerations. *Australian and New Zealand Journal of Criminology, 8,* 143–152.

Bastani, J.B., & Kentsmith, D.K. (1980). Psychotherapy with wives of sexual deviants. *American Journal of Psychotherapy, 34,* 20–25.

Batt, J.C. (1948). Homicidal incidence in the depressive psychoses. *Journal of Mental Science, 94,* 782–792.

Beauregard, E., & Martineau, M. (2012). A descriptive study of sexual homicide in Canada: Implications for police investigation. *International Journal of Offender Therapy and Comparative Criminology, 57,* 1454–1476.

Beauregard, E., & Martineau, M. (2016). Does the organized sexual murderer better delay and avoid detection? *Journal of Interpersonal Violence, 31,* 4–25.

Becker, R., & Veysey, N. (2018). *Doug Clark and Carol Bundy: The horrific true story behind the Sunset Strip slayers.* New York: Sea Vision.

Beebe, M., & Becker, M. (2009). *The bikepath killer.* New York: Pinnacle.

Beech, A.R., Fisher, D., & Ward, T. (2005). Sexual murderers: Implicit theories. *Journal of Interpersonal Violence, 20,* 1336–1389.

Begg, P., Fido, M., & Skinner, K. (1991). *Jack the Ripper A-Z.* London: Headline.

Bender, L. (1938). *A visual motor gestalt test and its clinical use.* American Orthopsychiatric Association. Research Monograph No. 3. New York.

Benedetti, J. (1972). *Gilles de Rais.* New York: Stein & Day.

Benezech, M. (1984). Homicides by psychotics in France: A five year study. *Journal of Clinical Psychiatry, 45,* 85–86.

Bennell, C., Jones, N., Taylor, P., & Snook, B. (2006). Validities and abilities in criminal profiling: A critique of the studies conducted by Richard Kocsis and his colleagues. *International Journal of Offender Therapy and Comparative Criminology, 50,* 344–360.

Beres, D. (1960). Perception, imagination, and reality. *International Journal of Psychoanalysis, 41,* 327–334.

Berkowitz, I.N. (1981). Feelings of powerlessness and the role of violent action in adolescents. *Adolescent Psychiatry, 9,* 477–492.

Berman, A.L. (1979). Dyadic death: Murder-suicide. *Suicide and Life-Threatening Behavior, 9,* 15–23.

Birnbaum, K. (1914). *Die psychopathischen verbrecker* (2nd ed.). Leipzig: Thieme.

Blackman, N., Lum, J.T., & Vanderpearl, R.J. (1974). Disturbed communications: A contributing factor in sudden murder. *Mental Health and Society, 1,* 345–355.

Blackman, N., Weiss, J., & Lamberti, J.W. (1963). The sudden murderer, III. Clues to preventative interaction. *Archives of General Psychiatry, 8,* 289–294.

Blake, P.Y., Pincus, J.H., & Buckner, C. (1996). Neurological abnormalities in murderers. *Neurology*, 45, 1641–1647.

Blanchard, G.T. (1995). Sexually addicted lust murderers. *Sexual Addiction and Compulsivity*, 2, 62–71.

Blau, T.H. (1998). *The psychologist as expert witness* (2nd ed.). New York: John Wiley.

Bleuler, E. (1922). *Textbook of psychiatry*. New York: Macmillan.

Bleuler, E. (1951). *Dementia praecox or the group of schizophrenias*. New York: International Universities Press. (Original work published 1911).

Bluglass, R., & Bowden, P. (Eds.). (1990). *Principles and practice of forensic psychiatry*. New York: Churchill Livingstone.

Bohannan, P. (1960). *African homicide and suicide*. Princeton, NJ: Princeton University Press.

Bornstein, R.F. (2001). Clinical utility of the Rorschach inkblot method: Reframing the debate. *Journal of Personality Assessment*, 77, 39–47.

Borum, R. (1996). Improving the clinical practice of violence risk assessment: Technology, guidelines, and training. *American Psychologist*, 51, 945–956.

Borum, R., & Grisso, T. (1995). Psychological test use in criminal forensic evaluations. *Professional Psychology: Research & Practice*, 26, 465–473.

Bourget, D., Gagne, P., & Moamai, J. (2000). Spousal homicide and suicide in Quebec. *Journal of the American Academy of Psychiatry and Law*, 28, 179–182.

Bourget, D., & Labelle, A. (1992). Homicide, infanticide, and filicide. *Psychiatric Clinics of North America*, 15, 661–673.

Bourguignon, A. (1997). Vampirism and autovampirism. In L.B. Schlesinger and E. Revitch (Eds.), *Sexual dynamics in anti-social behavior* (2nd ed., pp. 271–293). Springfield, IL: Charles C Thomas.

Bowman, K.M., & Blau, A. (1949). Psychotic states following head injury and brain injury in adults and children. In S. Brock (Ed.), *Injuries of the brain and spinal cord and their coverings* (pp. 47–71). Baltimore: Williams & Wilkins.

Bradford, J.M. (2000). The treatment of sexual deviation using a pharmacological approach. *Journal of Sex Research*, 37, 248–257.

Bradford, J.M., Greenberg, D.M., & Motayne, G.G. (1992). Substance abuse and criminal behavior. *Psychiatric Clinics of North America*, 15, 605–622.

Brancale, R. (1955). Problems of classification. *National Probation and Parole Association Journal*, 1, 118–125.

Brancale, R., Ellis, A., & Doorbar, R. (1952). Psychiatric and psychological investigation of convicted sex offenders. *American Journal of Psychiatry*, 102, 17–21.

Brancale, R., McNeil, D., & Vuocolo, A. (1965). Profile of the New Jersey sex offender. *Welfare Reporter*, 16, 3–9.

Brankley, A., Goodwill, A., & Reale, K. (2014). Escalation from fetish burglaries to sexual violence: A retrospective case study of former Col. D. Russell Williams. *Journal of Investigative Psychology and Offender Profiling*, 11, 115–135.

Briere, J., & Runtz, M. (1989). University males' sexual interest in children: Predicting potential indices of "pedophilia" in a non-forensic sample. *Child Abuse and Neglect*, 13, 65–75.

Briken, P., Habermann, N., Berner, W., & Hill, A. (2005). The influence of brain abnormalities on psychosocial development, criminal history, and paraphilias in sexual murderers. *Journal of Forensic Sciences*, 50, 1–5.

Briken, P., Hill, A., & Berner, W. (2003). Pharmacotherapy of paraphilias with long-acting agonists of luteinizing hormons releasing-hormone: A systematic review. *Journal of Clinical Psychiatry*, 64, 890–897.

Brinded, P.M.J. (1998). A case of acquittal following confession in a police videotaped interview. *Psychiatry, Psychology, and Law*, 5, 133–138.

Brinded, P.M.J., & Taylor, A.J. (1995). A mass killing in New Zealand. *Australian and New Zealand Journal of Psychiatry*, 29, 316–320.

Brittain, R.P. (1970). The sadistic murderer. *Medicine, Science, and Law, 10*, 198–207.

Brody, N. (1972). *Personality: Research and theory.* New York: Academic Press.

Bromberg, W. (1961). *The mold of murder: A psychiatric study of homicide.* New York: Grune & Stratton.

Brown, C.W.M. (1962). Sex chromosomes and the law. *Lancet, 1*, 503–509.

Brown v. Board of Education. 98 F. Supp. 797 (1951), 347 U.S. 483 (1954), 349 U.S. 294 (1955).

Brown, W. (1963). Murder rooted in incest. In R.E.L. Masters (Ed.), *Patterns of incest: A psychological study of incest based on clinical and historical data* (pp. 110–137). New York: Julian Press.

Brownmiller, S. (1976). *Against our will: Men, women and rape.* New York: Bantam.

Brussel, J.S. (1968). *Casebook of a crime psychiatrist.* New York: Grove.

Buckhout, R. (1974). Eyewitness testimony. *Scientific American, 231*, 23–31.

Bugliosi, V., & Gentry, C. (1975). *Helter skelter.* New York: Bantam.

Bull, R., & Clifford, B.R. (1999). Earwitness testimony. *Medicine, Science & the Law, 39*, 120–126.

Burgess, A.W., Hartman, C.R., Ressler, R.K., Douglas, J.E., & McCormack, A. (1986). Sexual homicide: A motivational model. *Journal of Interpersonal Violence, 1*, 151–272.

Bursten, B. (1972). The manipulative personality. *Archives of General Psychiatry, 26*, 318–321.

Burton, P., McNeil, D.E., & Binder, R.L. (2012). Firesetting, arson, pyromania, and the forensic mental health expert. *Journal of the American Academy of Psychiatry and Law, 40*, 355–365.

Busch, K.A., & Cavanaugh, J.L. (1986). The study of multiple murder: Preliminary examination of the interface between epistemology and methodology. *Journal of Interpersonal Violence, 1*, 5–23.

Butcher, J.N. (2000). Revising psychological tests: Lessons learned from the revision of the MMPI. *Psychological Assessment, 12*, 263–271.

Camie, P.M., Rhodes, J.E., & Yardley, L. (2003). *Qualitative research in psychology: Expanding perspectives in methodology and design.* Washington, DC: APA Press.

Campbell, J.L. (Ed.). (1995). *Assessing dangerousness: Violence by sexual offenders, batterers, and child abusers.* Thousand Oaks, CA: Sage.

Campion, J., Cravens, J., Rotholc, A., Weinstein, H., Covan, F., & Alpert, M.A. (1985). A study of 15 matricidal men. *American Journal of Psychiatry, 142*, 312–317.

Canter, D.V., Alison, L.J., Alison, E., & Wentink, N. (2004). The organized/disorganized typology of serial murder: Myth or model? *Psychology, Public Policy, and Law, 10*, 293–320.

Cantor, C.H., Mullen, P.E., & Alpers, P.A. (2000). Mass homicide: The civil massacre. *Journal of the American Academy of Psychiatry and Law, 28*, 55–63.

Carabellese, F., Manigilio, R., Greco, O., & Catanesi, R. (2011). The role of fantasy in a serial sexual offender: A brief review of the literature and a case report. *Journal of Forensic Sciences, 56*. 256–260.

Cartwright, D. (2001). The role of psychopathology and personality in rage-type homicide: A review. *South African Journal of Psychology, 31*, 12–19.

Casey-Owens, M. (1984). The anonymous letter-writer: A psychological profile? *Journal of Forensic Sciences, 29*, 816–819.

Cauldwell, D.O. (1948). *William Heirens, notorious sex maniac.* Girard, KS: Haldeman-Julius.

Causey, M., & Dempsey, J.M. (Eds.). (2000). *The Jack Ruby trial revisited.* Denton, TX: University of North Texas Press.

Cavaiola, A.A., & Schiff, M. (1988). Behavioral sequelae of physical and/or sexual abuse in adolescents. *Child Abuse and Neglect, 12*, 181–188.

Chan, H.C.O., & Heide, K.M. (2009). Sexual homicide: A synthesis of the literature. *Trauma, Violence, & Abuse, 10*, 31–54.

Chan, H.C.O., Heide, K.M., & Beauregard, E. (2011). What propels sexual murderers? A proposed integrated theory of social learning and routine activities theories. *International Journal of Offender Therapy and Comparative Criminology, 55*, 228–250.

Chancellor, A.S.,& Graham, G.D., Sr. (2014). Staged crime scenes: Crime scene clues to suspect misdirection of the investigation. *Investigative Sciences Journal, 6*,19–35

Chaney, M. (1976). *The co-ed killer.* New York: Walker.

Chertwood, D. (1988). Is there a season for homicide? *Criminology, 26,* 287–306.

Chow, S.L. (1998). Precis of statistical significance: Rationale, validity, and utility. *Behavioral and Brain Sciences, 21,* 169–194.

Clark, T. (1976). *Psychopath: The case of Patrick MacKay.* London: Routledge & K. Paul Publishers.

Clarke, J., & Carter, A.J. (2000). Relapse prevention with sexual murderers. In D.R. Laws & S.M. Hudson (Eds.). *Remaking relapse prevention with sex offenders: A sourcebook* (pp. 389–401). Thousand Oaks, CA: Sage.

Cleckley, H. (1941). *The mask of sanity.* St Louis MO: Mosby.

Cleckley, H. (1976). *The mask of sanity* (5th ed.). St. Louis, MO: Mosby. (Original work published 1941).

Cocores, J., & Cohen, R.S. (1996). Ganser's syndrome, prison psychosis and rare dissociative states. In L.B. Schlesinger (Ed.), *Explorations in criminal psychopathology* (pp. 238–254). Springfield, IL: Charles C Thomas.

Cocores, J., Schlesinger, L.B., & Mesa, V.B. (2007). Ganser's syndrome, prison psychosis, & rare dissociative states. In L.B. Schlesinger (Ed.), *Explorations in criminal psychopathy: Clinical syndromes with forensic implications* (2nd ed., pp. 236–252). Springfield, IL: Thomas.

Cohen, J. (1994). The earth is round (p <.05). *American Psychologist, 49,* 997–1003.

Cohen, L.E., & Felson, M. (1979). Social change and crime rate trends: A routine activity approach. *American Sociological Review, 44,* 588–608.

Coles, E.M. (1997). Impulsivity in major mental disorder. In C.D. Webster and M.A. Jackson (Eds.), *Impulsivity: Theory, assessment and treatment* (pp. 180–194). New York: Guilford Press.

Cook, G. (1980). *The role of the forensic psychologist in criminal and civil law.* Springfield, IL: Charles C Thomas.

Cormier, B.M. (1982). Psychodynamics of homicide committed in a marital relationship. *Corrective Psychiatry and Journal of Social Therapy, 8,* 187–194.

Cornwell, P. (2002). *Portrait of a killer: Jack the Ripper, Case closed.* New York: Putnam.

Cox, M. (1991). *The confessions of Henry Lee Lucas.* New York: Pocket Books.

Crabb, P.B. (2000). The material culture of homicide fantasies. *Aggressive Behavior, 26,* 225–234.

Crepault, C., & Couture, M. (1980). Mens' erotic fantasies. *Archives of Sexual Behavior, 9,* 565–581.

Crisp, R. (2002). *A crossing of paths: The true untold story of the Hillside Strangler case.* Weirsdale, FL: Old Flame Finders.

Cross, P.A., & Matheson, K. (2006). Understanding sadomasochism: An empirical examination of four perspectives. *Journal of Homosexuality, 50,* 133–166.

Cushing, H. (1933). Medicine at the crossroads. *Journal of the American Medical Association, 100,* 1567–1574.

Darjee, R., & Baron, E. (2018). Managing perpetrators of sexual homicide in the community. In J. Proulx, E. Beauregard, A.J. Carter, A. Mokros, R. Darjee, & J. James (Eds.). *Routledge International handbook of sexual homicide studies* (pp. 382–401). New York: Routledge.

Davidson, H. (1952). *Forensic psychiatry.* New York: Ronald Press.

Davidson, H. (1965). *Forensic psychiatry* (2nd ed.). New York: Ronald Press.

Davidson, M. (1994). Case report: Sadistically motivated offending in an individual with chromosome constitution 47 XXXY. *Journal of Forensic Psychiatry, 5,* 177–183.

Davis, J.A. (Ed.). (2001). *Stalking crimes and victim protection: Prevention, intervention, threat assessment, and case management.* Boca Raton, FL: CRC Press.

Davis, L.S., & Schlesinger, L.B. (2016). Animal cruelty, firesetting, and homicide. In M.P. Brewster, & C.L. Reyes (Eds.). *Animal cruelty: A multi-disciplinary approach to understanding* (2nd ed., pp. 301–321). Durham, NC: Carolina Academic Press.

De Bousingin, R. (1971). Essai de comparison entre l'historie clinique et les testes psychologigues en particulier les testes projectifs (Rorschach et TAT) chez l'adolescent et l'enfant meurtrier [A comparison between clinical history and psychological tests, in particular projective tests, with the adolescent and the child murderer]. *Revue de la Neuropsychiatrie Infantile, 19,* 219–223.

De Clue, G. (2005). Psychological consultation in cases involving interrogations and confessions. *Journal of Psychiatry and Law, 33*, 313–358.

Delgado-Escueta, A.V., Mattson, D., & King, L. (1981). The nature of aggression during epileptic seizures. *New England Journal of Medicine, 305*, 711–716.

De River, J.P. (1958). *Crime and the sexual psychopath*. Springfield, IL: Charles C Thomas.

De Sade, M. (1795/1990). *The complete justine, philosophy in the bedroom, and other writings* (A. Wainhouse & R. Seaver, Trans.). New York: Grove.

Deslauriers-Varin, N., Lussier, P., & St. Yves, M. (2011). Confessing their crime: Factors influencing the offender's decision to confess to the police. *Justice Quarterly, 28*, 113–145.

Deu, N. (1998). Executive function and criminal fantasy in the premeditation of criminal behavior. *Criminal Behavior and Mental Health, 8*, 41–50.

Devery, C.. (2010). Criminal profiling and criminal investigation. *Journal of Contemporary Criminal Justice, 26*, 393–409.

Dewey, L., Allwood, M., Fava, J., Arias, E., Pinizzotto, A., & Schlesinger, L.B. (2013). Suicide by cop. Clinical risks and subtypes. *Archives of Suicide Research, 17*, 448–461.

Dicke, J. (1994, Winter). Catathymic violence and mental status defenses. *Colorado Criminal Defense Bar, Rapsheet*, 10–13.

Dieker, T.E. (1973). WAIS characteristics of indicted male murderers. *Psychological Reports, 32*, 1066.

Dietz, P.E. (1986). Mass, serial, and sensational homicides. *Bulletin of the New York Academy of Medicine, 62*, 477–491.

Dietz, P.E., Harry, B., & Hazelwood, R.R. (1986). Detective magazines: Pornography for the sexual sadist. *Journal of Forensic Sciences, 31*, 197–211.

Dietz, P.E., Hazelwood, R.R., & Warren, J. (1990). The sexually sadistic criminal and his offenses. *Bulletin of the American Academy of Psychiatry and Law, 18*, 163–178.

Dinniss, S. (1999). Violent crime in an elderly demented patient. *International Journal of Geriatric Psychiatry, 14*, 889–891.

Doerner, W.G., & Lab, S.P. (2012). *Victimology* (6th ed.). New York: Elsevier.

Doerner, W.G., & Speir, J.C. (1986). Stitch and saw: The impact of medical resources upon criminally induced lethality. *Criminology, 24*, 319–330.

Dorpat, T.L. (1966). Suicide in murderers. *Psychiatry Digest, 27*, 51–55.

Dostoyevsky, F.M. (1886–1955). *Crime and punishment* (C. Garnett, Trans.). New York: Bantam.

Douglas, J., Burgess, A., Burgess, A.G., & Ressler, R. (1992). *Crime classification manual*. San Francisco: Jossey-Bass.

Douglas, J., Burgess, A., Burgess, A.G., & Ressler, R. (2013). *Crime classification manual* (3 rd ed). New York: Wiley.

Douglas, J.E., Burgess, A.W., Burgess, A.G., & Ressler, R.K. (2013). *Crime classification manual* (3rd ed.). New York: Wiley.

Douglas, J.E., & Olshaker, M. (1995). *Mind hunter*. New York: Pocket Books.

Douglas, J.E., Ressler, K.E., Burgess, A.W., & Hartman, C.R. (1986). Criminal profiling from crime scene analysis. *Behavioral Sciences and the Law, 4*, 401–421.

Douglas, K.S., Cox, D.N., & Webster, C.D. (1999). Violence risk assessment: Science and practice. *Legal and Criminological Psychology, 4*, 149–184.

Douglas, K.S., Hart, S.D., Webster, C.D., & Belfrage, H. (2013). *HCR-20: Assessing risk for violence*. Vancouver: Mental Health Law & Policy Institute.

Driver, E.D. (1968). Confession and the social psychology of coercion. *Harvard Law Review, 82*, 41–62.

Drob, S.L., Meehan, K.B., & Waxman, S.E. (2009). Clinical and conceptual problems in the attribution of malingering in forensic evaluations. *Journal of the American Academy of Psychiatry and Law, 37*, 98–106.

Drvota, S., & Student, V. (1975). Dangerous sexual aggressors. *Ceskoslovenska Psychiatrie, 71*, 33–37.

Du Plessix-Gray, F. (1998). *In the home of the Marquis de Sade*. New York: Penguin Putnam.

Dutton, D.G. (1998). *The abusive personality: Violence and control in intimate relationships.* New York: Guilford Press.

Dvorchak, R., & Howlewa, L. (1991). *Milwaukee massacre: Jeffrey Dahmer and the Milwaukee murders.* New York: Dell.

East, W.N. (1950). *Society and the criminal.* Springfield, IL: Charles C Thomas.

Egger, S.A. (1990a). Serial murder: A synthesis of literature and research. In S.A. Egger (Ed.), *Serial murder* (pp. 3–34). New York: Praeger.

Egger, S.A. (1990b). *Serial murder: An elusive phenomenon.* Westport, CT: Praeger.

Egger, S.A. (2002). *The killers among us* (2nd ed.). New York: Prentice Hall.

Eisler, R. (1953). Sadism and masochism in modern society. In I. Podolsky (Ed.), *Encyclopedia of aberrations* (pp. 74–93). New York: Philosophical Library.

Ellenberger, H. (1955). Psychological relationships between criminal and victim. *Archives of Criminal Psychodynamics, 1,* 257–291.

Englade, K. (1988). *Cellar of horror.* New York: St. Martin's Press.

Ennis, B.J., & Litwack, T.R. (1974). Psychiatry and the presumption of expertise: Flipping coins in the courtroom. *California Law Review, 62,* 693–752.

Enoch, M.D., Trethowan, W.N., & Bracher, J.L. (1967). *Some uncommon psychiatric syndromes.* Bristol: John Wright & Sons.

Estes, W.K. (1997). Significance testing in psychological research: Some persisting issues. *Psychological Science, 8,* 18–20.

Exner, J.E. (1974). *The Rorschach: A comprehensive system.* New York: John Wiley.

Fackler, S.M., Anfinson, T., & Rand, J.A. (1997). Serial sodium amytal interviews in the clinical setting. *Psychosomatics, 38,* 558–564.

Fagan, J. (1990). Intoxication and aggression. In M. Tonry & J.Q. Wilson (Eds.), *Crime and justice: A review of research* (pp. 241–320). Chicago, IL: University of Chicago Press.

Fedoroff, J.P. (2008). Sadism, sadomasochism, sex and violence. *Canadian Journal of Psychiatry, 53,* 637–646.

Feldman, M. (2004). *Playing sick? Untangling the web of Munchausen syndrome, Munchausen's by Proxy, malingering and factitious disorder.* New York: Brunner-Routledge.

Feliciano, S., Robins, C., Fletouris, S., Felps, M., Schlesinger, L.B., & Craun, S., (in press). Confessions in intimate partner homicide. *FBI Law Enforcement Bulletin.*

Felson, M., & Clarke, R.V. (1998). *Opportunity makes the thief: Practical theory for crime prevention.* London: Policing and Reducing Crime Unit.

Felthous, A.R. (1980). Aggression against cats, dogs, and people. *Clinical Psychiatry and Human Development, 10,* 169–177.

Felthous, A.R., & Bernard, H. (1979). Enuresis, firesetting, and cruelty to animals: The significance of the two thirds of this triad. *Journal of Forensic Sciences, 24,* 240–246.

Felthous, A.R., & Keller, S.R. (1987). Childhood cruelty to animals and later aggression against people: A review. *American Journal of Psychiatry, 144,* 710–717.

Fenichel, O. (1945). *The psychoanalytic theory of neurosis.* New York: Norton.

Feyerabend, K. (1969). *Langenscheidt pocket Greek dictionary.* New York: McGraw-Hill.

Fingerhut, L.A., & Kleinman, J.L. (1990). International and interstate comparison of homicide among young males. *Journal of the American Medical Association, 263,* 3292–3295.

Finkelhor, D., & Araji, S. (1986). Explanations of pedophilia: A four factor model. *Journal of Sex Research, 22,* 145–161.

Firestone, P., Bradford, J.M., Greenberg, D.M., & Larose, M.R. (1998). Homicidal sex offenders: Psychological, phallometric, and diagnostic features. *Journal of the American Academy of Psychiatry and Law, 26,* 537–552.

Florance, E. (1955). The neurosis of Raskolnikov: A study of incest and murder. *Archives of Criminal Psychodynamics, 1,* 344–396.

Flowers, R.B. (1996). *The sex slave murders: The true story of serial killers Gerald and Charlene Gallego.* New York: St. Martin's Press.

Ford, C.V. (1996). *Lies, lies, lies: The psychology of deceit.* Washington, DC: American Psychiatric Press.

Fox, B., & Farrington, D.P. (2018). What have we learned from offender profiling? A systematic review and meta-analysis of 40 years of research. *Psychological Bulletin, 144,* 1247–1274.

Fox, J.A., & Levin, J. (1994). *Overkill.* New York: Dell.

Fraboni, M., Cooper, D., Reed, T.L., & Saltstone, R. (1990). Offense type and two point MMPI code profiles: Discriminating between violent and non-violent offenders. *Journal of Clinical Psychology, 46,* 774–777.

Frank, L.K. (1948). *Projective methods.* Springfield, IL: Charles C Thomas.

Freedman, A.M., Kaplan, H.I., & Sadock, B.J. (1972). *Modern synopsis of comprehensive textbook of psychiatry.* Baltimore: Williams & Wilkins.

Freeman, L. (1956). *Catch me before I kill more.* New York: Pocket Books.

Freidman, A.F., Bollinskey, P., Nichols, D., & Levak, R.W. (2014). *Psychological assessment with the MMPI-2/MMPI-2RF.* New York: Routledge.

Freud, S. (1895). Obsession and phobias. In J. Strachey (Ed. and Trans.), *The standard edition of the complete psychological works of Sigmund Freud* (Vol. 3, pp. 71–84). London: Hogarth Press.

Freud, S. (1900). The interpretation of dreams. In J. Strachey (Ed. and Trans.), *The standard edition of the complete psychological works of Sigmund Freud* (Vol. 4, pp. 1–715). London: Hogarth Press.

Freud, S. (1905). Three essays on the theory of sexuality. In J. Strachey (Ed. and Trans.), *The standard edition of the complete psychological works of Sigmund Freud* (Vol. 7, pp. 130–243). London: Hogarth Press.

Freud, S. (1908). The sexual theories of children. In J. Strachey (Ed. and Trans.), *The standard edition of the complete psychological works of Sigmund Freud* (Vol. 9, pp. 207–226). London: Hogarth Press.

Freud, S. (1910). Contributions to the psychology of love. In J. Strachey (Ed. and Trans.), *The standard edition of the complete psychological works of Sigmund Freud* (Vol. 11, pp. 163–176). London: Hogarth Press.

Freud, S. (1914). From the history of an infantile neurosis. In J. Strachey (Ed. and Trans.), *The standard edition of the complete psychological works of Sigmund Freud* (Vol. 17, pp. 7–122). London: Hogarth Press.

Freud, S. (1916). Some character types met with in psychoanalytic work. In J. Strachey (Ed. and Trans.), *The standard edition of the complete works of Sigmund Freud* (Vol. 14, pp. 311–315). London: Hogarth Press.

Freud, S. (1920). Beyond the pleasure principle. In J. Strachey (Ed. and Trans.), *The standard edition of the complete psychological works of Sigmund Freud* (Vol. 18, pp. 3–64). London: Hogarth Press.

Freud, S. (1921). Group psychology and analysis of the ego. In J. Strachey (Ed. and Trans.), *The standard edition of the complete psychological works of Sigmund Freud* (Vol. 18, pp. 67–143). London: Hogarth Press.

Freud, S. (1923). The ego and the id. In J. Strachey (Ed. and Trans.), *The standard edition of the complete psychological works of Sigmund Freud* (Vol. 19, pp. 12–66). London: Hogarth Press.

Freud, S. (1925). Some psychical consequences of the anatomical distinctions between the sexes. In J. Strachey (Ed. and Trans.), *The standard edition of the complete psychological works of Sigmund Freud* (Vol. 19, pp. 248–258). London: Hogarth Press.

Freud, S. (1928). Dostoyevsky and parricide. In J. Strachey (Ed. and Trans.), *The standard edition of the complete psychological works of Sigmund Freud* (Vol. 21, pp. 175–196). London: Hogarth Press.

Freud, S. (1930). Civilization and its discontents. In J. Strachey (Ed. and Trans.), *The standard edition of the complete psychological works of Sigmund Freud* (Vol. 21, pp. 64–145). London: Hogarth Press.

Freud, S. (1932). *New introductory lectures on psychoanalysis.* New York: Norton.

Friedman, A.F., Bollinskey, P., Nichols, D., & Levak, R.W. (2014). *Psychological assessment with the MMPI-2/MMPl-2-RF*. New York: Routledge.

Friedman, L.M. (1993). *Crime and punishment in American history*. New York: Basic Books.

Friedmann, F.P. (1948). The legal disposition of the sexual psychopath. *University of Pennsylvania Law Review, 96*, 884–887.

Fujita, H. (1996). The TAT applied to an attempted murder suspect. *Japanese Journal of Criminal Psychology, 34*, 25–35.

Furby, L., Weinrott, M.R., & Blackshaw, L. (1989). Sex offender recidivism: A review. *Psychological Bulletin, 105*, 3–30.

Furio, J. (2001). *Team killers: A comparative study of collaborative criminals*. New York: Algora.

Gaarb, H.N. (1998). *Studying the clinician*. Washington, DC: American Psychiatric Association Press.

Gacono, C.B. (1992a). A Rorschach case study of sexual homicide. *British Journal of Projective Psychology, 37*, 1–21.

Gacono, C.B. (1992b). Sexual homicide and the Rorschach. *British Journal of Projective Psychology, 37*, 1–21.

Gacono, C.B., Evans, F.B., & Viglione, D.J. (2002). The Rorschach in forensic practice. *Journal of Forensic Psychology Practice, 2*, 33–53.

Gacono, C.B., & Meloy, J.R. (2013). *The Rorschach assessment of aggressive and psychopathic personalities*. New York: Taylor & Francis.

Gacono, L.B., Meloy, J.R., & Bridges, M.R. (2000). A Rorschach comparison of psychopaths, sexual homicide perpetrators, and non-violent pedophiles: Where angels fear to tread. *Journal of Clinical Psychology, 66*, 757–777.

Ganellen, R.J. (1996). *Integrating the Rorschach and the MMPI-2 in personality assessment*. Hillsdale, NJ: Lawrence Erlbaum.

Ganser, S.J. (1898). A peculiar hysterical state. *Archives für Psychiatrie & Neuen- Krankheiten, 30*, 633–640.

Garland, D. (1990). *Punishment and modern society: A study in social theory*. Chicago, IL: University of Chicago Press.

Garrison, A. (1996). The catathymic crisis: An explanation of the serial killer. *Journal of Police and Criminal Psychology, 11*, 4–12.

Gault, W. (1971). Some remarks on slaughter. *American Journal of Psychiatry, 128*, 450–454.

Gayral, L., Millet, G., Moron, P., & Turnin, J. (1956). Crises et paroxysmes catathymiques [Crises and catathymic paroxysms]. *Annales Médico Psychologiques, 114*, 25–50.

Geberth, V.J. (1981, September). Psychological profiling. *Law and Order*, 46–49.

Geberth, V.J. (1996). *Practical homicide investigation: Tactics, procedures, and forensic techniques*. Boca Raton, FL: CRC Press.

Geberth, V.J., & Turco, R.N. (1997). Antisocial personality disorder, sexual sadism, malignant narcissism, and serial murder. *Journal of Forensic Sciences, 42*, 49–60.

Geiser, L., & Stein, M.I. (1999). *Evocative images: The Thematic Apperception Test and the art of projection*. Washington, DC: APA Press.

Geller, L., Erlen, J., & Pinkus, L. (1986). A historical appraisal of America's experience with "pyromania": A diagnosis in search of a disorder. *International Journal of Law and Psychiatry, 9*, 201–229.

Gelles, R.J. (1973). Child abuse as psychopathology: A sociological critique and reformulation. *American Journal of Orthopsychiatry, 43*, 611–621.

Gibbons, D.C. (1968). *Society, crime, and criminal careers*. Englewood Cliffs, NJ: Prentice Hall.

Gibran, K. (1923). *The Prophet*. New York: Knopf.

Gil, D. (1970). *Violence against children*. Cambridge, MA: Harvard University Press.

Gilbert, G.M. (1947). *Nuremberg diary*. New York: Farrar, Straus.

Giorgi, A. (1977). The theory, practice, and evaluation of the phenomenological method as a qualitative research method. *Journal of Phenomenological Psychology, 28*, 235–260.

Gleyzer, R., Felthous, A.R., & Holzer, L.E. (2002). Animal cruelty and psychiatric disorder. *Journal of the American Academy of Psychiatry and Law, 30*, 257–265.

Glover, E. (1960). *The roots of crime.* New York: International Universities Press.

Godwin, G.M. (2000). *Hunting serial predators: A multivariate classification approach to profiling violent behavior.* Boca Raton, FL: CRC Press.

Godwin, M.G., & Canter, D. (1997). Encounter and death: The spatial behavior of US serial killers. *Policing: An International Journal of Police Strategy and Management, 20*, 24–38.

Gold, L.H. (2001). Clinical and forensic aspects of postpartum disorders. *Journal of the American Academy of Psychiatry and Law, 29*, 344–347.

Goldstein, N., Romaine, C.L., Zelle, H., Mesiarik, C., & Wolbransky, M. (2011). Psychometric properties of the Miranda Rights Comprehension Instruments with a juvenile justice sample. *Assessment, 18*, 428–441.

Goldstein, P., Brownstein, H.H., & Ryan, P.J. (1992). Drug-related homicides in New York: 1984–1988. *Crime and Delinquency, 38*, 459–476.

Goldstein, R.L. (1987). More forensic romances: De Clerambault's syndrome in men. *Bulletin of the American Academy of Psychiatry and Law, 15*, 267–274.

Goldstein, R.L. (2000). Serial stalkers: Recent clinical findings. In L.B. Schlesinger (Ed.), *Serial offenders: Current thought, recent findings* (pp. 167–186). Boca Raton, FL: CRC Press.

Gordon, R.M. (2001). *The American murders of Jack the Ripper.* Westport, CT: Praeger.

Gordon, R.M. (2003). *The American murders of Jack the Ripper.* Wesport CT: Praeger.

Goring, C. (1913). *The English convict.* London: Her Majesty's Stationery Office.

Gottfredson, S. (1987). Statistical and actuarial considerations. In F.N. Dutile & C.H. Foust (Eds.), *The prediction of criminal violence* (pp. 71–81). Springfield, IL: Charles C Thomas.

Gowers, W.R. (1885). *Epilepsy and other chronic convulsive disorders.* New York: William Wood & Co.

Grant, J.E., & Kim, S.W. (2007). Clinical characteristics and psychiatric co-morbidity of pyromania. *Journal of Clinical Psychiatry, 68*, 1717–1722.

Gratzer, T., & Bradford, J. (1995). Offender and offense characteristics of sexual sadists: A comparative study. *Journal of Forensic Sciences, 40*, 450–455.

Green, D., & Rosenfield, B. (2013). New and improved? A comparison of the original and revised versions of the Structured Interview Reported Symptoms. *Assessment, 20*, 210–218.

Greenall, P.V. (2012). Understanding sexual homicide. *Journal of Sexual Aggression, 18*, 338–354.

Greilsheimer, H., & Groves, J.E. (1979). Male genital self-mutilation. *Archives of General Psychiatry, 36*, 441–446.

Grendliner, V., & Byrne, D. (1987). Coercive sexual fantasies of college men as predic- tors of self-reported likelihood to rape and overt sexual aggression. *Journal of Sex Research, 23*, 1–11.

Grombach, J.V. (1982). *The giant liquidator.* Garden City, NY: Doubleday.

Grossman, L.S., Martis, B., & Fichtner, C.G. (1999). Are sex offenders treatable? A research review. *Psychiatric Services, 50*, 349–361.

Groth, A.N. (1979). *Men who rape: The psychology of the offender.* New York: Plenum.

Grubin, D. (1994). Sexual murder. *British Journal of Psychiatry, 165*, 624–629.

Grubin, D. (1997). Predictors of risk in serious sex offenders. *British Journal of Psychiatry, 170*, 17–21.

Grubin, D. (2010). The polygraph and forensic psychiatry. *Journal of the American Academy of Psychiatry and Law, 38*, 446–451.

Gudjonsson, G. (1990). One hundred alleged false confession cases: Some normative data. *British Journal of Clinical Psychology, 29*, 249–250.

Gudjonsson, G. (1995). "I'll help you boys as much as I can": How eagerness to please can result in a false confession. *Journal of Forensic Psychiatry, 6*, 333–342.

Gudjonsson, G. (1999). The making of a serial false confessor: The confessions of Henry Lee Lucas. *Journal of Forensic Psychiatry, 10*, 416–426.

Gudjonsson, G.H. (2018). *The psychology of false confessions: Forty years of science and practice.* New York: Wiley.

Gunn, J., & Bonn, J. (1971). Criminality and violence in epileptic prisoners. *British Journal of Psychiatry, 118,* 337–343.

Gunn, J., & Taylor, P.J. (1993). *Forensic psychiatry: Clinical, legal, and ethical issues.* Oxford: Butterworth-Heinemann.

Guttmacher, M.S. (1960). *The mind of the murderer.* New York: Farrar, Strauss & Cudahy.

Guttmacher, M.S. (1963). Dangerous offenders. *Crime and Delinquency, 9,* 381–390.

Guttmacher, M.S., & Weihoffer, H. (1952). *Psychiatry and the law.* New York: Norton.

Haapasalo, J., & Petaejae, S. (1999). Mothers who killed or attempted to kill their child: Life circumstances, childhood abuse, and types of killing. *Violence and Victims, 14,* 219–239.

Habermann, H., & Briken, B.W. (2007). Psychiatric disorders in single and multiple sexual murderers. *Psychopathology, 40,* 22–28.

Hagan, F.E. (1994). *Introduction to criminology* (3rd ed.). Chicago: Nelson-Hall.

Hain, J.D. (1964). The Bender-Gestalt test: A scoring method for identifying brain damage. *Journal of Consulting Psychology, 28,* 34–40.

Hale, R. (1994). The role of humiliation and embarrassment in serial murder. *Psychology: A Journal of Human Behavior, 31,* 17–23.

Halleck, S. (1971). *Psychiatry and the dilemmas of crime.* Los Angeles: University of California Press.

Halleck, S. (1978). Violence: Treatment versus correction. In I.L. Kutash, S.B. Kutash, & L.B. Schlesinger (Eds.), *Violence: Perspectives on murder and aggression* (pp. 377–393). San Francisco: Jossey-Bass.

Hammer, E.F. (1997a). *The clinical application of projective drawings* (6th ed.). Springfield, IL: Charles C Thomas.

Hammer, E.F. (1997b). The prediction of acting-out eruptions: Assault, rape, sexual abuse, homicide, suicide, exhibitionism. In E.F. Hammer (Ed.), *Advances in projective drawing interpretation* (pp. 45–78). Springfield, IL: Charles C Thomas.

Handler, L., & Thomas, A.D. (2013). *Drawings in assessment and psychotherapy.* New York: Routledge.

Hanson, R.K., & Bussiére, M.T. (1998). Predicting relapse: A meta-analysis of sexual offender recidivism studies. *Journal of Consulting and Clinical Psychology, 66,* 348–362.

Harcourt, B.E. (1998). Reflecting on the subject: A critique of the social influence conception of deterrence, the broken windows theory, and order-maintaining policing New York style. *Michigan Law Review, 97,* 292–386.

Hare, R.D. (1980). A research scale for the assessment of psychopathy in criminal populations. *Personality and Individual Differences, 1,* 111–119.

Hare, R.D. (1991). *Manual for the revised Psychopathy Checklist.* Toronto: Multi-Health Systems.

Hare, R.D. (1993). *Without conscience: The disturbing world of the psychopaths among us.* New York: Pocket Books.

Hare, R.D., Harpur, T.J., Hakstian, A.R., Forth, A.E., Hart, S.D., & Newman, J.P. (1990). The revised Psychopathy Checklist: Descriptive statistics, reliability, and factor structure. *Psychological Assessment, 2,* 338–341.

Harrer, G., & Kofler-Westergren, B. (1986). Depression and criminality. *Psychopathology, 19*(Suppl. 2), 215–219.

Hazelwood, R. (1989). Forward. In E. Revitch & L.B. Schlesinger (Eds.), *Sex murder and sex aggression.* Springfield, IL: Charles C Thomas.

Hazelwood, R.R., Dietz, P.E., & Warren, J.I. (1999). The criminal sadist. In R.R. Hazelwood & A.W. Burgess (Eds.), *Practical aspects of rape investigation* (2nd ed., pp. 361–371). Boca Raton, FL: CRC Press.

Hazelwood, R.R., & Douglas, J.E. (1980). The lust murderer. *FBI Law Enforcement Bulletin, 49,* 1–5.

Hazelwood, R.R., & Michaud, S.G. (2001). *Dark dreams: Sexual violence, homicide and the criminal mind.* New York: St. Martin's Press.

Hazelwood, R.R., & Warren, J.I. (1995). The relevance of fantasy in serial sexual crime investigation. In R.R. Hazelwood & A.W. Burgess (Eds.), *Practical aspects of rape investigation* (2nd ed., pp. 127–138). Boca Raton, FL: CRC Press.

Hazelwood, R.R., & Warren, J.I. (2000). The sexually violent offender: Impulsive or ritualistic? *Aggression and Violent Behavior, 5,* 267–279.

Hazelwood, R.R., & Warren, J. (2003). Linkage analysis: Modus operandi, ritual, and signature in serial sexual crime. *Aggression and Violent Behavior, 8,* 587–598.

Hazelwood, R.R., Warren, J.I., & Dietz, P.E. (1993). Compliant victims of the sexual sadist. *Australian Family Physician, 22,* 474–479.

Healey, J., Beauregard, E., & Beech, A. (2016). Is the sexual murderer a unique type of offender? A typology of violent sexual offenders using crime scene behavior. *Sexual abuse, 28,* 512–533.

Heath, S. (1986). Psychopathia sexualis: Stevenson's strange case. *Critical Quarterly, 28,* 93–108.

Hedaya, R.J. (1996). *Understanding biological psychiatry.* New York: Norton.

Heide, K.M., & Frei, A. (2009). Matricide: A critique of the literature. *Trauma, Violence, & Abuse, 11,* 3–17.

Heide, K.M., & Solomon, E. (2006). Biology, childhood trauma, and murder: Rethinking justice. *International Journal of Law and Psychiatry, 29,* 220–233.

Heilbrun, K. (1992). The role of psychological testing in forensic assessment. *Law and Human Behavior, 16,* 257–272.

Heilbrun, K., Rosenfeld, B., Warren, J., & Collins, S. (1994). The use of third party information in forensic assessments: A two state comparison. *Bulletin of the American Academy of Psychiatry and Law, 22,* 399–406.

Hein, S.F., & Austin, W.J. (2001). Empirical and hermeneutic approaches to phenomenological research in psychology: A comparison. *Psychological Methods, 6,* 3–17.

Hellman, D.D., & Blackman, N. (1966). Enuresis, firesetting, and cruelty to animals: A triad predictive of adult crime. *American Journal of Psychiatry, 122,* 1431–1435.

Hempel, A.G., Levine, R.E., Meloy, J.R., & Westermeyer, J. (2000). A cross-cultural review of sudden mass assault by a single individual in the oriental and occidental cultures. *Journal of Forensic Sciences, 45,* 582–588.

Hempel, A.G., Meloy, J.R., & Richards, T.C. (1999). Offender and offense characteristics of a non-random sample of mass murderers. *Journal of the American Academy of Psychiatry and Law, 27,* 213–225.

Hershman, D.J., & Lieb, J. (1994). *A brotherhood of tyrants: Manic-depression and absolute power.* Amherst, NY: Prometheus.

Hess, A.K., & Weiner, I.B. (1999). *Handbook of forensic psychology* (2nd ed.). New York: John Wiley.

Hickey, E.W. (1991). *Serial murderers and their victims.* Monterey, CA: Brooks/Cole.

Hickey, E.W. (1997). *Serial murderers and their victims* (2nd ed.). Belmont, CA: Wadsworth.

Higgs, T., Carter, A.J., Tully, R., & Browne, K.D. (2017). Sexual murder typologies: A systematic review. *Aggression and Violent Behavior, 35,* 1–12.

Hill, A., Rettenberger, M., & Haberman, N. (2012). The utility of risk assessment instruments for the prediction of recidivism in sexual homicide perpetrators. *Journal of Interpersonal Violence, 27,* 3553–3578.

Hill, D., & Williams, P. (1967). *The supernatural.* New York: Signet.

Hinsie, L.E., & Campbell, R.J. (1970). *Psychiatric dictionary* (4th ed.). New York: Oxford University Press.

Hirose, S. (1979). Depression and homicide: A psychiatric and forensic study of four cases. *Acta Psychiatrica Scandinavica, 59,* 211–217.

Holcomb, W.R., Adams, N.A., & Ponder, H.M. (1985). The development and cross- validation of an MMPI typology of murderers. *Journal of Personality Assessment, 49,* 240–244.

Holcomb, W.R., & Daniel, A.E. (1988). Homicide without an apparent motive. *Behavioral Sciences and the Law, 6,* 429–437.

Holinger, P.C. (1987). *Violent deaths in the United States.* New York: Guilford Press.

Holmes, R.M., & DeBurger, J.E. (1985). Profiles in terror: The serial murderer. *Federal Probation*, *49*, 29–34.

Horney, J. (1978). Menstrual cycles and criminal responsibility. *Law and Human Behavior, 2*, 25–36.

Howard, A.K. (2018). *His garden: Conversations with a sexual killer*: Denver: Wildblue Press.

Hunter, J.T. (2017). *Deadly deception: True story of Tampa's serial killer Bobby Joe Long*. Toronto: R. J. Parker Publisher.

Hutt, M.L. (1968a). *The Hutt adaptation of the Bender-Gestalt test: Revised*. New York: Grune & Stratton.

Hutt, M.L. (1968b). The projective use of the Bender-Gestalt test. In A.I. Rabin (Ed.), *Projective techniques in personality assessment* (pp. 397–452). New York: Springer.

Inbau, F., Reid, J.E., Buckley, J., & Jayne, B. (2004). *Criminal Interrogation and confessions* (4th ed.). Boston: Jones & Bartlett.

Irvine, L.M., & Brelje, T.B. (1972). *Law, psychiatry, and the mentally disturbed offender*. Springfield, IL: Charles C.Thomas.

Isenberg, S. (1991). *Women who love men who kill*. New York: Simon & Schuster.

Izner, S.M., Goldman, J., & Leiser, R. (1953). Hysterical amnesia treated by hypnosis. *Diseases of the Nervous System, 14*, 313–315.

Jackson, J.L., & Bekerian, D.A. (1997). *Offender profiling: Theory, research, and practice*. New York: John Wiley.

Jacobs, P.A., Brunton, M., & Melville, M.M. (1965). Aggressive behavior, mental subnormality, and the XYY male. *Nature, 208*, 1351–1352.

Jaffe, P.D., & DiCataldo, F. (1994). Clinical vampirism: Blending myth and reality. *Bulletin of the American Academy of Psychiatry and Law, 22*, 533–544.

Jameison, G.R. (1936). Suicide and mental disease: A clinical study of one hundred cases. *Archives of Neurology and Psychiatry. 36*, 1–12.

James, J., Lussier, P., & Proulx, J. (2018b). Serial and nonserial sexual murderers. In J. Proulx, E. Beauregard, A.L. Carter, A. Mokros, R. Darjee, & J. James (Eds.), *Routledge international handbook of sexual homicide studies* (pp. 70–91). New York: Routledge.

James, J., & Proulx, J. (2014). A psychological and developmental profile of sexual murders: A systematic review. *Aggression and Violent Behavior, 19*, 592–607.

James, J., & Proulx, J. (2016). The modus operandi of serial and nonserial sexual murderers: A systematic review. *Aggression and Violent Behavior, 31*, 200–218.

James, J. Proulx, J., & Lussier, P. (2018a). A cross-national study of sexual murderers in France and Canada. In J. Proulx, E. Beauregard., A.J. Carter, A Mokros, R. Darjee, & J. James (Eds.). *Routledge international handbook of sexual homicide studies* (pp. 171–195). New York: Routledge.

Jenkins, P. (1988). Serial murder in England, 1940–1985. *Journal of Criminal Justice, 16*, 1–15.

Jenkins, P. (1989). Serial murder in the U.S., 1900–1940: Historical perspective. *Journal of Criminal Justice, 17*, 377–391.

Jenkins, S.R. (2014). Thematic apperceptive techniques inform a science of individuality. *Rorschachiana, 35*, 92–102.

Jenkins, S.R. (2017). The narrative arc of TATs: Introduction to the JPA special section on thematic apperceptive techniques. *Journal of Personality Assessment, 99*, 225–237.

Jensen, A.R. (1957). Aggression in fantasy and overt behavior. *Psychological Monographs, 71* (whole No. 445), 1–13.

Jentzen, J., Palermo, G., Johnson, L.T., Ho, K.C., Stormo, K.A., & Teggatz, J. (1994). Destructive hostility: The Jeffrey Dahmer case: A psychiatric and forensic study of a serial killer. *American Journal of Forensic Medicine and Pathology, 15*, 283–294.

Johnson, B.R., & Becker, J.V. (1997). Natural born killers? The development of the sexually sadistic serial killer. *Journal of the American Academy of psychiatry and Law, 25*, 335–348.

Johnson, P.H. (1967). *On iniquity*. New York: Scribner.

Jones, S., Chan, H., Myers, W., & Heide, K. (2013). A proposed sexual homicide category: The psychopathic–sexually sadistic offender. In J.B. Helfgott (Ed.), *Criminal psychology (vol. 2: Typologies, mental disorders, and profiles*, pp. 403–422). Westport, CT: Praegar.

Justice, B., Justice, R, and Kraft, I. (1974). Early-warning signs of violence: Is a triad enough? *American Journal of Psychiatry, 131*, 457–459.

Kafka, M.P. (1995). Sexual impulsivity. In E. Hollander & D.J. Stein (Eds.), *Impulsivity and aggression* (pp. 212–223). New York: John Wiley.

Kahn, E. (1931). *Psychopathie*. Berlin: Gruyter.

Kahn, M.W. (1968). Superior performance IQ of murderers as a function of overt act or diagnosis. *Journal of Social Psychiatry, 76*, 113–116.

Kalichman, S.C. (1988). Empirically derived MMPI profile subgroups of incarcerated homicide offenders. *Journal of Clinical Psychology, 44*, 733–738.

Karaskasi, M.V., Vasilikos, E., Voultsos, P., Vlachaki, A., & Pavlidis, P. (2017. Sexual homicide: Brief review of the literature and case report involving rape, genital mutilation and human arson. *Journal of Forensic and Legal Medicine, 46*, 1–10.

Karmen, A. (2001). *Crime victims: An introduction to victimology* (4th ed.). Belmont, CA: Wadsworth.

Karmen, A. (2012). *Crime victims: An introduction to victimology* (8th ed). Belmont, CA: Wadsworth.

Karpman, B. (1935). *The individual criminal*. Washington, DC: Nervous and Mental Disease Publishing Co.

Karpman, B. (1948). The myth of psychopathic personality. *American Journal of Psychiatry, 104*, 523–534.

Karpman, B. (1954). *The sexual offender and his offenses*. New York: Julian Press.

Kassin, S.M. (1997). The psychology of confession evidence. *American Psychologist, 52*, 221–233.

Kassin, S.M. (1998). More on the psychology of false confession. *American Psychologist, 53*, 320–321.

Kassin, S.M. (2008). Confession evidence: Myths and misconceptions. *Criminal Justice and Behavior, 35*, 1309–1322.

Kassin, S.M., & Fong, C.T. (1999). "I'm innocent!" Effects of training on judgments of truth and deception in the interrogation room. *Law and Human Behavior, 23*, 499–516.

Kassin, S.M., & Kiechel, K.L. (1996). The social psychology of false confession: Compliance, internalization, and confabulation. *Psychological Science, 7*, 125–128.

Kassin, S.M., Tubb, V.A., Hosch, H.M., & Memon, A. (2001). On the "general acceptance" of eyewitness testimony research. *American Psychologist, 56*, 405–416.

Kassin, S.M., & Wrightsman, L. (1985). Confession evidence. In S. Kassin & L. Wrightsman (Eds.), *The psychology of evidence and trial procedure* (pp. 67–94). Beverly Hills, CA: Sage.

Kaufman, B., & Wohl, A. (1992). *Casualties of childhood: A developmental perspective on sexual abuse using projective drawings*. New York: Routledge.

Kavirajan, H. (1999). The amobarbital interview revisited: A review of the literature since 1966. *Harvard Review of Psychiatry, 7*, 153–165.

Kendrick, D.T., & Sheets, V. (1993). Homicidal fantasies. *Ethology and Sociobiology, 14*, 231–246.

Kennedy, F., Hoffman, H., & Haines, W.A. (1947). A study of William Heirens. *American Journal of Psychiatry, 104*, 113–121.

Kennedy, L. (1961). *Ten rollington place*. New York: Simon & Schuster.

Keppel, R.D. (1995). Signature murderers: A report of several related cases. *Journal of Forensic Sciences, 40*, 670–674.

Keppel, R.D. (1997). *Signature killers: Interpreting the calling cards of the serial murderer*. New York: Pocket Books.

Keppel, R.D. (2000). Investigation of the serial offender: Linking cases through M.O. and signature. In L.B. Schlesinger (Ed.), *Serial offenders* (pp. 121–134). Boca Raton, FL: CRC Press.

Kerr, K., Beech, A., & Murphy, D. (2013). Sexual homicide: Definition, motivation and comparison with other forms of sexual offending. *Aggression and Violent Behavior, 18*, 1–10.

Kienlen, K. (1998). Development and social antecedents of stalking. In J.R. Meloy (Ed.), *The psychology of stalking* (pp. 51–67). New York: Academic Press.

Kirschner, D., & Nagel, L. (1996). Catathymic violence, dissociative and adoption pathology: Implications for the mental status defense. *International Journal of Offender Therapy and Comparative Criminology, 40*, 204–211.

Klepfisz, A., & Racy, J. (1973). Homicide and LSD. *Journal of the American Medical Association, 22*, 429–439.

Klopfer, B., & Kelly, D.M. (1942). *The Rorschach technique*. Tarrytown, NY: World Press.

Knoll, J.L., & Hazelwood, R.R. (2009). Becoming the victim: Beyond sadism in serial sexual murderers. *Aggression and Violent Behavior, 14*, 106–114.

Koch, J.L. (1888). *The psychopathic inferiorities*. Ravensburg: Maier.

Koch, J.L. (1889). *Leitfaden der Psychiatrie*. Ravensburg: Dorn.

Kocsis, R.N. (2003). Criminal psychological profiling: Validities and abilities. *International Journal of Offender Therapy and Comparative Criminology, 47*, 126–144.

Kocsis, R.N. (2006). Validities and abilities in criminal profiling: The dilemma for David Canter's investigative psychology. *International Journal of Offender Therapy and Comparative Criminology, 50*, 458–477.

Koeppel, S., Schlesinger, L.B., Craun, S.W., Keel, T.G., Rubin, D., & Kum, J. (2019). Foreign object insertions in sexual homicide. *International Journal of Offender Therapy and Comparative Criminology, 63*, 1726–1737.

Kogan, N., & Wallach, M.A. (1964). *Risk taking: A study in cognition and personality*. New York: Holt, Rinehart & Winston.

Kogan, N., & Wallach, M. (1967). Risky shift phenomenon in small decision-making groups: A test of the information-exchange hypothesis. *Journal of Experimental Social Psychology, 3*, 75–84.

Koppitz, E.M. (1964). *The Bender-Gestalt test for young children*. New York: Grune & Stratton.

Kozol, H.L., Boucher, R.J., & Garofalo, R.F. (1972). The diagnosis and treatment of dangerousness. *Crime and Delinquency, 19*, 371–392.

Kozol, H.L., Cohen, M.I., & Garofalo, R.F. (1966). The criminally dangerous sex offender. *New England Journal of Medicine, 275*, 79–86.

Kraepelin, E. (1913). *Lectures on clinical psychiatry* (3rd ed.). New York: William Wood.

Krafft-Ebing, R. von. (1886). *Psychopathia sexualis* (C.G. Chaddock, Trans.). Philadelphia, PA: F.A. Davis.

Kretschmer, E. (1925). *Physique and character*. London: Kegan Paul.

Kretschmer, E. (1934). *A textbook of medical psychology*. London: Oxford University Press.

Krueger, R.B. (2009). The *DSM* diagnostic criteria for sexual sadism. *Archives of Sexual Behavior, 19*, 325–345.

Kundu, R., & Bhaumik, C. (1982). Some affective personality qualities of a murderer: A research note. *Personality Study and Group Behavior, 2*, 36–43.

Lamberti, J.W., Blackman, N., & Weiss, J. (1958). The sudden murderer: A preliminary report. *Journal of Social Therapy, 4*, 2–15.

Lane, R.C. (1984). Robert Lindner and the case of Charles, a teenage sex murderer: Songs my mother taught me. *Current Issues in Psychoanalytic Practice, 1*, 65–83.

Langevin, R. (1991). The sex killer. In A.W. Burgess (Ed.), *Rape and sexual assault, part III: A research handbook* (pp. 257–273). New York: Garland.

Langevin, R. (2003). A study of the psychosexual characteristics of sex killers: Can we identify them before it is too late? *International Journal of Offender Therapy and Comparative Criminology, 47*, 366–382.

Langfeldt, G. (1969). Schizophrenia: Diagnosis and prognosis. *Behavioral Science, 14*, 173–182.

Lanzkron, J. (1963). Murder and insanity. *American Journal of Psychiatry, 119*, 754–758.

Lassiter, G., & Meissner, C. (Eds.). (2010). *Police interrogation and false confession: Current research, practice and policy recommendations*. Washington, DC: American Psychological Association.

Lauerman, H. (2001). Klinefelter's syndrome and sexual homicide. *Journal of Forensic Psychiatry, 12*, 151–157.

Lavergne, G.M. (1998). *A sniper in the tower: The Charles Whitman murders.* New York: Doubleday.

LeBon, G. (1910). *La psychologie politique et la défense sociale.* Paris: Flammarion.

Lee, C.D. (1953). *The instrumental detection of deception — the lie test.* Springfield, IL: Charles C Thomas.

Lee, J., & Choi, K. (2014). Serial murder: An exploration and evaluation of theories and perspectives. *American International Journal of Contemporary Research, 4*, 99–106.

Leibowitz, M. (1999). *Interpreting projective drawings: A self psychological approach.* Philadelphia, PA: Brunner/Mazel.

Leitenberg, H., & Henning, K. (1995). Sexual fantasy. *Psychological Bulletin, 117*, 469–496.

Levi, J. (2019). *Inside Broadmoor: Up close and personal with Britain's most dangerous criminals.* London: Blink.

Levin, J., & Fox, J.A. (1985). *Mass murder.* New York: Plenum.

Lewis, B. (1987). *The assassins.* New York: Oxford University Press.

Lewis, D.O., Pincus, J.N., Feldman, M., Jackson, L., & Bard, B. (1986). Psychiatric, neurological, and psychoeducational characteristics of 15 death-row inmates in the Unites States. *American Journal of Psychiatry, 143*, 838–845.

Lewis, D.O., Shanok, S.S., & Pincus, J.N. (1979). Violent juvenile delinquents: Psychiatric, neurological, psychological, and abuse factors. *Journal of the American Academy of Child Psychiatry, 18*, 307–319.

Lewis, J.A. (1975). Violence and epilepsy. *Journal of the American Medical Association, 232*, 1165–1167.

Lewis, M., & Saarni, C. (Eds.). (1993). *Lying and deception in every day life.* New York: Guilford Press.

Lewis, N.D.C., & Yarnell, H. (1951). *Pyromania (pathological firesetting).* Nervous and Mental Disease Monographs No. 82. New York: Collidge Foundation.

Lieber, A.L. (1978). *The lunar effect.* New York: Doubleday.

Liebert, J.A. (1985). Contributions of psychiatric consultation in the investigation of serial murder. *International Journal of Offender Therapy and Comparative Criminology, 28*, 187–200.

Lifton, B.J. (1994). *Journey of the adopted self.* New York: Basic Books.

Lifton, R.J. (1986). *The Nazi doctors: Medical killing and the psychology of genocide.* New York: Basic Books.

Lindner, R.M. (1946). Content analysis in Rorschach work. *Rorschach Research Exchange, 10*, 121–129.

Lindner, R.M. (1950). Content analysis of the Rorschach protocol. In L.E. Abt & L. Bellak (Eds.), *Projective Psychology: Clinical approaches to the total personality* (pp. 68–82). New York: Knopf.

Lindner, R.M. (1982). *The fifty minute hour* (2nd ed.). Northvale, NJ: Aronson.

Lisak, D., Hopper, J., & Song, P. (1996). The relationship between child abuse, gender adjustment, and perpetration in men. *Journal of Traumatic Stress, 9*, 721–743.

Litwack, T.R. (2001). Actuarial versus clinical assessments of dangerousness. *Psychology, Public Policy, and Law, 7*, 409–443.

Litwack, T.R. (2002). Some questions for the field of violence risk assessment and forensic mental health: Or, "back to basics" revisited. *International Journal of Forensic Mental Health, 1*, 171–178.

Litwack, T.R., & Schlesinger, L.B. (1987). Assessing and predicting violence: Research, law, and applications. In I.B. Weiner & A.K. Hess (Eds.), *Handbook of forensic psychology* (pp. 205–257). New York: John Wiley.

Litwack, T.R., & Schlesinger, L.B. (1999). Dangerousness risk assessments: Research, legal, and clinical considerations. In A.K. Hess & I.B. Weiner (Eds.), *Handbook of forensic psychology* (2nd ed., pp. 171–217). New York: John Wiley.

Litzche, S., Horn, A., & Schinke, D. (2015). *Sexualmord in Bayern*. Frankfurt: Polizeiwissenschaft.

Lockwood, R. (2005). Cruelty toward cats: Changing perspectives. In D.J. Salem & A.N. Rowan (Eds.). *The state of the animals III* (pp. 15–26). Washington, DC: Humane Society Press.

Loftus, E.F. (2019). Eyewitness testimony. *Applied Cognitive Psychology, 33*, 498–503.

Loftus, E.F., & Doyle, J.M. (1976). *Eyewitness testimony: Civil and criminal*. Charlottesville, VA: Lexis Law.

Loftus, E.F., & Ketchman, K. (1991). *Witness for the defense: The accused, the eyewitness, and the expert who puts memory on trial*. New York: St. Martin's Press.

Loftus, G.R. (1996). Psychology will be a much better science when we change the way we analyze data. *Current Directions in Psychological Science, 5*, 161–171.

Lombroso, C. (1911). *Crime: Its causes and remedies* (H.P. Horton, Trans.). Boston: Little, Brown. (Original work published 1876).

Lourie, R. (1993). *Hunting the devil*. New York: Harper Collins.

Lowenstein, L.F. (1992). The psychology of the obsessed compulsive killer. *Criminologist, 16*, 26–38.

Lunde, D.T. (1976). *Murder and madness*. San Francisco: San Francisco Book Co.

Lundy, A. (1988). Instrumental set and Thematic Appreciation Test Validity. *Journal of Personality Assessment, 52*, 309–320.

Luntz, B.K., & Widom, C.S. (1994). Antisocial personality disorder in abused and neglected children growing up. *American Journal of Psychiatry, 151*, 670–674.

Lykken, D.T. (1998). *A tremor in the blood: Uses and abuses of the lie detector*. New York: Plenum Press.

Lyle, W.H. (Ed.). (1973). *Behavioral science and modern penology*. Springfield, IL: Charles C Thomas.

MacCulloch, M.C., Gray, N., & Watt, A. (2000). Brittain's sadistic murderer syndrome reconsidered: An associative account of the etiology of sadistic sexual fantasy. *Journal of Forensic Psychiatry, 11*, 401–418.

MacCulloch, M.C., Snowden, P.J., Wood, P., & Mills, H.E. (1983). Sadistic fantasy, sadistic behavior, and offending. *British Journal of Psychiatry, 143*, 20–29.

MacDonald, J.M. (1954). Narcoanalysis and the criminal law. *American Journal of Psychiatry, 111*, 283–288.

MacDonald, J.M. (1961). *The murderer and his victim*. Springfield, IL: Charles C Thomas.

MacDonald, J.M. (1963). The threat to kill. *American Journal of Psychiatry, 120*, 125–130.

MacDonald, J.M. (1967). Homicidal threats. *American Journal of Psychiatry, 124*, 475–482.

MacDonald, J.M. (1968). *Homicidal threats*. Springfield, IL: Charles C Thomas.

MacDonald, J.M. (1969). *Psychiatry and the criminal: A guide to psychiatric examination for the criminal court*. Springfield, IL: Charles C Thomas.

MacDonald, J.M. (1975). *Armed robbery*. Springfield, IL: Charles C Thomas.

MacDonald, J.M. (1986). *The murderer and his victims* (2nd ed.). Springfield, IL: Charles C Thomas.

MacLean, N., Neal, T., Morgan, R., & Murrie, D.C. (2019). Forensic clinicians' understanding of bias. *Psychology, Public Policy and Law, 25*, 323–330.

MacLean, P.D. (1962). New findings relevant to the evolution of psycho-sexual functions of the brain. *Journal of Nervous and Mental Disease, 135*, 289–301.

Maier, H.W. (1912). Katathyme Wahnbildung und Paranoia [On the subject of catathymic delusions and paranoia]. *Zeitschrift für die Gesamte Neurologie und Psychiatrie, 13*, 555–610.

Maier, H.W. (1923). Uebereinige arten der psychogenen Mechanismen [Regarding some types of psychogenic mechanisms: Catathymia, athymia, synthymia]. *Zeitschrift für die Gesamte Neurologie und Psychiatrie, 82*, 193–198.

Maier, H.W. (1987). *Cocaine addiction* (O.J. Kalant, Trans.). Toronto: Addiction Research Foundation. (Original work published 1926).

Malamuth, N.M. (1986). Prediction of naturalistic sexual aggression. *Journal of Personality and Social Psychology, 50*, 953–962.

Malmquist, C.P. (1996). *Homicide: A psychiatric perspective*. Washington, DC: American Psychiatric Press.

Maniglio, R. (2009). The impact of child sexual abuse on health: A systematic review of reviews. *Clinical Psychology Review, 29,* 647–657.

Maniglio, R. (2010). The role of deviant sexual fantasy in the etiopathogenesis of sexual homicide: A systematic review. *Aggression and Violent Behavior, 15,* 294–302.

Mark, V.M., & Ervin, F.R. (1970). *Violence and the brain.* New York: Harper & Row.

Mark, V.M., & Southgate, T.M. (1971). Violence and brain disease. *Journal of the American Medical Association, 216,* 1025–1034.

Marshall, W.L., Laws, D.R., & Barbaree, H.E. (1990). *Handbook of sexual assault: Issues, theories and treatment of the offender.* New York: Plenum.

Martin, S.E. (1992). The epidemiology of alcohol-related interpersonal violence. *Alcohol, Health, and Research World, 16,* 230–237.

Martinson, R. (1974). What works? Questions and answers about prison reform. *Public Interest, 35,* 22–54.

Mathis, G.L. (1971, January). The Madonna-prostitute syndrome. *Medical Aspects of Human Sexuality,* 202–209.

Matthews, J., & Wicker, C. (1996). *The eyeball killer.* New York: Kensington.

Mavromatis, M. (2000). Serial arson: Repetitive firesetting and pyromania. In L.B. Schlesinger (Ed.), *Serial offenders* (pp. 67–102). Boca Raton, FL: CRC Press.

Mayer-Gross, W., Stater, E., & Roth, M. (1969). *Clinical psychiatry* (3rd ed.). Baltimore: Williams & Wilkins.

Mayfield, D. (1976). Alcoholism, alcohol intoxication, and assaultive behavior. *Diseases of the Nervous System, 37,* 288–291.

McCall, W.V., Vaughn, W., Shelp, F.E., & McDonald, W.M. (1992). Controlled investigation of the amobarbital interview for catatonic mutism. *American Journal of Psychiatry, 149,* 202–206.

McCann, J. (1998). A conceptual framework for identifying various types of confessions. *Behavioral Science and the Law, 16,* 441–453.

McCarthy, J.B. (1978). Narcissism and the self in homicidal adolescents. *American Journal of Psychoanalysis, 38,* 19–29.

McConkey, K.M., & Sheehan, P.W. (1992). Ethical issues in forensic hypnosis. *Australian Psychologist, 27,* 150–153.

McDermaid, G., & Winkler, E.G. (1955). Psychopathology of infanticide. *Journal of Clinical and Experimental Psychopathology, 16,* 22–41.

McFarlane, J.M., Campbell, J.C., Wilt, S., Sachs, C.J., Ulrich, Y., & Xu, X. (1999). Stalking and intimate partner femicide. *Homicide Studies, 3,* 300–316.

McGrath, M.G. (2000). Criminal profiling: Is there a role for the forensic psychiatrist? *Journal of the American Academy of Psychiatry and Law, 28,* 315–324.

McGrath, R.J. (1991). Sex offender risk assessment and disposition planning: A review of empirical and clinical findings. *International Journal of Offender Therapy and Comparative Criminology, 35,* 328–350.

McKee, A., Stein, T., Nowjnski, C., Stern, R., Daneshvar, D., Alvarez, V., Lee, H., Hall, G., & Wojtowicz, S. (2013). The spectrum of disease in chronic traumatic encephalopathy, *Brain, 136,* 43–64.

McKenzie, C. (1995). A study of serial murder. *International Journal of Offender Therapy and Comparative Criminology, 39,* 3–10.

McKie, R.R. (1974). The mind of the murderer. In W.S. Willie (Ed.), *Citizens who commit murder* (pp. 71–90). St. Louis, MO: Warren Green.

Medlicott, R.W. (1966). Brief psychotic episodes (temporary insanity). *New Zealand Medical Journal, 65,* 966–972.

Mednick, S.A., Moffitt, T.E., & Stack, S.A. (Eds.). (1987). *The causes of crime: New biological approaches.* Cambridge: Cambridge University Press.

Meehl, P. (1954). *Clinical vs. statistical prediction.* Minneapolis, MN: University of Minnesota Press.

Megargee, E. (1966). Undercontrolled and overcontrolled personality types in extreme antisocial aggression. *Psychological Monographs, General and Applied, 80*, 1–29.

Meloy, J.R. (1988). *The psychopathic mind: Origins, dynamics and treatment.* Northvale, NJ: Aronson.

Meloy, J.R. (1992). *Violent attachments.* Northvale, NJ: Aronson.

Meloy, J.R. (1996a, Spring). Orestes in Southern California: A forensic case of matricide. *Journal of Psychiatry and Law,* 77–102.

Meloy, J.R. (1996b). Stalking (obsessional following): A review of some preliminary findings. *Aggression and Violent Behavior, 1*, 147–162.

Meloy, J.R. (1997). The psychology of wickedness: Psychopathy and sadism. *Psychiatric Annals, 27*, 630–633.

Meloy, J.R. (Ed.). (1998). *The psychology of stalking.* New York: Academic Press.

Meloy, J.R. (2000). The nature and dynamics of sexual homicide: An integrative review. *Aggression and Violent Behavior, 5*, 1–22.

Meloy, J.R. (2006). Empirical basis and forensic application of effective and predatory violence. *Australian and New Zealand Journal of Psychiatry, 40*, 539–547.

Meloy, J.R. (2010). A catathymic infanticide. *Journal of Forensic Sciences, 55*, 1393–1396.

Meloy, J.R., Gacono, L.B., & Kenney, L. (1994). A Rorschach investigation of sexual homicide. *Journal of Personality Assessment, 62*, 58–67.

Meloy, J.R. Hansen, T.L., & Weiner, I.B. (1997). Authority of the Rorschach: Legal citations during the past 50 years. *Journal of Personality Assessment, 69*, 53–62.

Meloy, J.R., & Mohandie, K. (2001). Investigating the role of screen violence in specific homicide cases. *Journal of Forensic Sciences, 46*, 1113–1118.

Melton, G.B., Petrila, J., Poythress, N., & Slobogin, C. (1997). *Psychological evaluations for the court* (2nd ed.). Ney York: Guilford.

Melton, G.B., Petrila, J., Poythress, N., Slobogin, C., Otto, R.., & Mossman, D. (2018). *Psychological evaluations for the courts* (4th ed.). New York: Guilford.

Mendelsohn, B. (1956, July). Victimology. *Etudes Internationales de Psycho-Sociologie Criminelle,* 23–26.

Mendelsohn, B. (1963). The origin of the doctrine of victimology. *Exerpta Criminologica, 3*, 239–244.

Menninger, K., & Mayman, M. (1956). Episodic dyscontrol: A third order of stress adaptation. *Bulletin of the Menninger Clinic, 20*, 153–163.

Menzies, R., Webster, C.D., McMain, S., Staley, S., & Scaglione, R. (1994). The dimensions of dangerousness revisited: Assessing forensic predictions about violence. *Law and Human Behavior, 18*, 1–29.

Merton, R.K. (1938). Social structure and anomie. *American Sociological Review, 3*, 672–682.

Merton, R.K. (1957). *Social theory and social structure.* New York: Free Press.

Meyerson, A. (1966). Amnesia for homicide. *Archives of General Psychiatry, 14*, 509–515.

Michaux, M.H., & Michaux, W.W. (1963). Psychodiagnostic follow-up of a juvenile sex murderer. *Psychoanalytic Review, 50*, 93–112.

Milgram, S. (1963). Behavioral study of obedience. *Journal of Abnormal and Social Psychology, 67*, 371–378.

Miller, D., & Looney, J. (1974). The prediction of adolescent homicide: Episodic dyscontrol and dehumanization. *American Journal of Psychoanalysis, 34*, 187–198.

Miller, H.A. (2001). *Miller Forensic Assessment of Symptoms Test.* Lutz, FL: Psychological Assessment Resources.

Miller, H.A. (2006). *Inventory of offender risks, needs, and strengths.* Lutz, FL: Psychological Assessment Resources.

Miller, L. (2000). The predator's brain: Neuropsychodynamics of serial killing. In L.B. Schlesinger (Ed.), *Serial offenders: Current thought, recent findings* (pp. 135–166). Boca Raton, FL: CRC Press.

Miller, P.A., & Eisenberg, N. (1988). The relation of empathy to aggressive and externalizing/antisocial behavior. *Psychological Bulletin, 103*, 324–344.

Milsom, J., Beech, A., & Webster, S. (2003). Emotional loneliness in sexual murderers: A qualitative analysis. *Sexual Abuse: A Journal of Research and Treatment, 15*, 285–296.

Miltenberger, R.G. (Ed.). (2001). *Tic disorders, trichotillomania, and other repetitive behavior disorders: Behavioral approaches to analysis and treatment.* New York: Kluwer.

Milton, R. (1992). Are you seeing a mass killer? *Australian Family Physician, 21*, 739–743.

Miron, M.S., & Douglas, J.E. (1979). Threat analysis: The psycholinguistic approach. *FBI Law Enforcement Bulletin, 48*, 5–9.

Mishima, Y. (1956). *The temple of the Golden Pavilion* (I. Morris, Trans.). New York: Berkley.

Mjanes, K., Beauregard, E., & Martineau, M. (2017). Revisiting the organized/disorganized model of sexual homicide. *Criminal Justice and Behavior, 44*, 1604–1619.

Monahan, J. (1981). *Predicting violent behavior: An assessment of clinical techniques.* Beverly Hills, CA: Sage.

Monahan, J. (1984). The prediction of violent behavior: Toward a second generation of theory and policy. *American Journal of Psychiatry, 141*, 10–15.

Monahan, J. (1996). Violence prediction: The past twenty years and the next twenty years. *Criminal Justice and Behavior, 23*, 107–130.

Monahan, J. (1997). The scientific status of research on clinical and actuarial predictions of violence. In D. Faigman, D. Kaye, M. Saks, & J. Sanders (Eds.), *Modern scientific evidence: The law and the science of expert testimony.* St. Paul, MN: West.

Money, J. (1990). Forensic sexology. Paraphiliac serial rape (biastophilia) and lust murder (erotophonophilia). *American Journal of Psychotherapy, 44*, 26–36.

Monroe, R.R. (1970). *Episodic behavioral disorders.* Cambridge, MA: Harvard University Press.

Monroe, R.R. (1974). Episodic behavioral disorder: An unclassified syndrome. In S. Arieti (Ed.), *American handbook of psychiatry* (2nd ed., Vol. 2, pp. 67–81). New York: Basic Books.

Monroe, R.R. (1978). *Brain dysfunction in aggressive criminals.* Lexington, MA: D.C. Heath.

Mora, G. (1975). Historical and theoretical trends in psychiatry. In A.N. Freedman, H.I. Kaplan, & B.J. Sadock (Eds.). *Comprehensive textbook of psychiatry* (6th ed., Vol. 1, pp. 1–75). Baltimore: Williams & Wilkins.

Moracco, K.E., Runyan, C.W., & Butts, J.B. (1998). Femicide in North Carolina, 1991–1993. *Homicide Studies, 2*, 422–446.

Morenz, B., & Herron, S. (2007). Morbid jealousy and criminal conduct. In L.B. Schlesinger (Ed.). *Explorations in criminal psychopathology: Clinical syndromes with forensic implications* (pp. 186–212). Springfield, IL: Charles C Thomas.

Morgan, D.L., & Morgan, R.K. (2001). Single participant research design. *American Psychologist, 56*, 119–127.

Morris, N., & Rothman, D.J. (Eds.). (1995). *The Oxford history of the prison: The practice of punishment in Western society.* New York: Oxford University Press.

Morris, S.B., Turner, C.W., & Szykula, S.A. (1988). Psychotherapy outcome research: An application of a new method for evaluating research methodology. *Psychotherapy, 25*, 18–26.

Morton, R., & Hilts, M. (2005). *Serial murder: Multi-disciplinary perspectives for investigators.* Washington, DC: U.S. Department of Justice.

Moskowitz, A. (2004). Dissociation and violence: A review of the literature. *Trauma, Violence & Abuse, 5*, 21–46.

Mulvey, E.P., & Lidz, L.W. (1995). Conditional prediction: A model for research on dangerousness to others in a new era. *International Journal of Law and Psychiatry, 18*, 129–143.

Muncie, W. (1939). *Psychobiology and psychiatry.* St. Louis, MO: Mosby.

Münsterberg, H. (1908). *On the witness stand.* New York: Doubleday.

Murray, H.A. (1938). *Explorations in personality.* New York: Oxford University Press.

Murray, H.A. (1943). *Thematic Apperception Test: Pictures and manual.* Cambridge, MA: Harvard University Press.

Murray, H.A. (1951). Uses of the T.A.T. *American Journal of Psychiatry, 107*, 577–581.

Myers, W., Chan, H.C., & Vo, E. (2010). Sexual sadism, psychopathy, and recidivism in juvenile sexual murderers. *Journal of Investigative Psychology & Offender Profiling, 7*, 49–58.

Myers, W.C. (2002). *Juvenile sexual homicide.* New York: Academic Press.

Myers, W.C., Beauregard, E., & Menard, W. (2019). An updated sexual homicide crime scene rating scale for sexual sadism. *International Journal of Offender Therapy and Comparative Criminology, 63*, 1766–1775.

Myers, W.C., & Blashfield, R. (1997). Psychopathology and personality in juvenile sexual homicide offenders. *Journal of the American Academy of Psychiatry and Law, 25*, 497–508.

Myers, W.C., Burgess, A.W., & Nelson, J.A. (1998). Criminal and behavioral aspects of juvenile sexual homicide. *Journal of Forensic Sciences, 43*, 340–347.

Myers, W., Chan, H.C., & Mariano, T. (2016). Sexual homicide in the USA committed by juveniles and adults, 1976–2007: Age of arrest and incidence trends over 32 years. *Criminal Behavior and Mental Health, 26*, 38–49.

Myers, W. Chan, H., Vo, E., & Lazarou, E. (2010). Sexual sadism, psychopathy and recidivism in juvenile sexual murderers. *Journal of Investigative Psychology and Offender Profiling, 7*, 49–58.

Myers, W.C., Husted, D., Safarik, M., & O'Toole, M.E. (2006). The motivation behind serial sexual homicide: Is it sex, power and control, or anger? *Journal of Forensic Sciences, 51*, 900–907.

Myers, W.C., Reccoppa, L., Burton, K., & McElroy, R. (1993). Malignant sex and aggression: An overview of serial sexual homicide. *Bulletin of the American Academy of Psychiatry and Law, 21*, 435–451.

Naoya, S. (1993). Han's crime. In S. Naoya (Ed.), *The paper door and other stories.* New York: Charles E. Tuttle.

Naples, M., & Hackett, T.P. (1978). The amytal interview: History and current uses. *Psychosomatics, 19*, 98–105.

Nash, J.R. (1973). *Bloodletters and badmen: A narrative encyclopedia of American criminals.* New York: Evans.

Nesca, M., & Kincel, R. (2000). Catathymic violence in a case of triple homicide. *American Journal of Forensic Psychiatry, 21*, 43–55.

Nestor, P.G. (1992). Neuropsychological and clinical correlates of murder and other forms of extreme violence in a forensic psychiatric population. *Journal of Nervous and Mental Disease, 180*, 418–423.

Nestor, P.G., & Haycock, J. (1997). Not guilty by reason of insanity of murder: Clinical and neuropsychological characteristics. *Journal of the American Academy of Psychiatry and Law, 25*, 161–171.

Neustatter, W.L. (1957). *The mind of the murderer.* London: Christopher Johnson.

Newton, M. (1992). *Serial slaughter: What's behind America's murder epidemic?* Port Townsend, WA: Loompanics.

Nichols, D.S. (2006). The trials of separating bath water from baby: A review and critique of the MMPI-2 restructured clinical scales. *Journal of Personality Assessment, 87*, 121–138.

Nitschke, J., Blendl, V., Ottermann, B., Osterheider, A., & Mokros, A. (2009). Severe sexual sadism: An underdiagnosed disorder? *Journal of Forensic Sciences, 54*, 685–691.

Norris, J. (1991). *Henry Lee Lucas.* New York: Kennington.

Norris, J. (1998). *Serial Killers: America's Growing Menace.* New York: Doubleday.

Oas, P. (1984). Validity of a Draw-a-Person and Bender Gestalt tests as measures of impulsivity with adolescents. *Journal of Consulting and Clinical Psychology, 52*, 1011–1019.

Olio, K., & Cornell, W.F. (1998). The facade of scientific documentation: A case study of Richard Ofshe's analysis of the Paul Ingram case. *Psychology, Public Policy, and Law, 4*, 1182–1197.

Olsen, J. (2002). *The creation of a serial killer.* New York: St. Martin's Press.

Olsson, N., Juslin, P., & Winman, A. (1998). Realism of confidence in earwitness versus eyewitness identification. *Journal of Experimental Psychology: Applied, 4*, 101–118.

Omalu, B., Dekosky, S., Minster, R., Kamboh, M., Hamilton, R., & Wecht, C. (2005). Chronic traumatic encephalopathy in a national football league player. *Neurosurgery, 57*, 128–134.

Orenstein, L., & Weisstein, A. (1958). A temporary insanity defense. *American Journal of Psychiatry*, *115*, 121–125.

Oshinsky, D. (2017). *Bellevue: Three centuries of medicine and mayhem at America's most storied hospital*. New York: Random House.

O'Toole, M.E. (1999). Criminal profiling: The FBI uses criminal investigative analysis to solve crimes. *Corrections Today*, *61*, 44–46.

Otto, R.K. (2000). Assessing and managing violence risk in outpatient settings. *Journal of Clinical Psychology*, *56*, 1239–1262.

Palermo, G.B., Smith, M.B., Jenzten, J.M., Henry, T.E., Konicek, P.J., Peterson, G.F., Singh, R.P., & Witek, M.J. (1997). Murder-suicide of the jealous paranoid type: A multi-center statistical pilot study. *American Journal of Forensic Medicine and Pathology*, *18*, 374–383.

Pallone, N.J. (1996). Sadistic criminal aggression: Perspectives from psychology, criminology, neuropsychology. In L.B. Schlesinger (Ed.), *Explorations in criminal psychopathology: Clinical syndromes with forensic implications* (pp. 187–211). Springfield, IL: Charles C Thomas.

Pallone, N.J., & Hennessey, J.J. (1993). Tinder box criminal violence: Neurogenic impulsivity, risk-taking, and the phenomenology of rational choice. In R.V. Clarke & M. Felson (Eds.), *Routine activity and rational choice: Advances in criminological theory* (pp. 127–158). New Brunswick, NJ: Transaction Press.

Pallone, N.J., & Hennessey, J.J. (1994). *Criminal behavior: A process psychology analysis*. New Brunswick, NJ: Transaction Press.

Palmer, C.T., & Thornhill, R. (2000). Serial rape. An evolutionary perspective. In L.B. Schlesinger (Ed.). *Serial Offenders: Current thought, recent findings* (pp. 51–65). Boca Raton, FL: CRC Press.

Pandina, R. (1996). Idiosyncratic alcohol intoxication: A construct that has lost its validity? In L.B. Schlesinger (Ed.), *Explorations in criminal psychopathology: Clinical syndromes with forensic implications* (pp. 142–148). Springfield, IL: Charles C Thomas.

Panton, I.H. (1960). Beta-WAIS comparison and WAIS subtest configuration within a state prison population. *Journal of Clinical Psychology*, *16*, 312–317.

Papachristos, A.V. (2009). Murder by structure: Dominance relations and the social structure of gang homicide. *American Journal of Sociology*, *115*, 74–128.

Park, J., Schlesinger, L.B., Pinizzotto, A.J., & Davis, E. (2008). Serial and single-victim rapists: Differences in crime-scene violence, interpersonal involvement, and criminal sophistication, *Behavioral Sciences and the Law*, *26*, 227–237.

Parker, R.N., & Rebhun, L. (1995). *Alcohol and homicide: A deadly combination of two American traditions*. Albany, NY: State University of New York Press.

Parwatikar, S.D., Holcomb, W.R., & Menninger, K.A. (1985). The detection of malingered amnesia in accused murderers. *Bulletin of the American Academy of Psychiatry and Law*, *13*, 97–103.

Patridge, G.D. (1928). A study of 50 cases of psychopathic personality. *American Journal of Psychiatry*, *7*, 953–974.

Paulhus, D., & Dutton, D.,G. (2016). Everyday sadism. In V. Zeigler-Hill & D. K Marcus (Eds.), *The dark side of personality: Science and practice in social, personality, and clinical psychology* (pp. 109–120). Washington, DC: American Psychological Association.

Pedneault, A., Beauregard, E., Harris, D., & Knight, R. (2015). Rationally irrational: The case of sexual burglary. *Sexual abuse: Journal Research and Treatment*, *27*, 376–397.

Pedneault, A., Harris, D., Knight, R. (2012). Toward a typology of sexual burglary: Latent class findings. *Journal of Criminal Justice*, *40*, 278–284.

Pennell, A., & Browne, K. (1999). Film violence and young offenders. *Aggression and Violent Behavior*, *4*, 13–28.

Perkins, D., & Carter, A.J. (2018). The treatment of sexual homicide offenders in secure psychiatric hospitals and prison settings for the purpose of risk reduction. In J. Proulx et al. (Eds.), *Routledge international handbook of sexual homicide studies* (pp. 370–381). New York: Routledge.

Pernanen, K. (1976). Alcohol and crimes of violence. In B. Kissin & H. Begleiter (Eds.), *The biology of alcoholism: Social aspects of alcoholism* (Vol. 4, pp. 351–344). New York: Plenum.

Perr, I.N. (1975). Psychiatric testimony and the *Rashomon* phenomenon. *Bulletin of the American Academy of Psychiatry and Law, 3*, 83–98.

Pillman, F., Rohde, A., Ullrich, S., Draba, S., & Sannemueller, U. (1999). Violence, criminal behavior, and the EEG: Significance of left hemisphere focal abnormalities. *Journal of Neuropsychiatry and Clinical Neuroscience, 11*, 454–457.

Pinel, P. (1806). *A treatise on insanity*. Sheffield: W. Todd.

Pinizzotto, A.J. (1984). Forensic psychology: Criminal personality profiling. *Journal of Police Science and Administration, 12*, 32–40.

Pinizzotto, A.J., & Davis, E.F. (1999). Suicide by cop: Implications for law enforcement management. *Law and Order, 47*, 95–98.

Pinizzotto, A.J., & Finkel, N.J. (1990). Criminal personality profiling: An outcome and process study. *Law and Human Behavior, 14*, 215–233.

Piotrowski, C., & Keller, J.W. (1992). Psychological testing in applied settings: A literature review from 1982–1992. *Journal of Training and Practice in Professional Psychology, 6*, 74–82.

Piper, A. (1993). "Truth serum" and "recovered memories" of sexual abuse: A review of the evidence. *Journal of Psychiatry and Law, 21*, 447–471.

Podolsky, E. (1966). Sexual violence. *Medical Digest, 34*, 60–63.

Pokorny, A.D. (1966). A follow-up study of 618 suicidal patients. *American Journal of Psychiatry, 122*, 1109–1116.

Pollock, P.H. (1995). A case of spree serial murder with suggested diagnostic options. *International Journal of Offender Therapy and Comparative Criminology, 39*, 258–268.

Pontius, A.A., & Yudowitz, B.S. (1980). Frontal lobe dysfunction in some criminal actions shown in the Narratives Test. *Journal of Nervous and Mental Disease, 168*, 111–117.

Pope, H.G. (1988). Affective and psychotic symptoms associated with steroid use. *American Journal of Psychiatry, 145*, 487–490.

Pope, K.S. (1996). Memory, abuse, and science: Questioning claims about the False Memory Syndrome epidemic. *American Psychologist, 51*, 957–974.

Porcerelli, J.H., Abramsky, M.F., Hibbard, S., & Kamoo, R. (2001). Object relations and defense mechanisms of a psychopathic serial sexual homicide perpetrator: A TAT analysis. *Journal of Personality Assessment, 77*, 87–104.

Power, D.J., & Selwood, D.H.P. (1987). *Criminal law and psychiatry*. London: Kluwer Law Publisher.

Powers, R.J., & Kutash, I.L. (1978). Substance induced aggression. In I.L. Kutash, S.B. Kutash, & L.B. Schlesinger (Eds.), *Violence: Perspectives on murder and aggression* (pp. 317–342). San Francisco: Jossey-Bass.

Prentky, R.A., Burgess, A.W., Rokous, R., Lee, A., Hartman, C., Ressler, R.K., & Douglas, J. (1989). The presumptive role of fantasy in serial sexual homicide. *American Journal of Psychiatry, 146*, 887–891.

Prentky, RA., Knight, PA., Sims-Knight, J.E., & Straus, H. (1989). Developmental antecedents of sexual aggression. *Developmental Psychopathology, 1*, 153–169.

Prichard, J.L. (1835). *A treatise on insanity and other disorders affecting the mind*. London: Sherwood, Gilbert & Pifer.

Proulx, J., Beauregard, E., Carter, A.J., Mokros, A., Darjee, R., & James, J. (2018). *Routledge international handbook of sexual homicide studies*: New York: Routledge.

Quinsey, V.L., Harris, G.T., Rice, M.E., & Cormier, C.A. (1999). *Violent offenders: Appraising and managing risk*. Washington, DC: APA Press.

Quinsey, V.L., Lalumiere, M.L., Rice, M.E., & Harris, G.T. (1995). Predicting sexual offenses. In J.L. Campbell (Ed.), *Assessing dangerousness: Violence by sexual offenders, batterers, and child abusers* (pp. 114–137). Thousand Oaks, CA: Sage.

Rabin, A.I. (1968). Projective methods: An historical introduction. In A.I. Rabin (Ed.), *Projective techniques in personality assessment* (pp. 3–17). New York: Springer.

Rada, R.T. (1978). Sexual psychopathology: Historical survey and basic concepts. In R.T. Rada (Ed.), *Clinical aspects of the rapist* (pp. 1–19). New York: Grune & Stratton.

Rado, S. (1959). Obsessive compulsive disorder: So-called obsessive compulsive neuro- sis. In S. Areiti (Ed.), *American handbook of psychiatry* (Vol. 1, pp. 317–343). New York: Basic Books.

Rae, G.W. (1967). *Confessions of the Boston Strangler.* New York: Pyramid Press.

Rafter, N. (2008). *The criminal brain.: Understanding biological theories of crime.* New York: New York University Press.

Raine, A. (1993). *The psychopathology of crime.* New York: Academic Press.

Raine, A. (2002). The biological basis of crime. In J.Q. Wilson & J. Petersilla (Eds.). *Crime: Public policies for crime control.* Oakland, CA: ICS Press.

Raine, A. (2014). *The anatomy of violence: The biological roots of crime.* New York: Random House.

Raine, A., Meloy, J.R., Bihrle, S., Stoddard, J., La Casse, L., & Buchsbaum, M.S. (1998a). Reduced prefrontal and increased subcortical brain functioning assessed using PET in predatory and affective murderers. *Behavioral Science and the Law, 16,* 319–332.

Raine, A., Phil, D., Stoddard, J., Bihrle, S., & Buchsbaum, M. (1998b). Prefrontal glucose defi-cits in murderers lacking psychosocial deprivation. *Neuropsychiatry, Neuropsychology, and Behavioral Neurology, 11,* 1–7.

Rajs, J., Lundström, M., Broberg, M., Lidberg, L., & Lindquist, O. (1998). Criminal mutilation of the human body in Sweden: A thirty year medico-legal and forensic psychiatry study. *Journal of Forensic Sciences, 43,* 563–580.

Ramsland, K. (2016). *Confessions of a serial killer: The untold story of Dennis Rader, the BTK killer.* Lebanon, NH: University Press of New England.

Raphael, A.J., Golden, C., & Cassidy-Feltgen, S. (2002). The Bernder-Gestalt Test (BGT) in forensic assessment. *Journal of Forensic Psychology Practice, 2,* 93–105.

Rappeport, J.R. (Ed.). (1967). *The clinical evaluation of the dangerousness of the mentally ill.* Springfield, IL: Charles C Thomas.

Rasmussen, J.G.C. (1997). Drug treatments for schizophrenia: Past, present, and future. *Journal of Clinical Psychopharmacology, 20,* 252–256.

Ratner, R.A., & Shapiro, D. (1979). The episodic dyscontrol syndrome and criminal responsibility. *Bulletin of the American Academy of Psychiatry and Law, 7,* 422–431.

Redlich, F., Ravitz, L.J., & Dession, G.A. (1951). Narcoanalysis and truth. *American Journal of Psychiatry, 107,* 586–593.

Reibman, J.E. (1990). The life of Dr. Fredric Wertham. In *The Fredric Wertham Collection* (pp. 11–22). Cambridge, MA: Harvard University Press.

Reich, P., & Hepps, R.B. (1972). Homicide during a psychosis induced by LSD. *Journal of the American Medical Association, 219,* 869–871.

Reid, S. (2017a). Compulsive criminal homicide: A new nosology for serial murder. *Aggression and Violent Behavior, 34,* 290–301.

Reid, S. (2017b). Developmental pathways to serial homicide: A critical review of the biological literature. *Aggression and Violent Behavior, 35,* 52–61.

Reinhardt, J.J. (1957). *Sex perversions and sex crimes.* Springfield, IL: Charles C Thomas.

Reinhardt, J.M. (1973). The dismal tunnel: Depression before murder. *International Journal of Offender Therapy and Comparative Criminology, 17,* 246–249.

Reiser, M. (1982, March). Crime-specific psychological consultation. *The Police Chief,* 53–56.

Relkin, N., Plum, F., Mattis, S., Eidelberg, D., & Tranel, D. (1996). Impulse homicide associated with an arachnoid cyst and unilateral fronto temporal cerebral dysfunction. *Seminars in Clinical Neuropsychiatry, 1,* 172–183.

Relinger, H., & Stern, T. (1983). Guidelines for forensic hypnosis. *Journal of Psychiatry and Law, 11,* 69–74.

Resnick, H.L.P. (1997). Eroticized repetitive hangings. In L.B. Schlesinger & E. Revitch (Eds.), *Sexual dynamics of anti-social behavior* (2nd ed., pp. 224–240). Springfield, IL: Charles C Thomas.

Ressler, R.K., Burgess, A.W., & Douglas, J.E. (1983). Rape and rape-murder: One offender and twelve victims. *American Journal of Psychiatry, 140,* 36–40.

Ressler, R.K., Burgess, A.W., & Douglas, J.E. (1988). *Sexual homicide: Patterns and motives.* New York: Free Press.

Ressler, R.K., Burgess, A.W., Douglas, J.E., & Depue, R.L. (1991). Criminal profiling research on homicide. In A.W. Burgess (Ed.), *Rape and sexual assault: A research handbook* (pp. 343–349). New York: Garland.

Ressler, R.K., Burgess, A.W., Douglas, J.E., Hartman, C.R., & D'Agostino, R.B. (1986). Sexual killers and their victims: Identifying patterns through crime scene analysis. *Journal of Interpersonal Violence, 1,* 288–308.

Ressler, R.K., Burgess, A.W., Hartman, C.R., & Douglas, J.E. (1986). Murderers who rape and mutilate. *Journal of Interpersonal Violence, 1,* 273–287.

Ressler, R.K., & Schachtman, T. (1992). *Whoever fights monsters.* New York: St. Martin's Press.

Ressler, R.K., & Schachtman, T. (1997). *I have lived in the monster.* New York: St. Martin's Press.

Retzlaff, P. (2010). MCMI-III diagnostic validity. Bad test or bad validity study. *Journal of Personality Assessment, 66,* 431–435.

Revitch, E. (1950). The concept of psychopathic personality. *Diseases of the Nervous System, 11,* 369–372.

Revitch, E. (1954). The problem of conjugal paranoia. *Diseases of the Nervous System, 15,* 271–277.

Revitch, E. (1957). Sex murder and sex aggression. *Journal of the Medical Society of New Jersey, 54,* 519–524.

Revitch, E. (1958). Psychomotor paroxysms of non-epileptic origin. *Diseases of the Nervous System, 19,* 562–585.

Revitch, E. (1964). Paroxysmal manifestations of non-epileptic origin: Catathymic attacks. *Diseases of the Nervous System, 25,* 662–670.

Revitch, E. (1965). Sex murder and the potential sex murderer. *Diseases of the Nervous System, 26,* 640–648.

Revitch, E. (1977). Classification of offenders for prognostic and disposition evaluation. *Bulletin of the American Academy of Psychiatry and Law, 5,* 41–50.

Revitch, E. (1978). Sexually motivated burglaries. *Bulletin of the American Academy of Psychiatry and Law, 6,* 277–283.

Revitch, E. (1979). Patients who kill their physician. *Journal of the Medical Society of New Jersey, 76,* 429–431.

Revitch, E. (1980). Gynocide and unprovoked attacks on women. *Corrective and Social Psychiatry, 26,* 6–11.

Revitch, E. (1997). Burglaries with sexual dynamics. In L.B. Schlesinger & E. Revitch (Eds.), *Sexual dynamics of antisocial behavior* (2nd ed., pp. 171–187). Springfield, IL: Charles C Thomas.

Revitch, E., & Schlesinger, L.B. (1978). Murder: Evaluation, classification, and prediction. In I.L. Kutash, S.B. Kutash, & L.B. Schlesinger (Eds.), *Violence: Perspectives on murder and aggression* (pp. 138–164). San Francisco: Jossey-Bass.

Revitch, E., & Schlesinger, L.B. (1981). *Psychopathology of homicide.* Springfield, IL: Charles C Thomas.

Revitch, E., & Schlesinger, L.B. (1989). *Sex murder and sex aggression.* Springfield, IL: Charles C Thomas.

Rhine, M.W., & Mayerson, P. (1973). A serious suicidal syndrome masked by homicidal threats. *Suicide and Life-Threatening Behavior, 3,* 3–10.

Richards, J., & Goodwin, J.M. (1994). Electra: Revenge fantasies and homicide in child abuse victims. *Journal of Psychohistory, 22,* 213–222.

Roesch, R., Zapf, P.A., Golding, S.L., & Skeem, J.L. (1999). Defining and assessing competency to stand trial. In A.K. Hess & I.B. Weiner (Eds.), *The handbook of Forensic Psychology* (2nd ed., pp. 327–349). New York: Wiley.

Rogers, R. (1984).Toward an empirical model of malingering and deception. *Behavioral Science and the Law, 2,* 93–106.

Rogers, R. (Ed.). (1988). *Clinical assessment of malingering and deception.* New York: Guilford Press.

Rogers, R., Bagby, R.M, & Dickens, S.E. (1992). *Structured interview of reported symptoms.* Odessa, FL: Psychological Assessment Resources.

Rogers, R., & Johansson-Love, J. (2009). Evaluating competency to stand trial with evidence-based practice. *Journal of the American Academy of Psychiatry and Law, 37,* 450–460.

Rogers, R., Sewell, K.W., & Gillard, N. (2010). *Structured interview of reported symptoms* (2nd ed.). Lutz, FL: Psychological Assessment Resources.

Rogers, R., Sewell, K., Harrison, K., & Jordan, M. (2006). The MMPI-2 restructured clinical scales: A paradigmatic shift in scale development. *Journal of Personality Assessment, 87,* 139–147.

Rorschach, H. (1947). *Psychodiagnostics* (P. Lemkau & B. Kronenberg, Trans.). New York: Grune & Stratton. (Original work published 1921).

Rosenbaum, M. (1990). The role of depression in couples involved in murder-suicide and homicide. *American Journal of Psychiatry, 147,* 1036–1039.

Rosenbaum, M., & Bennett, B. (1986). Homicide and depression. *American Journal of Psychiatry, 143,* 367–370.

Rosenthal, R.J., & Lesieur, H.R. (1996). Pathological gambling and criminal behavior. In L.B. Schlesinger (Ed.), *Explorations in criminal psychopathology: Clinical syndromes with forensic implications* (pp. 149–169). Springfield, IL: Charles C Thomas.

Rosenwald, G.L. (1968). The thematic apperception test. In A.I. Rabin (Ed.), *Projective techniques in personality assessment* (pp. 172–221). New York: Springer.

Rossi, D. (1982, January). Crime scene behavior analysis: Another tool for the law enforcement investigator. *The Police Chief,* 152–155.

Rossmo, D.K. (2000). *Geographic profiling.* Boca Raton, FL: CRC Press.

Rowe, D.C. (2002). *Biology and crime.* Los Angeles: Roxbury.

Rozeboom, W.W. (1970). The art of metascience, or, what should a psychological theory be? In J.R. Royce (Ed.), *Toward unification in psychology* (pp. 54–163). Toronto: University of Toronto Press.

Rule, A. (1983). *Lust killer.* New York: Signet.

Rule, A. (1988). *The stranger beside me.* New York: Signet.

Ruotolo, A. (1968). Dynamics of sudden murder. *American Journal of Psychoanalysis, 26,* 162–176.

Ruotolo, A. (1975). Neurotic pride and homicide. *American Journal of Psychoanalysis, 35,* 1–16.

Russell, M., Schlesinger, L.B., Leon, M., & Holdren, S. (2018). "Undoing" (or symbolic reversal) at homicide crime scenes. *Journal of Forensic Sciences, 63,* 478–483.

Ryzuk, M. (1994). *The Gainesville Ripper.* New York: St. Martin's Press.

Sadoff, R.L. (1975). *Forensic psychiatry: A practical guide for lawyers and psychiatrists.* Springfield, IL: Charles C Thomas.

Sadoff, R.L. (1995). Mothers who kill their children. *Psychiatric Annals, 25,* 601–605.

Safarik, M.E., & Jarvis, J.P. (2005). Examining attributes of homicide: Toward quantifying qualitative values of injury severity. *Homicide Studies, 9,* 183–203.

Safarik, M.E., & Ramland, K. (2020). *Spree killers: Practical classification for law enforcement and criminology:* Boca Raton, FL: CRC Press.

Saito, F. (1995). Characteristics of juvenile delinquents who produced cold-blooded aggressive fantasies in response to T.A.T. card 8BM. *Japanese Journal of Criminal Psychology, 33,* 29–40.

Samenow, S.E. (1984). *Inside the criminal mind.* New York: Times Book.

Sargent, D.A. (1979, January). Burglars who soil premises. *Medical Aspects of Human Sexuality,* pg. 97.

Sargent, W. (1957). *Battle for the mind: The mechanisms of indoctrination, brain washing, and thought control.* London: Pan Books.

Satten, J., Menninger, K., & Mayman, M. (1960). Murder without apparent motive: A study in personality disintegration. *American Journal of Psychiatry, 117,* 48–53.

Schaefer, R. (1959). Generative empathy in the treatment situation. *Psychiatric Quarterly, 28,* 342–373.

Schafer, J.A., Varano, S., Jarvis, J., & Cancino, J.M. (2010). Bad moon on the rise? Lunar cycles and incidents of crime. *Journal of Criminal Justice, 38,* 359–367.

Schechter, H. (1989). *Deviant.* New York: Pocket Books.

Schechter, H. (1990). *Deranged.* New York: Pocket Books.

Schechter, H., & Everitt, D. (1996). *The A to Z encyclopedia of serial killers.* New York: Pocket Books.

Scherl, D.J., & Mack, J.E. (1966). A study of adolescent matricide. *Journal of the American Academy of Child and Adolescent Psychiatry, 5,* 569–593.

Schlesinger, L.B. (1980). Distinction between psychopathic, sociopathic, and antisocial personality disorders. *Psychological Reports, 147,* 15–21.

Schlesinger, L.B. (1996a). The catathymic crisis, 1912-present: A clinical study. *Aggression and Violent Behavior, 1,* 307–316.

Schlesinger, L.B. (1996b). The catathymic process: Psychopathology and psychodynamics of extreme aggression. In L.B. Schlesinger (Ed.), *Explorations in criminal psychopathology: Clinical syndromes with forensic implications* (pp. 121–141). Springfield, IL: Charles C Thomas.

Schlesinger, L.B. (1998). Pathological narcissism and serial homicide: Review and case report. *Current Psychology, 17,* 212–221.

Schlesinger, L.B. (1999). Adolescent sexual matricide following repetitive mother-son incest. *Journal of Forensic Sciences, 44,* 746–749.

Schlesinger, L.B. (2000a). Serial homicide: Sadism, fantasy, and a compulsion to kill. In L.B. Schlesinger (Ed.), *Serial offenders: Current thought, recent findings* (pp. 3–22). Boca Raton, FL: CRC Press.

Schlesinger, L.B. (2000b). Serial burglary: A spectrum of behaviors, motives, and dynamics. In L.B. Schlesinger (Ed.), *Serial offenders: Current thought, recent findings* (pp. 187–206). Boca Raton, FL: CRC Press.

Schlesinger, L.B. (2000c). Familicide, depression, and catathymic process. *Journal of Forensic Sciences, 45,* 200–203.

Schlesinger, L.B. (2001a). Is serial homicide really increasing? *Journal of the American Academy of Psychiatry and Law, 29,* 294–297.

Schlesinger, L.B. (2001b). The potential sex murderer: Ominous signs, risk assessment. *Journal of Threat Assessment, 1,* 47–72.

Schlesinger, L.B. (2001c). The contract murderer: Patterns, characteristics, and dynamics. *Journal of Forensic Sciences, 46,* 108–112.

Schlesinger, L.B. (2002a). Stalking, homicide and catathymic process: A case study. *International Journal of Offender Therapy and Comparative Criminology, 46,* 64–74.

Schlesinger, L.B. (2002b). Understanding catathymic homicides: Clinical and forensic perspectives. *Journal of the New York State Psychological Association, 14,* 17–21.

Schlesinger, L.B. (2003a). Forensic psychology. In S.H. James & J.J. Nordby (Eds.), *Forensic science: An introduction to scientific and investigative techniques* (pp. 489–507). Boca Raton, FL: CRC Press.

Schlesinger, L.B. (2003b). A case study involving competency to stand trial: Incompetent defendant, incompetent examiner, or "malingering by proxy." *Psychology, Public Policy and Law, 9,* 381–399.

Schlesinger, L.B. (2005). Forensic psychology. In S.H. James & J.J. Norby (Eds.), *Forensic Science: An introduction to scientific and investigative techniques* (2nd ed., pp. 573–592). Boca Raton, FL: CRC Press.

Schlesinger, L.B. (2006). Celebrity stalking, homicide, and suicide: A psychological autopsy. *International Journal of Offender Therapy and Comparative Criminology, 50,* 39–46.

Schlesinger, L.B. (2017). *Psychiatric aspects of criminal behavior: Collected papers of Eugene Revitch.* Springfield, IL: Charles C Thomas.

Schlesinger, L.B. (2018). Psychopathic personality: Concept, disorder, diagnosis. In R.N. Kocsis (Ed.). *Applied criminal psychology: A guide to Forensic sciences* (pp. 49–67). Springfield, IL: Thomas.

Schlesinger, L.B., Gardenier, A., Jarvis, J., & Sheehan-Cook, J. (2014). Crime scene staging in homicide. *Journal of Police and Criminal Psychology, 29,* 44–51.

Schlesinger, L.B., Kassen, M., Mesa, V.B., & Pinizzotto, A. (2010). Ritual and signature in serial sexual homicide. *Journal of the American Academy of Psychiatry and Law, 38,* 239–246.

Schlesinger, L.B., & Kutash, I.L. (1981). The criminal fantasy technique: A comparison of sex offenders and substance abusers. *Journal of Clinical Psychology, 37,* 210–218.

Schlesinger, L.B., & Mesa, V.B. (2008). Homicidal celebrity stalkers: Dangerous obsessions with nonpolitical public figures. In J.R. Meloy, L. Sheridan, & J. Hoffmann (Eds.)., *Stalking, threatening, and attacking public figures* (pp. 83–104). New York: Oxford University Press.

Schlesinger, L.B., Pinizzotto, A.J., & Pakhomou, S. (2004). Burglary and sexually motivated homicide. *Sex Offender Law Report, 5,* 21–36.

Schlesinger, L.B., Ramirez, S., Tusa, B., Jarvis, J., & Erdberg, P. (2017). Rapid-sequence serial sexual homicides. *Journal of the American Academy of Psychiatry and Law, 45,* 72–80.

Schlesinger, L.B., & Revitch, E. (1980). Stress, violence, and crime. In I.L. Kutash & L.B. Schlesinger (Eds.), *Handbook on stress and anxiety* (pp. 134–188). San Francisco: Jossey-Bass.

Schlesinger, L.B., & Revitch, E. (1990). Outpatient treatment of the sex murderer and potential sex murderer. *Journal of Offender Counseling, Services, and Rehabilitation, 15,* 163–178.

Schlesinger, L.B., & Revitch, E. (1997a). Sexual dynamics in homicide and assault. In L.B. Schlesinger & E. Revitch (Eds.), *Sexual dynamics of antisocial behavior* (2nd ed., pp. 203–223). Springfield, IL: Charles C Thomas.

Schlesinger, L.B., & Revitch, E. (Eds.). (1997b). *Sexual dynamics of antisocial behavior* (2nd ed.). Springfield, IL: Charles C Thomas.

Schlesinger, L.B., & Revitch, E. (1999). Sexual burglaries and sexual homicide: Clinical, forensic, and investigative considerations. *Journal of the American Academy of Psychiatry and Law, 27,* 227–238.

Schneck, J.M. (1962). Pseudomalingering. *Diseases of the Nervous System, 23,* 396–398.

Schneck, J.M. (1966). Dostoyevsky and Freud on criminal psychopathology. In *Psychiatric Quarterly Supplement, Part 2* (pp. 1–5). Utica, NY: State Hospitals Press.

Schneider, K. (1959). *Clinical psychopathology.* New York: Grune & Stratton.

Schreiber, F.R. (1984). *The shoemaker: The anatomy of a psychotic.* New York: Signet Books.

Schretlen, D.J. (1988). The use of psychological tests to identify malingered symptoms of mental disorder. *Clinical Psychology Review, 8,* 451–469.

Schroer, J., & Puschel, K. (2007). Special aspects of crime scene interpretation and behavioral analysis. The phenomena of undoing. *Forensic Pathology Review, 4,* 193–202.

Schwartz, A.E. (1992). *The man who could not kill enough.* Secaucus, NJ: Carol.

Sedman, G. (1966). A comparative study of pseudohallucinations, imagery and true hallucinations. *British Journal of Psychiatry, 112,* 9–17.

Shah, I. (1972). *The exploits of the incomparable Mullah Nasrudin.* New York: Dutton.

Sheldon, W.H. (1940). *The varieties of human physique.* New York: Harper & Row.

Shenken, L.I. (1966). The implications of ego-psychology for a motiveless murder. *Journal of the Academy of Child Psychiatry, 5,* 741–751.

Sigal, M., Altmark, D., Alfici, S., & Gelkopf, M. (1992). Ganser's syndrome: A review of 15 cases. *Comprehensive Psychiatry, 32,* 134–138.

Silva, J.A., Harry, B.E., Leong, G.B., & Weinstock, R. (1996). Dangerous delusional misidentification and homicide. *Journal of Forensic Sciences, 41,* 641–644.

Silverman, D. (1943). Clinical and EEG studies on criminal psychopaths. *Archives of Neurology and Psychiatry, 50,* 18–33.

Silverman, D. (2011). *Qualitative research* (3rd ed.). Thousand Oaks, CA: Sage.

Silverstein, M.L., & Nelson, L. (2000). Clinical and research implications of revising psychological tests. *Psychological Assessment, 12,* 298–303.

Simon, R.E. (1977). Type A, AB, and B murderers. *Bulletin of the American Academy of Psychiatry and Law, 5,* 344–362.

Simpson, M.A. (1973). Female genital self-mutilation. *Archives of General Psychiatry, 29,* 808–810.

Sinnamon, G. (2015). Psychopathology and criminal behavior. In W. Petherick (Ed.). *Applied crime analysis. A social science approach to understanding crime, criminals, and victims* (pp. 208–252). Cambridge, MA: Academic Press.

Sinnamon, G., & Petherick, W. (2017). Catathymia and compulsive homicide: A psychological perspective. In G. Sinnamon & W. Petherick (Eds.). *The psychology of criminal and antisocial behavior: Victim and offender perspectives* (pp. 51–78). Cambridge: Academic Press.

Siomopoulos, V., & Goldsmith, J. (1976). Types of sadism. *Medical Aspects of Human Sexuality, 10,* 82–83.

Skeem, J., Douglas, K.S., & Lilienfield, S.. (Eds.). (2009). *Psychological science in the courtroom: Consensus and controversy.* New York: Guilford.

Skrapec, C.A. (2001). Phenomenology and serial murder: Asking different questions. *Homicide Studies, 5,* 46–63.

Smith, B.M. (1967). The polygraph. *Scientific American, 216,* 25–31.

Socarides, C.W. (1988). *The preoedipal origin and psychoanalytic therapy of sexual perversions.* New York: International Universities Press.

Society for Personality Assessment. (2005). The status of the Rorschach in clinical and forensic practice: An official statement by the Board of Trustees of the society for personality assessment. *Journal of Personality Assessment, 85,* 219–237.

Spitzberg, B., & Cupach, W. (1994). *The dark side of close relationships.* Mahwah, NJ: Lawrence Erlbaum.

Spunt, B., Brownstein, H., Goldstein, P., Fendrich, M., & Liberty, H.J. (1995). Drug use by homicide offenders. *Journal of Psychoactive Drugs, 27,* 125–134.

Steadman, H. (1982). A situational approach to violence. *International Journal of Psychiatry and Law, 5,* 171–186.

Steadman, H., & Cocozza, J. (1974). *Careers of the criminally insane.* Lexington, MA: D.C. Heath.

Stefanska, E., Nitschke, J., Carter, A., & Mokros, A. (2019). Sadism among sexual homicide offenders: Validation of the Sexual Sadism Scale. *Psychological Assessment, 31,* 132–137.

Stekel, W. (1924). *Peculiarities of behavior* (Vol. 2). New York: Boni & Liveright.

Stekel, W. (1953). *Sadism and masochism.* New York: Liveright.

Stone, A. (1993). Murder with no apparent motive. *Journal of Psychiatry and Law, 21,* 175–189.

Stone, A. (1998a). Sadistic personalities in murderers. In T. Millon & E. Simonson (Eds.), *Psychopathy: Antisocial, criminal, and violent behavior* (pp. 12–38). New York: Guilford Press.

Stone, M.H. (1998b). The personalities of murderers: The importance of psychopathy and sadism. In A.E. Skodol (Ed.), *Psychopathology and violent crime* (pp. 29–52). Washington, DC: American Psychiatric Press.

Storr, A. (1972). *Human destructiveness.* New York: Basic Books.

Strentz, T., & Hassel, C.V. (1970). The sociopath: A criminal enigma. *Journal of Police Science and Administration, 6,* 135–140.

Strupp, H.H. (1973). *Psychotherapy: Clinical, research and theoretical issues.* New York: Jason Aronson.

Sutherland, A.E. (1965). Crime and confession. *Harvard Law Review, 79,* 21–41.

Sutherland, E.H. (1937). *The professional thief.* Chicago, IL: University of Chicago Press.

Sutherland, E.H. (1949). *While collar crime.* New York: Dryden Press.

Sutherland, E.H., & Cressey, D.R. (1939). *Principles of criminology.* Philadelphia, PA: Lippincott.

Svalastoga, K. (1956). Homicide and social contact in Denmark. *American Journal of Sociology, 62,* 37–53.

Swanson, D.W., Bohnert, P.J., & Smith, J.A. (1970). *The paranoid.* Boston: Little, Brown.

Swigert, V.L., Farrell, R.A., & Yoels, W.L. (1976). Sexual homicide: Social psychological and legal aspects. *Archives of Sexual Behavior, 5,* 391–401.

Tanay, E. (1969). Psychiatric study of homicide. *American Journal of Psychiatry, 125,* 1252–1258.

Tanay, E. (1972). Psychiatric aspects of homicide prevention. *American Journal of Psychiatry, 128*, 49–52.

Tanay, E. (1975). Dangerousness in psychiatry. *Current Concepts in Psychiatry, 1*, 17–26.

Tanay, E. (1978). Psychodynamic differentiation of homicide. *Bulletin of the American Academy of Psychiatry and Law, 6*, 364–373.

Tang, H., Sun, Y., Li, C., Fang, M., & Fan, G. (1999). Clinical features and psychopathology of depressive patients involved in homicide. *Chinese Mental Health Journal, 13*, 123–125.

Tapia, F. (1971). Children who are cruel to animals. *Child Psychiatry and Human Development, 2*, 70–77.

Tarasoff v. Regents of the University of California. 17 Cal. 3d 425, 551 P.2d 334, 131 Cal. Rpt. 14 (1976).

Tarescavage, A.M., & Glassmire, D.M. (2016). Differentiation between Structured Interview of Reported Symptoms (SIRS) and SIRS-2 sensitivity estimates among forensic inpatients: A criterion group comparison. *Law and Human Behavior, 40*, 488–502.

Templeman, T.L., & Stinnett, R.D. (1991). Patterns of sexual arousal and history in a "normal" sample of young men. *Archives of Sexual Behavior, 20*, 137–150.

Thornberry, T.P., & Jacoby, J.E. (1979). *The criminally insane: A community follow- up of mentally ill offenders.* Chicago, IL: University of Chicago Press.

Tombaugh, T.N. (1996). *Test of memory malingering.* New York: MHS.

Uhlin, D.M. (1978). The use of drawings for psychiatric evaluation of a defendant in a case of homicide. *Mental Health and Society, 4*, 61–73.

Urschel, H.C., & Woody, G.E. (1994). Alcohol idiosyncratic intoxication: A review of the data supporting its existence. In W. Widiger (Ed.), *DSM-IV sourcebook* (Vol. 1, pp. 117–128). Washington, DC: American Psychiatric Press.

U.S. Department of Justice. (2000). *Intimate partner violence.* Bureau of Justice Statistics Special Report, May. No. 178247.

Valle, R.S., King, M., & Halling, S. (1989). An introduction to existential-phenomenological thought in psychology. In R.S. Valle & S. Halling (Eds.), *Existential- phenomenological perspectives in psychology* (pp. 3–16). New York: Plenum.

Vanderkolk, B.A. (1989). Compulsion to repeat the trauma: Re-enactment, re-victimization, and masochism. *Psychiatric Clinics of North America, 12*, 389–411.

Vicary, A.M., & Fraley, C. (2010). Captured by true crime. Why are women drawn to tales of rape, murder, and serial killers? *Social Psychological and Personality Science, 1*, 81–86.

Vinas-Racionero, R., Schlesinger, L.B., Scalora, M.J., & Jarvis, J. (2017). Youthful familicidal offenders: Targeted victims, planned attacks. *Journal of Family Violence, 32*, 535–542.

Volavka, J. (1995). *Neurobiology of violence.* Washington, DC: American Psychiatric Press.

Volavka, J. (2002). *Neurobiology of violence* (2nd ed.). Washington, DC: American Psychiatric Press.

Von Hentig, H. (1941). Remarks on the interaction of perpetrators and victims. *Journal of Criminal Law, Criminology, and Police Science, 31*, 303–309.

Vronsky, P. (2015). *Paul Bernardo and Karla Homolka: The Ken and Barbie killers.* Toronto: R.J. Parker.

Vuocolo, A.B. (1969). *The repetitive sex offender.* Menlo Park, NJ: Quality Printing.

Wagner, E.E., & Klein, I. (1977). WAIS differences between murderers and attackers referred for evaluation. *Perceptual and Motor Skills, 44*, 125–126.

Ward, B. (1994). *Innocent prey.* New York: Windsor.

Warren, J., Hazelwood, R.R., & Dietz, P.E. (1996). The sexually sadistic serial killer. *Journal of Forensic Sciences, 41*, 970–974.

Wax, D.E., & Haddox, V.G. (1974a). Enuresis, firesetting and animal cruelty. *Child Psychiatry and Human Development, 4*, 151–156.

Wax, D.E., & Haddox, V.G. (1974b). Enuresis, firesetting, and animal cruelty in male adolescent delinquents: A triad predictive of violent behavior. *Journal of Psychiatry and Law, 2*, 45–71.

Webster, C.D., & Jackson, M.A. (1997). *Impulsivity: Perspectives, principles, and practice.* New York: Guilford Press.

Wedgewood, C.V. (1957). *The thirty years war.* Harmondsworth: Penguin Books.

Weinberg, T., & Levi, G.W. (1983). *S & M: Studies in sadomasochism.* New York: Prometheus.

Weiner, I.B., Exner, J.E., Jr., & Sciara, A. (1996). Is the Rorschach welcome in the courtroom? *Journal of Personality Assessment, 67,* 422–424.

Weins, A.W., Matarazzo, J.D., & Gavor, K.D. (1959). Performance and verbal IQ in a group of sociopaths. *Journal of Clinical Psychology, 15,* 191–193.

Wells, G.L., Malpass, R.S., Lindsay, R.C.L., Fisher, R.B., Turtle, J.W., & Fulero, S.M. (2000). From lab to the police station: A successful application of eyewitness research. *American Psychologist, 55,* 581–598.

Werfel, F. (1920). *Not the assassin but the victim is guilty.* Munich: Kurt Wolff Verlag.

Wertham, F. (1934). *The brain as an organ: Its postmortem study and interpretation.* New York: Macmillan.

Wertham, F. (1937). The catathymic crisis: A clinical entity. *Archives of Neurology and Psychiatry, 37,* 974–977.

Wertham, F. (1941). *Dark legend: A study in murder.* New York: Duell, Sloan & Pierce.

Wertham, F. (1949). *Show of violence.* Garden City, NY: Doubleday.

Wertham, F. (1954). *Seduction of the innocent.* New York: Rinehart.

Wertham, F. (1956). *The circle of guilt.* New York: Rinehart.

Wertham, F. (1966). *A sign for Cain: An exploration of human violence.* New York: Macmillan.

Wertham, F. (1968). What do we know about mass media effects? *Corrective Psychiatry and Social Therapy, 14,* 196–199.

Wertham, F. (1978). The catathymic crisis. In I.L. Kutash, S.B. Kutash, & L.B. Schlesinger (Eds.), *Violence: Perspectives on murder and aggression* (pp. 165–170). San Francisco: Jossey-Bass.

West, D.J. (1967). *Murder followed by suicide.* Cambridge, MA: Harvard University Press.

West, D.J. (1987). *Sexual crimes and confrontation: A study of victims and offenders.* Brookfield, VT: Gower.

Weston, W.A. (1996). Pseudologia fantastica and pathological lying. In L.B. Schlesinger (Ed.), *Explorations in criminal psychopathology* (pp. 98–115). Springfield, IL: Charles C Thomas.

Wetmore, S. Neuschatz, J., & Gronlund, S. (2014). On the power of secondary confession evidence. *Psychology, Crime & Law, 20,* 339–357.

Widom, C.S. (1989a). Child abuse, neglect, and adult behavior: Research design and findings on criminality, violence, and child abuse. *American Journal of Orthopsychiatry, 59,* 355–367.

Widom, C.S. (1989b). The cycle of violence. *Science, 244,* 160–166.

Widom, C.S., & Massey, M. (2015). A prospective examination of whether childhood sexual abuse predicts subsequent sexual offending. *JAMA Pediatrics, 169,* 1433–1457.

Wilcox, D.E. (1985). The relationship of mental illness to homicide. *American Journal of Forensic Psychiatry, 6,* 3–15.

Wilding, J., Cook, S., & Davis, J. (2000). Sound familiar? *Psychologist, 13,* 558–562.

Wille, W. (1974). *Citizens who commit murder.* St. Louis: Warren Greene.

Williams, A.H. (1964). The psychopathology and treatment of sexual murderers. In I.Rosen (Ed.), *The pathology and treatment of sexual deviation* (pp. 351–377). London: Oxford University Press.

Williams, E. (1967). *Beyond belief.* New York: Random House.

Wilson, C. (2000). *The history of murder.* New York: Carroll & Graf.

Wilson, C., & Pitman, P. (1962). *Encyclopedia of murder.* New York: Putnam.

Wilson, D., & Harrison, P. (2010). *The lost British serial killer.* London: Sphere.

Wilson, D., Tolputt, H., Howe, N., & Kemp, D. (2010). When serial killers go unseen: The case of Trevor Joseph Hardy. *Crime, Media, Culture: An International Journal, 6,* 153–167.

Wilson, M., Daly, M., & Daniele, A. (1995). Familicide: The killing of spouse and children. *Aggressive Behavior, 21,* 275–291.

Witt, P.H., Del Russo, J., Oppenheim, J., & Ferguson, G. (1996, Fall). Sex offender risk assessment and the law. *Journal of Psychiatry and Law*, 343–377.

Woddis, G.M. (1957). Depression and crime. *British Journal of Delinquency*, 8, 85–94.

Wolfgang, M.E. (1958). *Patterns of criminal homicide*. Philadelphia: University of Pennsylvania Press.

Wolfgang, M.E. (1969). Who kills whom? *Psychology Today*, 3, 55–75.

Woods, S.M. (1961). Adolescent violence and homicide. *Archives of General Psychiatry*, 5, 528–534.

World Health Organization. (2018). *International classification of diseases* (11th Revision). Retrieved from https://icd.who.int/browse11/1-m/en

Wright, J., & Hensley, C. (2003). From animal cruelty to serial murder: Applying the graduation hypothesis. *International Journal of Offender Therapy and Comparative Criminology*, 47, 71–88.

Yallop, D.A. (1980). *Deliver us from evil*. New York: Coward, McCann, & Geoghegan.

Yalom, I.D. (1960). Aggression and forbiddenness in voyeurism. *Archives of General Psychiatry*, 3, 305–319.

Yankee, W.J. (1995). The current status of research in forensic psychophysiology and its application in the psychophysiological detection of deception. *Journal of Forensic Sciences*, 40, 137–150.

Yarmey, A.D. (1995). Earwitness speaker identification. *Psychology, Public Policy, and Law*, 1, 792–816.

Yarvis, R.M. (1990). Axis I and axis II diagnostic parameters of homicide. *Bulletin of the American Academy of Psychiatry and Law*, 18, 249–269.

Yochelson, S., & Samenow, S.E. (1976). *The criminal personality: The change process*. New York: Jason Aronson.

Yronwode, C. (1983). *The comic buyer's guide*. Iola, WI: Krause Publications.

Zahn, M.A., & Sagi, P.C. (1987). Stranger homicides in nine American cities. *Journal of Criminal law and Criminology*, 78, 377–397.

Zhou, X. (2011). *Wechsler Abbreviated Scale of Intelligence (2nd ed.)*. Bloomington, MN: Pearson.

Zimbardo, P. (1973). Interpersonal dynamics in a simulated prison. *International Journal of Criminology and Penology*, 1, 69–97.

Zona, M., Sharma, K., & Lane, J. (1993). A comparative study of erotomania and obsessional subjects in a forensic sample. *Journal of Forensic Sciences*, 38, 894–903.

Zonana, H.V. (1979). Hypnosis, sodium amytal, and confession. *Bulletin of the American Academy of Psychiatry and Law*, 7, 18–28.

Index

Page numbers in *italics* refer to Tables and Figures.

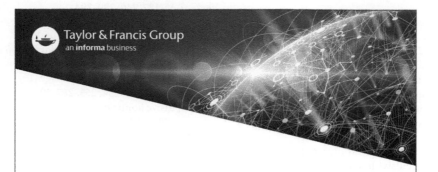